COCONUTS &
KETTLEBELLS

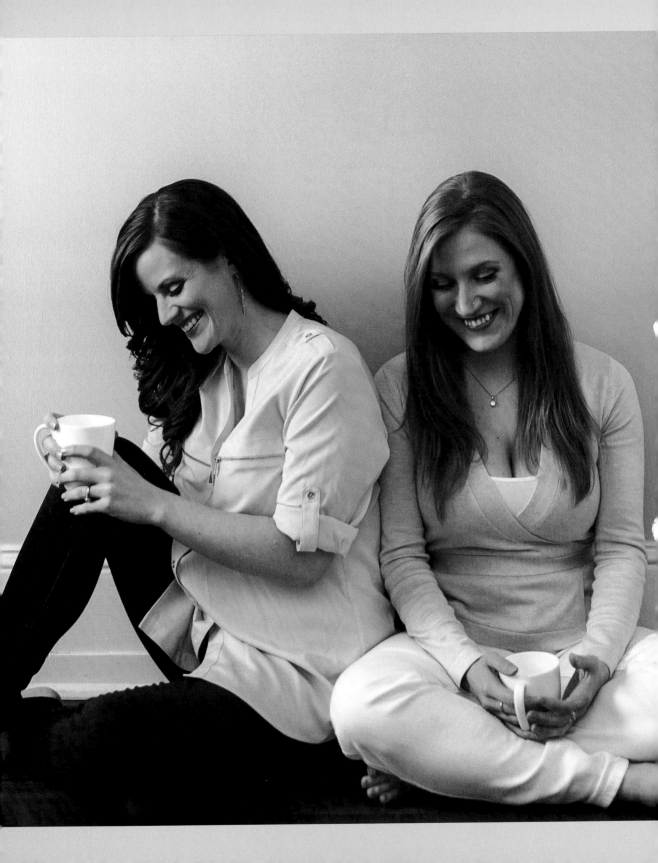

COCONUTS &
KETTLEBELLS

A PERSONALIZED
4-WEEK FOOD AND FITNESS PLAN
FOR LONG-TERM HEALTH,
HAPPINESS, AND FREEDOM

NOELLE TARR AND STEFANI RUPER

WILLIAM MORROW
An Imprint of HarperCollinsPublishers

COCONUTS AND KETTLEBELLS. Copyright © 2018 by Coconuts and Kettlebells, LLC and Stefani Ruper Enterprises, LLC. All rights reserved. Printed in the United States of America. No part of this book may be used or reproduced in any manner whatsoever without written permission except in the case of brief quotations embodied in critical articles and reviews. For information address HarperCollins Publishers, 195 Broadway, New York, NY 10007.

HarperCollins books may be purchased for educational, business, or sales promotional use. For information please e-mail the Special Markets Department at SPsales@harpercollins.com.

FIRST EDITION

Designed by Diahann Sturge
Fitness photography by Matt Godfrey
Food photography by Alena Haurylik
Lifestyle photography by Teresa Robertson

Library of Congress Cataloging-in-Publication Data has been applied for.

ISBN 978-0-06-269029-6

18 19 20 21 22 LSC 10 9 8 7 6 5 4 3 2 1

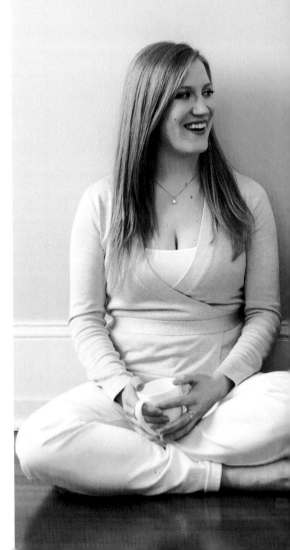

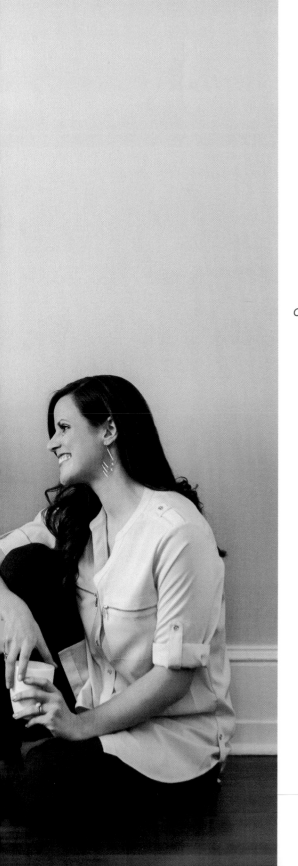

For Ken
Thank you for all the late-night grocery
store runs to get more ingredients,
for testing (and retesting) workouts,
and for supporting Stella and me so I
could pursue my dreams. You are the best
thing that has ever happened to me.
—*Noelle*

For Dorothy
—*Stef*

CONTENTS

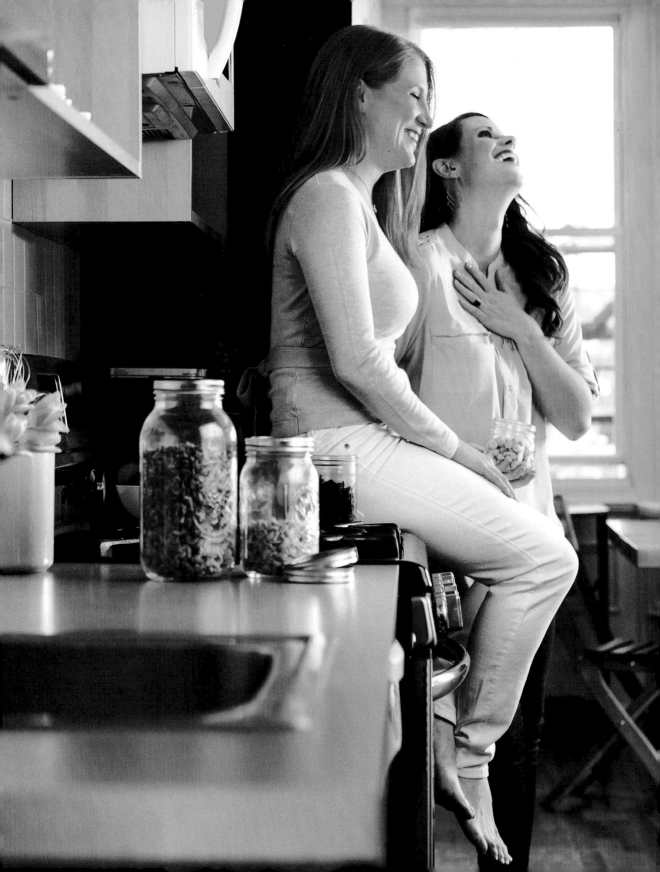

INTRODUCTION

Back in 2008, we were both struggling with a number of health conditions, including anxiety, fatigue, digestive issues, weight fluctuations, infertility, and hormonal imbalances—to name a few. Despite doing everything *right*, our health continued to decline. We did detoxes and cleanses, tracked calories, and never missed workouts. It seemed the more we followed the conventional health and fitness advice to "eat less and exercise more," the worse things got. According to all the experts, we should have been the happiest, fittest, healthiest women on the planet.

But we were not.

Both of us were lost in a sea of frustration, confusion, and doubt. Instead of finding freedom in each new diet we tried, we felt more and more restricted. We assumed there must be something wrong with our bodies and were desperate to figure out what we were missing. After years of obsessively trying to maintain the "perfect" diet, we hit our breaking points. There had to be more to the story—and we were determined to figure it out.

This was well before the two of us had met and become besties, so we carried out our searches independently. We spent months deep in research looking at medical journals and textbooks, exploring the evolution of the human diet, and scrutinizing the weight-loss and dieting industry. Eventually, we both came to discover one important, life-changing truth:

today's culture demands that we eat *less*. But that is backward. What we really need to do is eat *more*.

The more we learned about the biochemistry of human bodies—and especially female bodies—the more we realized what we needed was totally opposite from what society had been telling us. We had been told we needed to eat less to be healthy. We had been told 1,200 calories a day was a magical number that would make the pounds melt off and our worries melt away. We had been told we needed to restrict the quantity of food we ate in order to make our bodies lean, energetic, beautiful, and healthy.

But this advice was completely detrimental to our well-being. After all of our research, we realized we needed to stop obsessing over the *quantity* of food we ate and instead shift our focus to the *quality*. In fact, the more we erred on the side of eating more rather than less, the healthier we got. So instead of setting maximum limits on the amount of food we ate, we set *minimums*. No longer did we force ourselves to follow dieting "rules." Instead, we made sure to eat at least 2,000 calories a day and filled our plates with nutrient-dense foods that worked best for our bodies. Even better, we dropped the guilt and shame that so often accompany weight-loss diets and stopped associating our worth with our ability to cut calories and restrict certain foods.

And we got better.

Once we ditched the diets and gave our bodies the nourishment they needed to heal, we felt happy, healthy, and free. Our mental and emotional health improved, our fertility returned, our hormones rebalanced, and we were no longer obsessed with tracking our food or fearful of what would happen if we didn't follow all the rules. We learned how to eat with freedom, with peace, and with joy. We developed plans for ourselves that not only made us feel amazing, but ended up being sustainable in the long run.

What we've discovered isn't rocket science. While we've both spent many, *many* years conducting experiments on our own bodies, the strategies we developed—and still follow—are quite simple. After making our discoveries, we were eager to spread the word. We left our jobs, started our own blogs, and began writing articles that challenged conventional health and fitness advice. Eventually, we were not only helping hundreds of thousands of people through our websites, we were also working with countless clients one-on-one to help them restore their health, happiness, and relationships with their bodies.

In 2013, we met through the community of health bloggers online and decided to join forces. We started our podcast, *Well-Fed Women* (formerly known as *The Paleo Women Podcast*), which quickly rose to the top of the charts, and launched a number of successful programs that took the holistic health world by storm. It became readily apparent that people were desperate to ditch diet dogma and pursue health with an entirely different mind-set.

We wrote this book to help you do exactly that.

Coconuts and Kettlebells is your way to achieve the same successes we've enjoyed. It's a comprehensive guide that pioneers a new era in achieving long-term health and happiness. It's not a weight loss gimmick, quick fix, or restrictive protocol that requires you stay on the wagon at all times. It's a solid, reasonable plan built off concrete science and unchanging truths about how the body's physiology works. Best of all, it's a way forward that puts you in the driver's seat. By following a few key guidelines, you'll create a food and fitness plan that perfectly fits your needs. There's no second-guessing. No feeling guilty. No nagging little "shoulds." At the end of the day, there's only one plan to follow: the one that works for you.

WHAT'S IN THIS BOOK

It's no secret—most of us are stressed, short on time, and juggling multiple responsibilities. Struggling with complicated recipes and long, exhausting workouts does nothing more than add more stress to your life. Knowing this, we've packed this book with easy, actionable tips that you can start incorporating into your life right now. This book is designed to be your all-in-one solution to making sustainable health changes and figuring out what is right for *your* body. Each part of the book combines knowledge with customized tools to meet your needs. Using simple and straightforward guidelines, we walk you step-by-step through a comprehensive plan that will tackle your health concerns and get you to your goals.

In Part I, you'll get all the know-how you need to make educated decisions about food. You'll learn why it's important to achieve goal minimums rather than maximums and whether you should eat more carbs or more fat. This brings up one of our favorite questions: Are you a *bread* lover like Stef or are you a *butter* lover like Noelle? (Don't worry if you're not sure—we show you exactly how to figure it out!) Then we'll guide you through our foundational program, the 4x4. For four weeks, you'll eliminate the four foods that are most often problematic for people: grains, dairy, vegetable oils, and refined sugar. By eliminating these foods for a set period of time, you'll be able to observe the effect they have on your body. This knowledge will empower you to know what your own special dietary needs and preferences are. We then walk you through reintroducing these foods and how to manage your health long-term. Importantly, there is no need to be fearful of food or consider certain ones to be "bad"—even if you've discovered they don't work for you. We show you simple mind-set changes that will help you let go of the dieting mentality, eat with freedom and peace, and celebrate your body.

Part II is where the fun begins. To help you implement the 4x4 with ease, there are two simple meal plans to choose from: one for bread lovers and one for butter lovers. Each meal plan includes a shopping list so you know exactly what is needed each week during your 4x4. You also have access to seventy-five easy and delicious recipes that can be prepared during your 4x4 and beyond. Recipes range from quick and simple snacks to one-pot weeknight meals, and they all require minimal time in the kitchen. We've also included a guide to kitchen essentials and quick tips about how to stock your pantry. From buying to cooking to eating, you've got all the resources you need to put your plan into action.

The final piece of Part II is the Coconuts and Kettlebells Fitness Plan. Despite what you may have learned from the latest fitness trend, workouts don't have to be depleting, time-consuming, or unenjoyable to be effective. In fact, you can build your fitness just about anywhere using workouts that easily fit into your schedule. To help you incorporate movement into your life, you'll learn how to create a fitness template using four key elements: frequency, dose, type, and rest. If you'd like to get started immediately, try one of our three targeted four-week plans.

Included in the plan are twenty-four do-anywhere-style workouts that you can complete in thirty minutes or less. To keep it simple, the workouts require only two different tools: your body and a kettlebell. There are easy-to-follow photos showing how to complete each exercise, plus answers to common fitness-related questions, such as how to know when to take a rest day, what to eat before and after your workouts, and how to track your progress. In other words—this book is like having your own personal trainer in the palm of your hand.

What you are about to read is the start of a revolution in how we approach health and fitness. Our lives have been radically transformed by the principles we share in this book. We can't tell you how excited we are that your life is about to be, too.

Noelle and Stef

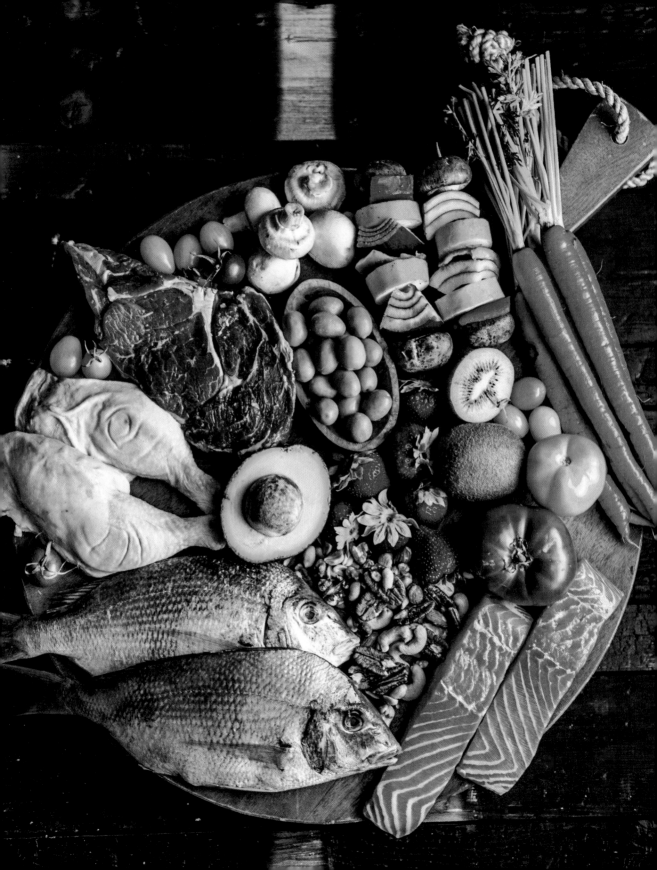

PART I

EATING

for a

VIBRANT,
HEALTHY LIFE

1

NOURISH YOUR BODY WITH *MORE* PROTEIN, CARBS, AND FATS

hances are, you've been on a diet before. According to the Boston Medical Center, an estimated 45 million Americans go on a diet each year and spend $33 billion on weight-loss products. Maybe you counted points (you could eat about 20). Maybe you counted meals (you could have three a day—but remember, *no snacking!*). Or maybe you counted calories (you could eat 1,500 if you wanted to lose weight slowly, but 1,200 was better if you were *really* serious about weight loss).

No matter what you've tried, we've been in your shoes. Between the two of us, we have been on pretty much every diet around the block: Atkins, Weight Watchers, SlimFast, Lean Cuisine, Special K, vegetarian, low-fat, low-carb, low-calorie, and various kinds of undereating. We kept trying new diets because we were certain that one of them was going to be the ticket—the thing we were missing. We thought if we could just eat a little more perfectly, we'd arrive at the promised land.

Only we didn't.

Western culture is obsessed with the idea that calories—that is, the amount of energy in the food you eat—are all that matter for weight loss and health. The basic idea is this: *the more energy you eat, the more weight you gain.* People who believe this argue that health is about eating a specific amount of calories every day. If you consume *fewer* calories than your body needs, you'll lose weight, and if you consume *more*, you'll gain weight. This is why people are obsessed with eating *less*. They think that if they consume less, they'll weigh less.

Unfortunately, this is an oversimplified formula. Yes, calories *do* matter. But they don't matter as much as you might think. This is because your health plays a role in how well your body processes energy.

The more healthful a food is, the more it will contribute to a well-functioning body. Consider a candy bar. A normal-size candy bar has 230 calories. For the same number of calories, you could have an avocado. You could also have two and a half bananas or a leafy green salad with two tablespoons of dressing. Let's say that Noelle eats six candy bars a day and Stefani eats some fruit, avocado, a salad, and oven-roasted spareribs (see page 232 for this scrumptious recipe). We eat exactly the same amount of calories. But because the food that Stefani eats contains a variety of macronutrients and micronutrients, she will feel a lot more energetic than Noelle, and undoubtedly be healthier, too.

Quality matters. The more nourishing your diet is, the better your body is able to process the food you eat. The better you enrich your diet with vitamins, minerals, plants, and nutrient-dense animal products, the more you will heal. When you eat well, you provide your body with the nutrients it needs to repair damage and become strong and vibrant. If you predominantly eat nutritionally empty foods, your body simply won't have the building blocks it needs to operate well. *All* the systems in your body will be at risk of malfunctioning. This could result in conditions such as fatigue, hormonal imbalances, high blood pressure, heart disease, osteoporosis, mental health disorders, acne, autoimmune diseases, joint pain, gut distress, and metabolic dysfunction, which affects how your body burns energy.

THE PROBLEM WITH UNDEREATING

When it comes to caloric intake, many diets fail to recognize one important fact: the less food you eat, the fewer nutrients you give your body. For example, because Noelle avoided dietary fat for quite some time, she was deficient in the fat-soluble vitamins A, D, E, and K. As a result, she had very dry skin and suffered from keratosis pilaris—otherwise known as "chicken skin"—on her arms. Because Stefani wasn't eating sufficient protein, she was deficient in iron. As a result, she became anemic and weak. These are just two examples of ways in which we deprived our bodies of nutrients because we simply didn't eat enough.

Many health conditions can be linked to deficiencies in specific nutrients. A deficiency in B vitamins—in particular, B12—can cause anxiety, fatigue, and mood problems. B vitamins are found in high-quality animal products such as beef, poultry, and fish, and in leafy greens. Another nutrient many people are deficient in is vitamin D, which is found dietarily in eggs (yes, *with* the yolk), fish, and beef liver. Low vitamin D has been linked to a number of health issues, including osteoporosis, autoimmune disorders, and depression.

Perhaps the most detrimental consequence of undereating is the hormone response. The thing about human bodies—and especially female bodies—is that they like to have fat on them. They like to know that they have ample energy stored up so they can support reproduction. Throughout the vast majority of human history, pregnancy was a very precarious thing. If you became pregnant during a time of famine, you very well might have died.

In order to prevent this sad end, the female body evolved a mechanism to protect itself. In situations in which the body experiences excessive stress, whether that be from undereating, overexercising, or too much work, it triggers a process known as the pregnenolone steal. Pregnenolone is the precursor from which nearly all other steroid hormones are made, including progesterone, testosterone, estrogens, and cortisol. In times of stress, the body shuttles all its pregnenolone toward the production of cortisol and away from the sex hormones. In other words, it turns off the systems in the body that support reproduction for the sake of making stress hormones.

Now, you might be thinking, *This was all well and good for those prehistoric ladies of the savannah, but I live in the twenty-first century! I have bountiful access to food!* Yes, this is true. But if you don't actually *feed* your body, and if you regularly eat less than what your body needs, then your body is going to think you are starving.

The thing about these hormone systems is that they don't just operate for the sake of reproduction. Estrogen, progesterone, testosterone, luteinizing hormone (LH), follicle-stimulating hormone (FSH), prolactin, and other reproductive hormones play important roles in the rest of the body. If hormone levels fall, you may lose the ability to sleep, feel calm, feel happy, have a libido, have clear skin, have strong bones, menstruate, and do many other things, including have children.

One unique and important hormone that suffers as a result of undereating is the thyroid hormone. The thyroid gland is responsible for regulating cell metabolism, or the way your body uses energy. When the thyroid is functioning well and properly releasing the hormones it produces (T3 and T4), you feel energetic, your organs perform as they should, and your metabolism hums along quickly and smoothly.

Unfortunately, if you undereat, your body decreases its production of thyroid hormone in an effort to conserve energy. (Again, this is especially the case for women—the female body *really* wants to preserve as much energy and fat as possible.) When you undereat, the production of thyroid hormones decreases, and with them, your ability to burn fat.

That's right. It's so important, we'll say it again: undereating causes production of thyroid hormones to slow, which can damage the body's ability to burn fat, instead causing it to *store* fat.

THE SHAME CYCLE

There is a common pattern among people who regularly restrict their food. It goes like this:

You feel bad about yourself, so you forbid yourself from eating certain foods. Let's say you decide to completely avoid a particular food, such as a cheeseburger.

But then, all of a sudden, everywhere you look you're seeing cheeseburgers.

You crave them. You dwell on them. You can't stop thinking about them.

Then you cave to the pressure you've put on yourself and eat a cheeseburger. Maybe you eat two, or even three. While you're eating, you're in heaven. But the second you stop, you feel guilt, shame, and despair. You had *promised* yourself you wouldn't eat any more. But you did anyway! You feel awful. And you torture yourself over your failure. This torture might come simply in the form of negative self-talk. Or you might make yourself go for a 5-mile run when you wake up in the morning, or force yourself to avoid cheeseburgers yet again. Attempting to erase or correct your wrongs makes you feel worn out, hungry, and restricted. And eventually, you succumb to your desire to have a cheeseburger again.

We call this the shame cycle. And for many women, it's a loop that never stops.

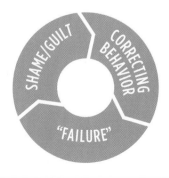

If you've experienced this, or something like it, you are not alone, and it's not your fault. This is how human beings are wired. Millions of people around the world today are stuck in this kind of cycle. People at the gym, people in line behind you at the supermarket, people thick and people thin.

Everyone assumes that the way out of it is to just finally marshall enough willpower to successfully restrict themselves down to a perfect weight. But the answer—the *only* answer—is actually the opposite.

The answer is to freely and lovingly give yourself permission to eat as much as you feel you need. The answer is to focus on the quality of food you consume and not restrict the quantity. The answer, we know from experience, is to stop thinking about food in terms of *maximums* and start thinking in terms of *minimums*.

EAT AT LEAST 2,000 CALORIES A DAY (OR AS MUCH AS YOU NEED)

You have likely been told your whole life that you should eat no more than a certain number of calories a day. Wherever that number came from, it's likely always been in the back of your head. For years, you've idolized being able to maintain a specific calorie intake with ease: 1,600 calories a day, 1,400 calories a day, or the magical 1,200 calories a day (which, by the way, is the recommended calorie intake for a three-year-old). The reason most diets default to recommending a set calorie intake is that it's easy. And while conventional diets keep telling people all they have to do is eat less and exercise more, no one is getting any slimmer or healthier.

Our solution may sound radical, but it isn't. It's just *unfamiliar* because of the diet industry BS you've been exposed to your entire life. Our solution is literally the only way that is healthy and sustainable. And once you decide to embrace it, it's exciting—and liberating.

We say:

Eat *at least* 2,000 calories a day.

When in doubt, err on the side of eating more rather than less.

Choose nourishment. Choose to give your body the bountiful vitamins and minerals that it's been craving its whole life. Choose to give your body the energy and nutrients it needs to heal, rebuild its systems, and provide you with life, energy, and vitality.

THE BENEFITS OF A 2,000-CALORIE MINIMUM

Setting a calorie minimum for yourself can do wonders for you physically. The more you fill up on nutrient-dense foods, the more your body has the opportunity to absorb nutrients and heal. When you give your body the nutrients it needs to function properly, it will reward you with all the things you are hoping for: clearer skin, easier sleep, improved mental health and clarity, more energy, less struggle with your weight or fitness, fertility, stronger sex drive, and stronger bones.

By eating enough, you can also heal your metabolism and thyroid function. If you have Hashimoto's thyroiditis, an autoimmune condition in which the body attacks the thyroid gland, your path to thyroid health may require more interventions. But if you are suffering from decreased thyroid function in any capacity, you can boost your thyroid production by eating more. The less your body thinks it is starving and the more it thinks you live in a period of bounty and plenty, the happier it will be to run smoothly and burn energy with ease.

Finally, eating enough can also help regulate your appetite. If you feel chronically hungry, or like you always "could eat," it's likely due to the fact that your satiety signals have gone haywire. This is common for people who have a history of yo-yo dieting or regularly restricting access to food. You may have struggled with "cravings" your whole life. This is normal, and something that often resolves when you give yourself the freedom to eat intuitively, and when you want to.

Unfortunately, this is not always a *simple* fix. Appetite-signaling problems can be caused by neurotransmitter imbalances or nutrient deficiencies, which can take longer to resolve. There are also many physical and psychological aspects of cravings that can take longer to work through. But actually *eating when your body wants you to* is the critical first step to finally beating cravings and feeling at peace with food, for good.

MAKING THE 2,000-CALORIE-A-DAY MINIMUM WORK FOR YOU

For most women, a 2,000-calorie-a-day minimum is a great place to start. However, there may be instances where 2,000 calories a day is too many. If you feel overfed or overstuffed, you can slowly scale down your caloric intake until you no longer feel too full but also don't feel hungry. It's perfectly acceptable for you to need less, and your caloric requirements may decrease at different points in your life according to your specific situation. You may feel more comfortable at a lower calorie intake if you are exceptionally short or of a smaller build, have been sedentary for a prolonged amount of time, have gone through menopause, or are a mature woman of advanced age.

There are also cases in which a 2,000-calorie-a-day minimum may not be a sufficient. If you are pregnant, breastfeeding, experiencing chronic stress, recovering from an eating disorder, attempting to regain fertility or get pregnant, or have a high activity level, you may benefit from bumping up your minimum to at least 2,500 calories a day.

It's important to note that a minimum is just that—a *minimum*. It's not a set number of calories you must stick to each day. Bodies are dynamic and ever-changing, and the energy you need each day can fluctuate dramatically. Each day, shoot to achieve your minimum, then add more calories according to your hunger and activity level.

MACRONUTRIENT MINIMUMS

Just as you've been told you need to restrict your overall food intake to be healthy, you've also probably been told you need to cut back on carbs or fat. There is no shortage of websites, books, magazines, and Netflix documentaries advocating for one side or the other.

Is fat causing all your health problems? Many people who adhere to the USDA guidelines think so, especially when it comes to saturated fat. They argue that a low-fat diet is best for avoiding or alleviating the symptoms of chronic health conditions such as diabetes, obesity, and heart disease.

Are carbs causing all your health problems? Many people who advocate a low-carb, paleo, primal, or ketogenic diet would say so. Like low-fat dieters, people who advocate a low-carb diet believe reducing carbohydrates is best for avoiding or alleviating the symptoms of chronic health conditions such as diabetes, obesity, and heart disease.

The reality is that both are right, and both are wrong. The research on low-carb and low-fat diets is conflicting. Some studies show that low-carb diets are better for certain health conditions and weight loss, and other articles demonstrate that low-fat diets are better. This brings us to one simple conclusion: the problem isn't that carbs are unhealthy or that fats are unhealthy. The problem is that there are poor-quality carbs and poor-quality fats, and when these "bad" carbs and fats get used in studies, it confounds the variables

What Are Macronutrients?

$\mathcal{M}$acronutrients are the three main types of energy that people consume: protein, carbohydrate, and fat.

Protein is predominantly found in animal products, though smaller amounts can be found in plant foods. Protein is composed of molecules called amino acids. Animal proteins contain all nine essential amino acids the human body needs but can't produce for itself. Plant sources of protein, including most beans and nuts, do not, which is why vegetarians and vegans need to be careful about where and how they get their protein.

Carbohydrates are the sugars, starches, and fiber found in plant products. Typically, people think of "carbs" as bread and pasta. While bread and pasta *are* made nearly entirely of carbohydrates, so are many whole foods, such as fruits and vegetables.

Fats are the oily, densely energetic components of foods. They are present in both plant and animal products. In animal products, fat can be found in fatty cuts of meat and poultry, eggs, and fatty fish such as salmon. Plants that contain high quantities of fat include olives, coconuts, avocados, and nuts.

and makes it impossible to tell what is actually causing the problem being addressed, such as obesity, diabetes, or systemic inflammation.

In other words, when you compare people who drink soda and eat processed sugar and grains regularly to those who don't, the people who eat more carbs are worse off. Likewise, when you compare people who are eating deep-fried chicken and fast food regularly to those who don't, the people who eat more fat are worse off. When we look at more nutrient-dense versions of carbs and fat, such as sweet potatoes and olive oil, we get a completely different result.

The other thing that both sides fail to recognize is that there is no one specific diet that works for everyone all the time. We all have our own bioindividuality, meaning we've all grown up in different environments and have varying genetics and histories. As a result, there is a great diversity of body types, so people naturally react differently to different ratios of macronutrients.

Because of this, you may find that you function better with a higher percentage of carbs or fat in your diet, based on your own situation and preferences. This is perfectly normal. Stefani finds that she functions better on carbohydrates. She feels more mentally clear, she has more energy, she sleeps better at night, and, importantly, she simply likes them better. She is what we lovingly (and somewhat ironically, since she eats very little bread) call a *bread* lover.

Noelle finds that she functions better on fats. She has better focus and mental clarity, her digestion is better, she has more energy, and she is much more satisfied at the end of a meal. She is what we lovingly (if also ironically, since she doesn't eat much butter) call a *butter* lover.

Defining "Bread Lover" and "Butter Lover"

It may be a touch ironic, but Stefani doesn't eat much bread and Noelle doesn't eat much butter. This is just a fun play on words that we use to define our differences. Stefani does *like* bread and other carbs, and Noelle does *like* butter and other fats. We simply do not eat them all that much, since bread isn't the most nutrient-dense food and we both react negatively to dairy.

ALL ABOUT FAT—WHY FAT IS YOUR FRIEND

Fat is essential to the body for several reasons. First, many vitamins and micronutrients are *fat-soluble*, which means they need to be eaten with fat to be properly absorbed in the digestive tract. The fat-soluble vitamins, which include vitamins A, D, E, and K, play a key role in immune system function, heart and bone health, and fertility. Studies show when vegetables are eaten with fat, there is significantly more absorption in the small intestine of the vitamins and micronutrients in those vegetables. Research also suggests that unless fruits and vegetables are consumed with fat, they do not lower the risk of coronary heart disease. In short, to get the most from your salad, you'll want to add plenty of avocado slices and olive oil, which are rich in fat (and delicious—you're welcome).

Second, fats serve as the building blocks for cell membranes and hormones. The adult human body is made up of *trillions* of cells, and fatty acids make up the structural component of every cell in the body. Fatty acids are also used to make hormones—specifically, sex hormones—and hormone-like substances that control inflammation. Without sufficient fat intake, these systems do not function appropriately.

Fat is incredibly important, particularly for women, because having fat stores in the hips, breasts, buttocks, and thighs tells the brain the body is healthy, well fed, and capable of reproduction. Without fat—both in the diet and on the body—hormone production shuts down and reproductive function falters. As a result, hormonal symptoms like irregular or absent menstrual cycles, low libido, acne, poor sleep, mood swings, depression, and anxiety can occur.

In short, fat is your friend. Don't fear it—use it with gusto and pride.

ALL ABOUT CARBOHYDRATES—WHY CARBS ARE YOUR FRIEND

In recent years, many health gurus have warned that consumption of carbs leads to negative health consequences, disease, and "insidious" weight gain, regardless of quality or source. They worry that carbohydrates cause insulin levels to rise and eventually cause insulin resistance.

As it turns out, carbohydrates *do* elevate insulin levels, but that isn't bad for you in the context of a healthy body that isn't suffering from diabetes or insulin resistance. In fact, while removing carbohydrates from the diet can help minimize the insulin response, it will *not* cure the underlying problem causing the insulin resistance. What does help to increase insulin sensitivity is reducing inflammation, managing stress, and healing the gut. This can be done with a diet that includes any amount of carbohydrates, within reason.

Carbohydrates actively promote good health in many instances. For one thing, they are an important source of energy. The body needs carbohydrates when performing high-intensity (or anaerobic) activity. While athletes' bodies can adapt to burning fat for fuel during activity, carbohydrates are the most readily available fuel source in the body; this makes carbohydrates great for optimizing athletic performance. Sufficient carbohydrates, in combination with protein, are needed post-workout to stimulate muscle growth.

Carbohydrates are also necessary for women's health, particularly for women of reproductive age. Carbohydrates play an important role in leptin signaling. Leptin is a hormone that controls hunger and feelings of satiety, signaling to the brain that the body has been fed. Drastically cutting carb intake for too long can potentially mess with leptin signaling, which can result in poor appetite regulation, fatigue, a sluggish metabolism, impaired hormone production, and infertility.

Worse still, if you're already overloaded with stress, eating too low-carb can add fuel to the fire by increasing the demand on the adrenals to provide glucose. This can cause your body to produce too much or too little stress hormone, or at the wrong time, which interferes with pretty much all of the body's systems and can especially affect sleep, mental health, and energy.

Just as with calories, instead of setting maximum amounts, the best way to pursue eating the appropriate amount of macronutrients is to set a minimum amount of protein, carbs, and fat to consume each day. From there, you can fill in whatever you'd like. This enables you to get the requisite nourishment from each macronutrient while providing you with tons of flexibility based on your own needs and wants.

For most people, a good minimum carbohydrate intake is 100 grams. This is equal to approximately four pieces of fruit or two medium sweet potatoes. For fat, a great starting point is 50 grams. This is about 4 tablespoons (¼ cup) of oil or two medium avocados.

For protein, your minimum intake will vary depending on your body size, gender, age, and the type and amount of activity you do. Women may require anywhere between 50 and 125 grams of protein a day and men between 75 and 150 grams. A typical can of tuna or palm-size portion of meat, poultry, or fish will give you 25 grams of protein. Twice that amount would be the minimum for women and three times that amount would be the minimum for men.

It's important to note that when you add up your minimums, your total calorie intake will be much less than you need. Minimums are your baseline, and from there, you should add the foods that work best for you to get to your daily caloric intake. Play with varying the amount of carbohydrates or fat in your diet to see what works best for you. For example, you may want to eat a higher-carbohydrate diet for a month or two and then shift to a high-fat diet. Be conscious of how it makes you feel. Do you notice a difference in your energy levels, athletic performance, fat mass, muscle mass, mood, libido, sleep, PMS, menstrual cycle, or appetite? These are important qualities of life that may shift depending on the ratio of carbohydrates to fat in your diet.

You may also simply want to eat more carbohydrates because you feel like it. Or more fat. That's great! You'll get no arguments here. Taste is a perfectly good reason to eat more of one kind of food than another. Simply make sure to get in your minimum requirements of all the macronutrients, then eat according to your body's needs. Repeat.

Sample "More Fat" Day for Noelle

BREAKFAST: 2 eggs, 1 large Pink Lady apple, 2 to 3 tablespoons almond butter

LUNCH: 1 or 2 servings Apple, Avocado, and Chicken Salad (page 177), handful of macadamia nuts

SNACK: ½ cup Slow Cooker Bison Chili (page 226)

DINNER: Large salad with nuts, raisins, and olive oil, 1 or 2 servings Zucchini-Beef Taco Skillet (page 214)

SNACK: 2 or 3 squares dark chocolate

PROTEIN: 120 grams (480 calories)

CARBS: 140 grams (560 calories)

FAT: 130 grams (1,170 calories)

TOTAL CALORIES: 2,210

MINIMUM VS. ADDED INTAKE IN CALORIES

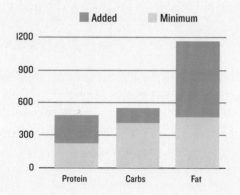

TOTAL PERCENTAGE OF CALORIES FROM PROTEIN, CARBS, AND FAT

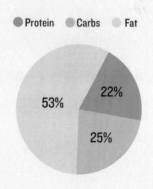

Sample "More Carb" Day for Stefani

BREAKFAST: 2 servings Twice-Baked Breakfast Sweet Potatoes (page 142), 2 hard-boiled eggs

LUNCH: Roasted Beets and Berries Salad (page 180), 2 cups diced fruit

SNACK: Palm-size serving beef jerky, 1 cup banana chips

DINNER: 2 servings Rosemary Roasted Potatoes (page 164), ¼ cup lean ground beef sautéed with kale

SNACK: 1 pint blackberries with 1 tablespoon honey

PROTEIN: 77 grams (308 calories)

CARBS: 243 grams (972 calories)

FAT: 89 grams (801 calories)

TOTAL CALORIES: 2,081

MINIMUM VS. ADDED INTAKE IN CALORIES

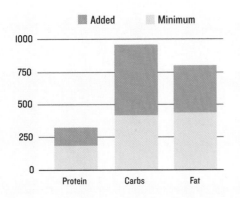

TOTAL PERCENTAGE OF CALORIES FROM PROTEIN, CARBS, AND FAT

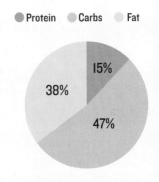

ARE YOU A BREAD LOVER OR A BUTTER LOVER?

You may find, for a variety of reasons, that you prefer eating more carbs or more fat. It could be because you feel better and have better health following a particular approach, or simply because you feel more satisfied and less restricted. The decision is entirely up to you and should be based on your experience and preferences.

You can figure out if you're one, the other, or both by paying attention to your body.

To help you figure out if you might be *physically* inclined one way or the other, we've compiled a list of various health components of both choices. Will you thrive as a bread lover or a butter lover? Check the following reasons to see if you fit one of the categories.

ARE YOU A BREAD LOVER? REASONS FOR A HIGHER-CARB DIET

HIGH ACTIVITY LEVEL

People who are highly active require more carbohydrates to burn as fuel than those who are not. If you are constantly on the move or exercise regularly, bump up the lower limit of your carbohydrate intake to 150 grams a day. If you are *highly* active, such as if you have a labor-intensive job or are a serious athlete, or both, you may need at least 200 grams of carbohydrate each day.

INSOMNIA

Carbohydrates have been shown to help improve sleep, especially if consumed two to four hours before bedtime. If you struggle with falling asleep, staying asleep, and/or having restful sleep, consider consuming a minimum of 150 grams a day. Note that while most people typically benefit from eating their carb dose later in the day, some people need to have carbohydrates throughout the entire day to sleep well.

FERTILITY

A woman's fertility can be greatly affected by carbohydrate intake. Without adequate carbohydrates, the body may believe that it does not have access to enough energy, which can result in reduced sex hormone output. If you are trying to conceive, have trouble with your menstrual cycle, or especially if you have a history of undereating or dieting, then it may be important for you to eat a minimum of 150 grams of carbohydrates a day.

PREGNANCY AND BREASTFEEDING

If you are growing another human being inside of your body or feeding it with your milk supply, it's no time for deprivation! Carbohydrates are an important source of energy for feeding your baby. Kick up your minimum carb intake to at least 150 grams a day, especially if you are noticing fatigue or struggling with your milk supply. Of course, your appetite can be very particular at this point in time, so it's also important to let your food intake wax and wane with your body's signals.

GENETICS

Some people have several copies of a gene called AMY1 that codes for an enzyme called amylase in their saliva. This makes starch break down faster. If you have this, shifting your diet toward carbohydrates can result in better weight management and improved health. To figure out if you have this enzyme, you'd need to get a genetic test done by a company such as 23andMe, and the results would be listed in their report. You could also make an educated guess by trying a higher-carbohydrate diet and seeing if it works well for your weight maintenance.

ARE YOU A BUTTER LOVER? REASONS FOR A HIGHER-FAT DIET

DIABETES/INSULIN RESISTANCE

If you have diabetes, are insulin resistant, or suspect that you are insulin resistant, a lower-carbohydrate approach will likely be a helpful way for you to manage your symptoms.

Type 1 diabetes, an autoimmune disease in which the body attacks the cells of the pancreas that are responsible for producing insulin, is, unfortunately, intractable. For many people, eating a low-carbohydrate diet makes type 1 diabetes easier to manage because it keeps insulin injections to a minimum and it's easier to match insulin to carbohydrate intake.

People with type 1 diabetes who are concerned about thyroid health or fertility can typically increase their carb intake up to 75 to 100 grams a day by spacing out their carbohydrate intake throughout the day and pairing carbs with a good dose of fiber and fat, as fiber and fat blunt blood sugar spikes.

Type 2 diabetes and prediabetes (insulin resistance), on the other hand, can often be treated with diet and lifestyle choices. The most effective way to overcome insulin resistance and even type 2 diabetes is to work on gut health. Restoring gut flora populations, healing the intestinal lining, and reducing inflammation are the keys to helping cells become more insulin sensitive and thus easing the burden on the pancreas to produce so much insulin (see page 71 for more on optimizing digestion and gut health). In the meantime, however—while that healing is taking place—a lower-carbohydrate diet reduces the amount of insulin your pancreas makes. This helps manage symptoms such as extreme hunger or thirst, increased urination, fatigue, and difficulty losing weight.

If you suffer from insulin resistance, a low-carb diet can halt the progression from insulin resistance to diabetes. Importantly, however, *this is not a cure.* A low-carbohydrate diet keeps insulin levels from rising but doesn't solve the underlying problem. In fact, being on a very low-carbohydrate diet for a long period of time can actually *worsen* insulin sensitivity. For that reason, it's best to focus on fixing underlying problems (such as poor gut flora health, intestinal permeability, and inflammation) for a long-term solution and to use a low-carbohydrate diet as *part* of the solution.

REACTIVE HYPOGLYCEMIA

Reactive hypoglycemia is a condition in which the body clears sugar out of the bloodstream quickly and precipitously. When people (often women) with reactive hypoglycemia eat carbohydrates, their blood sugar levels drop very low.

Symptoms of reactive hypoglycemia include rapid heartbeat, headaches, shaking, sweating, fatigue, difficulty sleeping, blurry vision, sudden mood changes, fainting, and head rushes, as when you stand up too fast.

A lower-carbohydrate approach can help keep blood sugar levels from going too high and therefore prevent these precipitous drops.

BLOOD SUGAR SWINGS

Blood sugar swings (essentially, when your blood sugar fluctuates from too high to too low and vice versa) can happen to anybody, with any degree of frequency. They can result in symptoms of both low and high blood sugar: Low blood sugar can result in fainting, blurry vision, fatigue, and shaking. High blood sugar can result in excitability, jitteriness, mania, and high energy.

If you struggle with blood sugar issues, consider experimenting with limiting carbohydrates to around 100 grams a day (spaced as evenly throughout the day as possible), while focusing mostly on fat in the diet. If you refrain from eating large amounts of carbohydrates, your body may have an easier time keeping a steady amount of glucose in your blood.

MENOPAUSE

Many women in menopause will do great with a higher-carbohydrate diet—so we're not saying that you *must* eat high-fat if you're going through menopause. We simply know that many women struggle with a shift in body composition at this time as fat moves from more "female" areas such as the hips and thighs into the abdomen.

Menopausal abdominal fat (as well as other testosterone-related symptoms such as acne and facial hair growth) occurs because the body produces fewer female sex hormones at this time. The fewer female sex hormones you have, the less fat your body will shuttle to areas such as the breasts and hips. You can help keep testosterone levels to a minimum by keeping carbohydrate intake on the low end, as insulin is one of the primary drivers of testosterone production.

GENETICS

Some people are genetically inclined to be better at burning fat for fuel (perhaps 2.5 times faster than others). If this is you, you may tend to do better on a higher-fat diet. To figure this out, you can get your genes analyzed by a company such as 23andMe and check your results for the genes FABP2, PPARG, ADRB2, and PPARG (don't worry—the company will tell you in its report if you're an efficient fat burner, so you don't necessarily have to learn about and hunt for these genes yourself). You may also, if you wish, make an educated guess based on your experience.

WHICH ARE *YOU*?

And now for the million-dollar question: Are you a bread lover or are you a butter lover? One of our favorite parts about our approach to health is that it's *totally okay* to be one or the other . . . or both! Your body has its own specific needs. Any time you hear a proclamation that "low-carb is best for everyone" or "you must be low-fat or else," alarm bells should go off. Yes, for some people, low-carb is better. But for others, it's not. Perhaps what's been holding you back (as was the case for us) was trying to fit your needs into these cookie-cutter molds.

To figure out what is going to work best for you, you'll need to experiment with each approach. Start with your minimums and add either more carbs or more fat. You can shift your carbs down and fats up (or vice versa) until you hit your sweet spot. Do your best to forget "diet rules," and pay attention to how your body and mind feel instead. Over time you'll find a balance that works best for you.

Also keep in mind that what works for you now may not work for you later—if you do best as a bread lover right now, in a few years, you may find you thrive as a butter lover. Keep your options open, remain flexible, and make changes according to how your body responds.

Good Sources of Carbohydrates

LESS DENSE

Broccoli	Eggplant	Spinach
Brussels sprouts	Kale	Parsnips
Carrots	Mushrooms	Peppers
Chard	Onions	Zucchini

MORE DENSE

Vegetables

Acorn squash	Sweet potatoes	Yucca
Beets	Taro	
Potatoes	Winter squash	

Fruits

Apple	Grapes	Pear
Apricot	Kiwi	Pineapple
Banana	Mango	Plantain
Blackberries	Orange	Plum
Blueberries	Papaya	Raspberries
Cherries	Passion fruit	Starfruit
Grapefruit	Peach	Strawberries

Good Sources of Fat

Avocados

Coconut (coconut oil, coconut milk, coconut meat)

Cooking fats and oils (see page 40 for a list of high-quality cooking fats)

Fatty cuts of grass-fed/pasture-raised meats (cow, bison, lamb, pork)

Fatty cuts of pasture-raised poultry (turkey, chicken, duck)

Fatty fish (salmon, tuna, mackerel)

Ghee (clarified butter)

Nuts and seeds

Pasture-raised eggs

2

THE BIG FOUR INFLAMMATORY FOODS

The way we engage with food has changed in profound ways in the last few hundred years. Before the Industrial Revolution, most people grew their own vegetables, kept livestock, hunted, and processed food by hand using small tools. If you wanted bread, you harvested the grain, ground it up, and used it to make homemade bread. If you wanted butter, you milked the cow, separated the cream from the milk, and churned the cream into butter. Now if you want food, you simply go to the drive-through or press a button, and it's delivered to your doorstep.

While we are both absolutely *thrilled* we don't have to churn our own butter, food that is cheap, fast, and easy typically isn't high quality. Thanks to industrial processing, many ingredients unknown to our ancestors, such as refined grains and sugars, vegetable oils, trans fat, high-fructose corn syrup, artificial sweeteners, and food additives, now dominate packaged and prepared foods. Unfortunately, most of these ingredients make food hyper-palatable (translation: unnaturally tasty) while being completely devoid of nutrients.

To distinguish nutrient-dense foods from ones that aren't, Western culture tends to separate food into two categories: whole foods and processed foods. Whole foods are foods that can be found in nature, such as apples, eggs, and potatoes. They have been processed or refined as little as possible and are free from additives and other substances. As a result, they are more nutrient-dense and contain vitamins and minerals in the exact ratios nature intended.

While most of the food we consume goes through some sort of processing to get it from farm to store, when we talk about "processed foods," we mean foods that are not in their original form. They are typically made from ingredients that are highly refined and devoid of nutrients, and have additives like artificial colors and flavors. In general, foods that are heavily processed look nothing like the food they came from. Examples include chicken nuggets, breakfast cereals, and baked goods.

So what happens when your diet is centered on foods that are processed and devoid of nutrients? Your body stops functioning optimally. You are much more likely to experience things like nutrient deficiencies, blood sugar dysregulation, gut flora disruption, digestive distress, and inflammation. For some people, this means sleep problems, hormonal imbalances, and weight gain. For others, it means fatigue, brain fog, and joint pain. For you it could be any mix of various symptoms. By eating *more* whole foods and *fewer* processed foods, you are treating the root cause of those symptoms. This is why many people find the health problems they experience on a day-to-day basis completely resolved when they make the shift to eating more whole foods.

THE BIG FOUR

We're not going to sugarcoat it (pun intended): reducing the amount of processed food you consume can seem incredibly hard, unenjoyable, and restrictive. You may think you're doomed to ordering salads at restaurants for the rest of your life, but we have no intention of letting that happen to you. Being healthy isn't about eating perfectly or obsessing over the small things. In fact, strict rules and restrictions can often be detrimental to your overall health. So we want you to focus only on what we call the Big Four: grains, dairy, vegetable oils, and refined sugar.

By reducing or removing the Big Four, you'll get the biggest return on your investment. This is because these foods tend to be the most problematic for people and can be significant contributors to chronic, low-grade inflammation. While inflammation is the immune system's normal and healthy response to injury and infection, *chronic* inflammation is like a fire that never gets put out. Over time, this incessant immune response can lead to a long list of health problems, including cancer, cardiovascular disease, asthma, Alzheimer's, autoimmune conditions, and diabetes (to name a few).

GRAINS

A *grain* is a small, dry, hard seed harvested from various types of plants. The grain is the reproductive force of the plant, so it has a lot of responsibility in the life cycle of the plant. Grain in its raw state is toxic to the human digestive tract, meaning it has to be processed in some way before we are able to consume it. The most common grains include millet, corn, sorghum, barley, rye, oats, rice, spelt, teff, triticale, wheat, buckwheat, amaranth, chia, and quinoa. These can be found in a vast and diverse number of food products, including dietary staples. Breads, breakfast cereals, bagels, desserts, and various pastas are all very high in grains, and many sauces contain flour.

Grains have typically been touted as some of the most valuable and healthful foods. But more and more science is beginning to reveal that grains are problematic. As it turns out, grains are at best pretty nutritionally empty, and at worst—for many people—a significant factor in the development and recurrence of serious health conditions.

Much of the current discussion on grains focuses on potential problems with the protein gluten, found in most grains. Unfortunately, nutritionists who focus on gluten to the exclusion of other problems with grain products miss the point. It's not just gluten that is cause for concern, and not just for people who test positive for celiac disease; grains have a lot more potential for harm. It's important, therefore, to investigate very seriously the claims that people make about grains. Do grains really live up to the hype?

CLAIM #1: GRAINS CONTAIN FIBER

Plenty of experts will tell you that grains are important because they are an excellent source of fiber in the diet. This is true, to an extent. Grains *do* contain significant amounts of fiber. However, vegetables and fruits contain fiber, too, and consuming a moderate amount of fruits and vegetables is more than enough to meet the body's fiber needs.

Moreover, the kind of fiber in vegetables and fruits is gentler on the gut than the fiber in grains. Vegetables and fruits contain mostly soluble fiber, which feeds good gut bacteria and does not abrade the intestinal lining. Grains, on the other hand, contain a significant amount of insoluble fiber, which passes through the body undigested and can abrade the intestinal walls along the way. This can contribute to gut-related conditions, such as irritable bowel syndrome (IBS).

CLAIM #2: WHOLE GRAINS ARE A RICH SOURCE OF VITAMINS AND MINERALS

Grains do contain some vitamins and minerals, but not all that much. Grains contain some B vitamins, magnesium, and trace amounts of minerals such as iron and selenium.

The overall amount of vitamins and minerals in grain products depends on the quality of the soil in which the grains are grown. Unfortunately, most grains today are grown on mineral-depleted stretches of overfarmed soil. Plus, almost all grain products, including breads, cereals, and pasta, are *fortified* with synthetic vitamins and minerals. Recent evidence shows that synthetic forms of vitamins aren't absorbed or assimilated well because nutrients need other nutrients present in very specific ratios to be properly digested and absorbed.[1] These ratios are found in perfect balance in whole foods, which can't be reproduced in a lab.

Grains also contain a high amount of compounds called antinutrients, such as gluten and lectin (fruits and vegetables contain antinutrients, too, but fewer than grains). Because plants don't have arms or legs to run away from predators, antinutrients are their built-in defense mechanism. They act like barbed wire around the grain to protect it from overconsumption, contamination, and digestion. When we consume grains, antinutrients make it more difficult for the body to absorb the nutrients within the grain to which the antinutrients are bound.

Even more concerning, antinutrients can disrupt the villi, the small, fingerlike projections that line the intestines through which our bodies absorb nutrients. Studies also show that certain grains can cause the tight junctions that hold the gut together to become loose, allowing food to actually permeate the gut lining and filter into the body without being properly broken down and absorbed. This is most widely known as leaky gut syndrome.[2]

Although the causes of autoimmune diseases, such as rheumatoid arthritis, Hashimoto's thyroiditis, and multiple sclerosis, are complex and still being researched, leaky gut syndrome has been shown to activate autoimmunity, and all autoimmune diseases that have been tested show the presence of intestinal permeability.

CLAIM #3: GRAINS ARE "HEART HEALTHY"

The USDA loves to refer to whole grains as "heart healthy" because they contain fiber. Fiber, they say, is important for heart health because a diet rich in fiber has been correlated with lower cholesterol levels.

There are a lot of problems with this claim. First, people can get ample fiber from consuming fruits and vegetables. Second, there are *many* reasons that fiber is associated with lower cholesterol levels that have nothing to do with grains. Since most diets low in fiber are also very nutritionally poor (think: pizza, mac and cheese, and French fries), it is actually much more likely that people who eat a low-fiber diet have a greater incidence of heart disease because their diet is full of unhealthful foods.

It is also important to be aware that the biochemistry of cholesterol is not as simple as it may seem. While the claim "grains reduce cholesterol and incidence of heart disease" is enticingly simple and easy to craft a diet around, it is incredibly flawed. There are many different kinds of cholesterol, including high-density lipoprotein, or HDL and low-density lipoprotein, or LDL. Reducing the "good" cholesterol, HDL, isn't necessarily a good thing, as cholesterol is used by the body to promote healing. Eating dietary cholesterol from whole foods isn't "bad," and foods that don't contain cholesterol aren't necessarily good.

And then there's the pervasive myth that dietary cholesterol is bad for you. Most medical professionals used to believe that consuming dietary cholesterol (such as that found in eggs) was a big problem for health. However, recent research has demonstrated that the vast majority of the body's cholesterol does not come from what you *eat,* but is rather produced by the body itself in times of stress. *This* is why cholesterol rises when you eat poorly; the body is experiencing stress and trying to heal itself.

Instead of claiming that grains are intrinsically heart healthy, it would be more accurate to state that whole grains contain *some* fiber (nutritionally no better or worse than the fiber found in fruits and vegetables) and that consuming fiber has been linked to improved health.

CLAIM #4: WHOLE GRAINS ARE AN EXCELLENT SOURCE OF PROTEIN

It's a common misconception that whole grains are an excellent source of protein. Compared to animal products, grains contain significantly less protein per gram. In one slice of whole-grain bread, there are 100 calories and 4 grams of protein. In a 100-calorie portion of lean meat, there are 25 grams of protein. In other words, you'd have to eat 600 calories' worth of bread to get the same amount of protein available in 100 calories of meat. Additionally, a calorie-by-calorie comparison shows that high-quality animal products are far more nutrient-dense than grains. A single serving of high-quality meat will contain many more nutrients than a single serving of grains.

When it comes to quality, grains (except for quinoa) are an "incomplete" protein, meaning they don't contain all nine essential amino acids (see page 9 for more on protein and amino acids). Long-term, if you were to rely on grains for the majority of your protein, it could lead to nutrient deficiencies and health problems.

DAIRY

Dairy is anything that is derived from or contains milk. Dairy is the most complex of the Big Four because it can be incredibly problematic for some people and not at all for others. There are also many different kinds of dairy, and while some kinds of dairy (such as milk) may cause issues for you, other kinds (such as butter or ghee) may not.

Dairy can cause health problems for three reasons. First, industrialized dairy cattle often receive antibiotics and added growth hormones and produce milk throughout their pregnancy. This results in high levels of hormones, such as estrogen and progesterone, in the milk they produce. Studies show that people who drink milk regularly have increased levels of hormones in their blood, which can suppress the body's own hormonal regulation.[3] Consuming milk can also can stimulate growth hormones, such as insulin-like growth factor (IGF). Unfortunately, these growth-oriented hormones can wreak havoc on the skin. If you suffer from acne, and *especially* if you are female and struggle with hormone balance, dairy may play a role.

Second, many people are unable to properly digest lactose, which is a naturally occurring sugar found in dairy products. If the body stops producing an enzyme called lactase, which it needs to digest lactose, consuming foods that contain lactose can cause digestive distress, bloating, and gas and lead to conditions such as small intestinal bacterial overgrowth (SIBO).

While some people may experience an immediate, run-to-the-bathroom reaction to lactose, others may react inconsistently and develop symptoms over time, which can make it hard to know if lactose is a problem. In fact, it's estimated that 65 percent of the human population (and up to 90 percent of people in certain cultures) have a reduced ability to digest lactose. People who are sensitive to lactose may tolerate butter and cultured dairy products such as yogurt just fine, as both have minimal lactose.

Third, many people react negatively to whey and casein, two proteins found in dairy. While both proteins can cause similar issues, casein is more often the cause of protein-related problems. For some people, these proteins can provoke an excessive inflammatory immune response, which can manifest as acne or other skin conditions, asthma, allergies, congestion, or sinus problems. It can also lead to gut disruption, both to the intestinal wall and to the gut microbiome, which can trigger symptoms for those struggling with digestive issues or autoimmune disease(s).

What Is Ghee?

*G*hee (or clarified butter) is butter from which the milk solids have been removed. This means ghee doesn't contain lactose or casein. When you're eliminating dairy, ghee is perfectly okay to keep in your diet. (Please proceed with caution and discuss this with your doctor if you have a severe intolerance or allergy.) One special exception is people who struggle with hormonal imbalance and/or have sensitive skin (Stefani is one of those people). Because ghee contains hormones, you may want to eliminate it to see if it has any effect on you. You can make your own ghee by boiling butter, letting it cool, and scraping the solids off the top. If you prefer to buy ghee, look for brands that do additional testing to certify that their ghee is lactose- and casein-free, such as Pure Indian Foods and Tin Star Foods.

DON'T PASS ON GRASS

While dairy can be a healthful food for people who do not react negatively to it, most of the dairy products available in stores today are, unfortunately, highly processed and from poor-quality sources. Conventional dairy comes from cows that are grain-fed and confined to very tight living quarters to maximize their milk production with the least amount of human labor. Grain-fed cows produce milk that is much higher in omega-6 fatty acids and lower in omega-3 fatty acids, a combination that can trigger inflammation in the body. And while many health experts consider milk to be full of nutrients, many dairy products, such as reduced-fat and fat-free milk, must be fortified with synthetic vitamins such as vitamins A and D because removing the fat removes many of the nutrients it naturally contains.

Studies show dairy products from grass-fed cows are significantly richer in fatty acids and fat-soluble vitamins, including vitamins A and D, and two rare nutrients, conjugated linoleic acid and vitamin K2.[4, 5] Conjugated linoleic acid may reduce tumor growth, improve immune function, and help with both diabetes and weight maintenance. Vitamin K2 is necessary for a wide array of cellular functions, including supporting healthy skin. Both of these nutrients are found in the fat of dairy products, which is why grass-fed butter and ghee can be beneficial foods to include in your diet long-term.

Cultured dairy products, which are foods that have been fermented with lactic acid bacteria, can also be beneficial. Examples of these products are yogurt and kefir. They are full of gut-building beneficial bacteria and are enriched with additional vitamins and enzymes relative to milk.

VEGETABLE OILS

Vegetable oils are oils that have been extracted from various plants and are in liquid form at room temperature. The most common vegetable oils include soybean, canola, corn, peanut, palm kernel, rapeseed, cottonseed, grapeseed, safflower, sesame, sunflower, and rice bran oil.

Since entering the American food supply in the early 1900s, vegetable oils have dominated as the primary fat source.[6] They are found in nearly every product that comes in a package and are used to cook most meals in American restaurants because they are cheap and easy to use.

Vegetable oils can be problematic for people because they are very high in polyunsaturated fats (also known as PUFAs). Due to their structure, PUFAs are highly unstable and oxidize when exposed to heat, light, and air. Oxidized fats are incredibly destructive to the human body because they cause free-radical damage and inflammation and are linked to all sorts of major degenerative diseases, such as cancer and heart disease. In short, oxidation is *not* your friend.

To be extracted, vegetable oils must go through high-heat processing (usually with a chemical solvent known as a hexane) and be degummed, bleached, and chemically deodorized before being packaged for sale. Many vegetable oils are sold in clear plastic bottles and sit on store shelves for long periods of time; they are then used to cook, bake, or fry foods, which exposes them to heat. This means that when you consume and cook with vegetable oils, it is *very* likely you are consuming oxidized fats.

The two most widely known polyunsaturated fats are omega-3 fatty acids and omega-6 fatty acids. Both omega-3 and omega-6 fats are essential fatty acids (EFAs), meaning our bodies can't make them on their own.

Omega-3 fats are known for their incredible ability to fight systemic inflammation, support brain function, and even reduce symptoms associated with ADHD, depression, and autoimmune conditions. You can find them in high concentrations in wild fish (salmon, sardines, cod), grass-fed and pasture-raised meats, eggs, and some nuts and seeds. Omega-6 fats help brain function, support the immune system, and help with overall growth and development. They can be found in a wide variety of food sources, including grains, nuts and seeds, vegetables, and meats. While some vegetable oils contain minimal amounts of omega-3 fats, they are all *very* high in omega-6 fats.

In recent years, the amount of omega-6 fats Westerners consume has skyrocketed. The ratio of omega-6 to omega-3 fats in the Western diet has gone from 8:1 in 1935 to 10:1 in 1985 to anywhere from 15:1 to 17:1 today.[7, 8] In the 1960s, omega-6 fats comprised about 8 percent of fat tissue in the average American body; the most recent estimates put it at around 23 percent of fat tissue.[9] Intake of omega-6 fats has more than doubled, and its levels in the human body have tripled.

Many experts now agree that keeping your ratio of omega-6 to omega-3 fats in balance is crucial to overall health. Since omega-6 fats help to stimulate inflammation, without sufficient omega-3 fats, chronic inflammation occurs. Even worse, a wide swath of studies across different countries and research groups has shown that diets high in vegetable oils raise death rates by 50 to 350 percent. Even at the low end, 50 percent is an enormous increase in mortality.[10]

Studies show a ratio of 4:1 is associated with a 70 percent decrease in total mortality.[11] The easiest way to improve your ratio of omega-6 to omega-3 fats is to reduce your overall consumption of omega-6 fats. This is best done by eliminating or reducing foods high in omega-6 fats, such as vegetable oils, refined grains, and factory-farmed meats, and to eat whole-food sources of omega-3 fats, including wild fish, grass-fed meats, and eggs, two or three times a week.

Just a Couple of Nuts

*A*ll nuts (except for macadamias) are composed in large part of omega-6 fats. This means it's probably best to refrain from making nuts a staple in your diet. But it's okay to eat them from time to time; nuts are a whole food, which means the fats do not oxidize as easily as they do when they are extracted from their source (as with oils). When purchasing nuts, look for nuts that are raw and unsalted. Feel free to snack on nuts—just don't *go nuts* with them.

REFINED SUGAR

According to the USDA's Economic Research Service, the average American consumes almost 3 pounds of sugar *a week*, which adds up to a whopping 150 pounds of sugar annually. While you may only think of Twinkies and cupcakes as being high in sugar, sugar can be found in a variety of foods, including bottled salad dressing, canned soup, French fries, frozen dinners, "unsweetened" cereal, ketchup, and prepared pasta sauce. Manufacturers add sugar to just about everything because it makes food taste really, *really* good, and the more you like something, the more you'll buy it.

Refined sugar, which has been extracted from its natural source and stripped of nutrients, can be problematic for a number of reasons. First, when the body processes carbohydrates, it needs vitamins and minerals—specifically B vitamins, phosphorous, magnesium, iron, copper, manganese, zinc, and chromium—to metabolize it. Because refined sugar has no nutritional value, when you consume foods high in refined sugar, you are continually depleting your cells of these important nutrients. On the contrary, whole-food sources of carbohydrates, such as sweet potatoes, contain the exact nutrients they need to be processed in the body, *plus* some.

Foods high in refined sugar also spike blood sugar and insulin levels. The pancreas is responsible for secreting the hormone insulin to clear sugar (glucose) out of the blood and deposit it into cells, as too much sugar in the blood is toxic. When the body is continually responding to an overload of sugar in the blood, it can develop issues regulating blood sugar. This can lead to constant blood sugar crashes, which can cause brain fog, dizziness, irritability, and fatigue. Excess blood glucose also puts the body in a proinflammatory state and has been shown to cause significant oxidative stress—one of the most prominent causes of tissue damage and inflammation.[12] Where there is excess inflammation and oxidative stress, there's an increased risk of developing most major chronic and degenerative diseases.

Studies also show that sugar suppresses the ability of white blood cells to respond to pathogens that make us sick.[13] This means that a diet high in refined sugar can result in a weakened immune system, which makes us more susceptible to infectious disease.

The final issue with refined sugar is that it makes food hyperpalatable. Eating food that tastes delicious is all well and good—we are 100 percent about having satisfying and enjoyable meals. The problem with *hyperpalatability* is that it confuses the body's natural appetite signaling. Hyperpalatable foods are *so good* that they override the body's ability to regulate appetite. Your body fails to feel full when it normally would, so you get hungry more easily.

While the chemical effects of sugar on the brain and body are not the same nor as potent as those of addictive substances such as cocaine, heroin, or alcohol, they can still be incredibly powerful. For example, research has shown that rodents will repeatedly push a buzzer that gives them pain to get access to sugar.[14] Humans, of course, are not rodents, though Stefani would argue that she has gone to similar lengths to get a sugar hit at certain points in her past. In short, the biochemistry of sugar's potency is very real, and should also be taken into consideration when evaluating how sugar impacts your overall health.

Sugar: Natural Options for Sweetness

These natural sweeteners are refined or processed as little as possible and contain all of their naturally occurring beneficial compounds, such as vitamins, minerals, and antioxidants. While we do not recommend eating copious amounts of these sweeteners, they can be used judiciously to sweeten foods, as we demonstrate with our recipes and meal plans. They include:

Dates
Fruit juices
Molasses

Pure maple syrup (dark)
Raw honey

A Note About Artificial Sweeteners

Artificial sweeteners are "zero calorie" sugar substitutes that are 200 to 600 times sweeter than sugar. They are made through chemical reactions where synthetic molecules are either combined or added to existing molecules. The body doesn't recognize these new combinations, so artificial sweeteners *pass through* the body without being metabolized into energy. While this seems like a great idea, studies show that when we consume something super sweet yet provide the body with no calories, psychological changes can occur that dissociate sweet-tasting food with energy intake.[15, 16] This can lead to an increase in appetite and a decrease in feelings of satiety.

Artificial sweeteners have also been found to negatively impact gut flora, and cause gas, bloating, and diarrhea, especially when consumed too much or too often (we speak from experience on this one).[17] As a result, we recommend avoiding all artificial sweeteners, including acesulfame potassium (also called acesulfame K), aspartame, saccharin, sucralose, neotame, and advantame.

If you're looking for a no-calorie sugar substitute, stevia leaf is a great option. Stevia is an herb that has a sweet taste but doesn't raise blood sugar levels. When using stevia, make sure to use either whole dried stevia leaves or stevia powder or liquid extract, which only contains stevia extract and no other artificial sweeteners or sugar substitutes.

3

THE 4X4: DROP THE BIG FOUR FOR FOUR WEEKS (DEPRIVATION *NOT* INCLUDED)

To help you figure out which foods affect you personally, we've create the 4x4. For four weeks, you'll drop the Big Four from your diet, then reintroduce them individually to see how your body responds.

Removing the Big Four from your diet removes the potential risk they pose of disrupting your body. If a specific food is the culprit behind your fatigue, hormonal imbalance, high blood pressure, anxiety, or digestive issues, for example, the 4x4 will give you clarity on how to move forward.

After removing the Big Four, some people notice a dramatic difference in how they feel. For others, the improvements are subtler. How your body responds to the 4x4 will be different from others, and from both of ours. The 4x4 is designed to be a tool you can use today, and throughout your life, to better understand *your* needs. Once you do, you'll be able to create an individualized plan that is sustainable and specific to your body.

ELIMINATE THE BIG FOUR

For exactly four weeks, you'll eliminate the Big Four: grains, dairy, vegetable oils, and refined sugar (if you need a refresher on these, see chapter 2). To help you do this, we've created two meal plans (see chapter 6)—one for bread lovers and one for butter lovers—and crafted seventy-five simple and delicious recipes (starting on page 134) that are free of the Big Four.

Because getting ready for this four-week phase may take some additional time and preparation, we recommend starting your 4x4 on a Monday. Take the weekend before to go grocery shopping, plan out your meals, and remove items that contain the Big Four from your house.

It's also best to do the 4x4 during a time where you feel ready to take on the task physically, mentally, and emotionally. Trying to implement the 4x4 during a high-stress time, such as when you're traveling a lot for work or there's a new baby at home, will make it much harder. Stress can impact how your body responds to certain foods and make it more difficult to know which foods are causing your symptoms.

Once you begin your 4x4, do your best to stick to it. It is important to do this elimination phase for the entire four weeks so your body has the appropriate time to rebalance and heal. Even the smallest amount of grains or dairy can set off health problems for people who are sensitive to them. One of the only ways to find out if you are—and to get started overcoming the issues they cause—is to remove them from your diet completely and observe how your body responds.

MAKE OBSERVATIONS

Before starting the 4x4, it's important to take a full inventory of your body. To do this, write down your answers to these three questions:

1. *What current health conditions do I have?* (This could include things like diabetes, heart disease, and hypothyroidism.) On a scale of 1 to 10, with 1 being the least and 10 being the most, what would you rate the overall pain/disruption you experience on a daily basis with each health condition?

2. *What chronic symptoms do I have that are not identified with a health condition?* (This could include things like insomnia, joint pain, skin conditions, dental issues, digestive problems, headaches, fatigue, brittle hair and nails, depression, anxiety, brain fog, cravings, hot flashes, menstrual cramps, low libido, and high blood pressure, to name a few.)

3. *How do I feel right now, in my body, at this moment?* Do you feel confident? Are you happy? What is your mental and emotional state?

Take your time when answering these questions so you can honestly assess and explore your current state. Then, when you begin your 4x4, check in with yourself and answer these questions again on a weekly basis. We recommend doing this every Sunday evening before the start of the next week. Assess what symptoms are still present and how you are feeling physically, mentally, and emotionally. Have any of your symptoms decreased or resolved? If so, good. If not, make note of what you *are* feeling. It is common to go through an adjustment period when doing the 4x4. Some people experience brain fog and grumpiness for a few days when they remove sugar from their diets, for example, so it is *very* possible you will need to get through the first week before experiencing any positive changes.

Going through the 4x4 with full notes of your symptoms each week will demonstrate to you, with concrete evidence from your own experience, how removing these foods affects you. Then, when you start reintroducing foods, you will be able to map out exactly which foods are causing certain symptoms.

Noelle's Experience

Since age ten, I struggled with digestive issues, including IBS. While I could always tell that my symptoms were aggravated by food, it seemed random and hard to identify. Sometimes I would eat ice cream and be fine, and other times, I would be running to the bathroom. It wasn't until I completely eliminated potentially problematic foods (both dairy and gluten) that my symptoms disappeared. Writing my symptoms down ahead of time allowed me to really see how things changed during my elimination phase. I went from having terrible cramping and gas once or twice a week to having almost no digestive issues at all.

Stefani's Experience

$\mathcal{I}$ used to have acne so bad I was afraid to leave the house. Eliminating grains, dairy, seed oils, and sugar from my diet (as well as making sure I ate at least 2,000 calories a day!) finally healed my skin enough that I could begin to figure out which foods were good for my skin and which were causing harm. Nowadays I still have to steer clear of dairy and a few other foods that have the potential to irritate the skin (goji berries, who knew!), but it's totally worth it. Without the 4x4 and Noelle's and my reintroduction practices, I never would have been able to walk out the door with so much freedom and confidence.

GET IN THE KNOW

During your 4x4, it's important to know how to spot the Big Four, and to be prepared with quick and easy foods you can eat in the event that your favorites don't make the cut.

When shopping for food, always check the ingredients list on any packaged or prepared foods. If the food has an ingredients list, it *very* likely contains grains, dairy, vegetable oils, or refined sugar—or all four. Everything from pasta sauces to canned soups to soy sauce to ketchup contain at least one of the Big Four, so it's important to make yourself aware of what to look for.

A good place to start is the Foods to Eliminate During Your 4x4 guide on page 37. While you may see these exact names listed in the ingredients, often the names will be slightly different because they are derived from one of the Big Four. For example, Enriched Wheat Flour and Malted Barley Flour (grains), Reduced Lactose Whey (dairy), and Expeller-Pressed Sunflower Oil (vegetable oil) are ingredients that should all be avoided.

The first time you venture out to explore what's in packaged and prepared foods at the grocery store, give yourself ample time and patience. It can be frustrating to discover that many foods contain these added ingredients. The good news is, many stores are now carrying brands that provide high-quality alternatives to common convenience foods. A list of our favorite brands can be found on page 333.

It's All in the Marketing

*W*hile many foods are labeled "whole," "real," and "natural," they're often not. There is absolutely no regulation on these terms, which means manufacturers can use them on any packaged foods they chose to. This is why it's important to look beyond the fancy label and check the ingredients list to see what's inside.

EATING AT RESTAURANTS

While we are all for enjoying a meal with family or friends at your favorite restaurant, during your 4x4, it's best to avoid restaurants altogether. This is because almost all restaurants use vegetable oils to cook food, and it can be very hard to know exactly what's in the food you are ordering. Many restaurants have become more accommodating to people with food intolerances, so it *is* possible to work with your server to figure out what dishes would be best to order. But to get the best results from the 4x4, the safest bet is to wait until after your 4x4 is over to patronize your favorite restaurants again.

That being said, if a big restaurant event comes up during your 4x4 and you don't want to miss it, do *not* stress yourself out over whether you should go. Relax, go, and have a good time—just do your best to avoid the Big Four while you are there. You can prepare by checking the menu ahead of time to see what's available and eating a small meal beforehand so you don't show up super hungry. Sides like salads (ask for olive oil for dressing) and steamed vegetables, and entrées that are broiled or baked are a great place to start. When dining out during your 4x4, it's important to avoid alcohol, as it can cause inflammation and disrupt gut flora, which can interfere with your reintroduction results. (See more about alcohol during your 4x4 on page 61.)

Foods to Eliminate During Your 4x4

GRAINS

Amaranth	Oats	Spelt
Barley	Quinoa	Teff
Buckwheat	Rice	Triticale
Corn	Rye	Wheat
Millet	Sorghum	

DAIRY

Butter	Cream	Whey protein
Cheese	Milk	Yogurt

VEGETABLE OILS

Canola oil	Margarine	Sesame oil
Corn oil	Palm kernel oil	Soybean oil
Cottonseed oil	Peanut oil	Sunflower oil
Grapeseed oil	Rapeseed oil	Vegetable oil spreads
Hydrogenated or partially hydrogenated oils	Rice bran oil	Vegetable shortening
	Safflower oil	

REFINED SUGAR*

Agave nectar	Date sugar	Maltose
Barley malt	Dehydrated cane juice	Muscovado sugar
Beet sugar	Dextrose	Palm sugar
Brown rice syrup	Evaporated cane juice	Panela sugar
Brown sugar	Fructose	Raw sugar
Buttered syrup	Glucose	Rice syrup
Cane juice crystals	Grape sugar	Sorghum syrup
Cane sugar	High-fructose corn syrup	Sucanat
Coconut sugar	Invert sugar	Sucrose
Confectioners' sugar	Lactose	Treacle sugar
Corn syrup	Malt syrup	Turbinado sugar

*These are just *some* of the ways refined sugar can be listed on an ingredients label.

While it's important to know what foods to eliminate during the 4x4, it's *just* as important to know what foods to include. And the good news is, there's still plenty to eat. For a complete list of the foods available to you, check out the 4x4 Friendly Foods on page 39.

During your 4x4, you should be providing yourself with a plethora of nutrient-dense foods and meeting your 2,000-calorie-a-day minimum as described in chapter 1. You should also be meeting your macronutrient minimums (50 grams of protein, 100 grams of carbs, 50 grams of fat; see page 9 for a macronutrient refresher) and eating *more* protein, carbs, and fat depending on your individual needs and what works best for you.

Remember: This is *not* some crash diet that involves strict rules and calorie limits. Cutting out the Big Four is a *big* deal, and it takes quite a bit of focus, time, and preparation. By eliminating the Big Four for four weeks, you are reducing or removing potentially disruptive substances from your body and giving it the chance to function optimally. So focus on meeting your minimums and eating enough. Your body will heal in the presence of a ton of nutrient-dense food—and for many people, maybe even *especially* because you're eating more food. The more you eat, the more nutrients you get, so don't focus on restricting the quantity of your food. That's not productive. Focus on enriching the quality, and go ahead and eat to your heart's content.

A Special Note on Legumes

*L*ike grains, legumes such as lentils, beans, and peanuts contain antinutrients called lectins and phytic acid. While these are not inherently bad and can be found in high concentrations in many different foods, including spinach and Swiss chard, we recommend keeping legumes to a minimum during your 4x4. Legumes aren't the most nutrient-dense food, and this is especially the case given that phytic acid binds to certain minerals and prevents their absorption. Legumes also can cause digestive problems such as gas and bloating for people with poor gut function. For this reason, the recipes in this book do not contain legumes. If you choose to include them in your diet, keep your consumption to two or three times a week during the 4x4 and make sure to include other nutrient-dense foods with your meal.

4x4 Friendly Foods

VEGETABLES

Acorn squash
Artichokes
Arugula
Asparagus
Beets
Bok choy
Broccoli
Brussels sprouts
Butternut squash
Cabbage
Carrots
Cauliflower
Celery
Collard greens
Cucumber
Dandelion greens
Eggplant*

Fennel
Garlic
Green onion
Jicama
Kale
Leeks
Lettuce
Mushrooms
Mustard greens
Okra
Onions
Parsnips
Peppers*
Potatoes*
Pumpkin
Radish
Rutabaga

Seaweed
Shallots
Spaghetti squash
Spinach
Sprouts
Summer squash
Sweet potatoes
Swiss chard
Tomatillos*
Tomatoes*
Turnips
Watercress
Zucchini squash
Yams
Yuca

*Nightshades (see page 56)

FRUITS

Apples
Apricots
Avocado
Bananas
Blackberries
Blueberries
Cherries
Coconut
Cranberries
Figs
Grapefruit
Grapes
Guavas

Kiwi
Lemon
Lime
Longon
Lychees
Mango
Melon
Nectarines
Oranges
Papaya
Passion fruit
Peaches
Pears

Persimmon
Pineapple
Plantains
Plums
Pomegranate
Rambutan
Raspberries
Rhubarb
Star fruit
Strawberries
Tangerines
Watermelon

ANIMAL FOODS

Land

Bacon
Beef

Bison
Boar

Buffalo
Chicken

(continued)

Land (*continued*)

Duck
Eggs
Elk
Goat
Goose

Lamb
Ostrich
Pork
Quail
Rabbit

Turkey
Veal
Venison
Wild Boar

Water

Anchovy
Catfish
Clams
Cod
Conch
Crab
Eel
Flounder
Grouper
Halibut
Herring

Lobster
Mackerel
Mahimahi
Mussels
Octopus
Oysters
Prawns
Salmon
Sardines
Scallops
Sea bass

Shark
Shrimp
Snails
Snapper
Squid
Swordfish
Tilapia
Trout
Tuna

FATS AND OILS

Avocado oil
Beef tallow
Coconut oil

Duck fat
Ghee (clarified butter)
Lard

Nut oils (cold-pressed)
Olive oil (extra-virgin)

NUTS AND SEEDS

Almonds
Brazil nuts
Cashews
Chestnuts
Chia seeds
Flaxseed

Hazelnuts
Hemp seed
Macadamia nuts
Pecans
Pine nuts
Pistachios

Pumpkin seeds (pepitas)
Sesame seeds
Sunflower seeds
Walnuts

FERMENTED FOODS

Kimchi
Kvass

Kombucha
Sauerkraut

LEGUMES*

Beans
Lentils

Peanuts
Peas

*Keep consumption of legumes to a minimum, as they are not a nutrient-dense food and can cause digestive issues for people with poor gut function (for more information, see page 38).

BE MINDFUL

We know that eliminating the Big Four can be overwhelming. It can seem like a huge change, and a huge challenge.

Can you really give up four pretty major types of food for four weeks?

You absolutely can. We know that you can.

Elimination diets are pretty common. Many people follow ones such as Paleo, auto-immune protocols, or the Whole 30 for different reasons. Some of them are incredibly popular and are used by millions of people every year. However, we have also personally experienced and witnessed how much people can struggle with them. When you are given "just because" rules, precise portion sizes, specific windows of time in which you are allowed to eat, and specific macronutrient ratios to eat, it can be exhausting. For many people, it is simply too much. It is mentally taxing and demands too much willpower. We don't blame them. We don't like it, either.

For that reason, we set out to make the 4x4 the most psychologically satisfying elimination diet possible. We focused on the foods that give you the biggest bang for your buck, and got rid of every rule we possibly could. Fretting over the small things does you absolutely no good. We refused to compromise on this standard. The 4x4 is about *healing* you, not punishing you.

Your ability to go through these four weeks, feel good, and heal is actually quite dependent on your mind-set. The more you enjoy what you are doing and see it for what it is—a choice—the more likely you will be to stick to it. This means you will be much more likely to embrace what works for you and overcome your health conditions in the long run.

MAKE CHOICES, NOT RULES

It's no secret—the more you feel you *can't* have something, the more you want it. Giving up a specific food because you think it is "bad" or wrong to eat will always lead to cravings, feelings of deprivation, and eventually indulging (or overindulging) in the very food you are trying to avoid. It's a phenomenon both of us have experienced with a variety of foods depending on the diet we were following at the time or the latest trending "problematic" foods. Whether it was all sweets and desserts, high-carb foods, bread, or peanut butter, once we deemed a food "bad," we started obsessing over it.

Now our approach to how we engage with food is completely different. We know that food does *not* have morality, and therefore, it is neither "good" nor "bad." Of course, there are foods that are more nutrient-dense than others, and there may be specific foods that are detrimental to your health and don't make you feel well. But this does not mean a food is inherently bad, and you are not a bad person because of what you do or don't eat.

Understanding this truth frees you up to see food for what it is: neutral. Each day when you wake up, you get to decide what foods you are going to eat. It is a *choice*. Even if you choose to eat something that doesn't make you feel very well, there is no need to feel shame about it—you haven't done anything wrong.

Shifting your mind-set and understanding that *all* foods are available to you is incredibly freeing and empowering. You stop feeling drawn to the "bad" foods and can better follow your intuition and what works best for you. Instead of making choices based on what some diet said to do, you start making choices because you *want* to. Whether it's to keep your digestion feeling good (very important for Noelle), to keep your skin clear (very important for Stefani), or to figure out if removing a food is healthy for you, it is a choice that has a purpose.

Now that you're *in the know* about how the Big Four can affect your body, you can make the choice to do the 4x4 to see how your body responds. By eliminating these foods for four weeks, you'll have a pretty solid idea of how it would feel to eliminate them from your life. After the four weeks, you can experiment with bringing the Big Four back into your diet—we'll address this in the next chapter. They do not have to be gone forever. What you're doing right now is conducting an experiment. It is a choice you are making. Don't let yourself feel deprived or rule-bound. Relax into your role. It's just four weeks, and it's a four-week-long choice that could literally change *everything*.

4

BRING BACK THE BIG FOUR
OVER FOUR WEEKS
(IF YOU WANT TO)

A s many allowances as there are on the 4x4, it still requires you to eliminate a lot of foods you might have really enjoyed throughout your life. You may be itching to have some nice, rich, fatty yogurt again. Or maybe you really miss the occasional sorbet, or a slice of sourdough bread with your morning coffee.

Thankfully, the 4x4 isn't a way of eating you *must* implement for the rest of your life. The purpose of the 4x4 isn't to get you used to doing it forever. Instead, it's to reset. It's to start fresh. It's to show you how your body functions when you remove potentially problematic foods. Once you experience this, you can play around with bringing the Big Four back into your diet (if you want to).

To figure out which foods might be causing specific symptoms for you, we've created a step-by-step protocol for bringing back the Big Four. Over the course of four weeks, you'll reintroduce each of the Big Four individually, independent of one another, in specific amounts. Doing so will allow you to see exactly which foods are problematic for you, and if your reactions are dose-dependent. We get you started with dairy, as it is the most complex of the Big Four and can be an incredibly healthful food for some people. Then we have you reintroduce grains, refined sugars, and vegetable oils to see how you feel with those foods back in your diet.

To help you keep track of everything, we've included a Reintroduction Worksheet for you to use throughout the reintroduction phase (see page 47). To download a printable form, go to coconutsandkettlebells.com/book downloads.

BEFORE YOU REINTRODUCE THE BIG FOUR

Before reintroducing the Big Four, it's important to recognize how you are feeling and understand the changes that happened during your 4x4. On the last day of your 4x4, answer the three questions on pages 33–34 again. Because you answered these questions at the end of each week, you should have some solid information about the improvements that occurred throughout your 4x4. Take special note of any symptoms you listed in question 2, and make a list of any symptoms that improved or completely resolved at the top of your Reintroduction Worksheet.

THE BASICS OF REINTRODUCTION

To reintroduce each of the Big Four, you'll simply bring one category back into your diet for one day only, then monitor your body for any symptoms for two days afterward. We recommend adding one serving of the category you're testing to each meal on day 1. For example, if you are reintroducing dairy, you could put cream in your coffee with breakfast, have some full-fat yogurt with lunch, and top your cooked vegetables with butter at dinner. If all goes well and you don't have any major reactions during your two days of monitoring, you'll bring back dairy (or whichever of the Big Four you're testing) on day 4, except this time you'll include two servings at each meal, then monitor your symptoms for the next three days. This process will take exactly one week. After week 1 is complete, you'll move on to the next Big Four category.

Reintroduction Day by Day

DAY 1: Reintroduce Big Four category #1 (1 serving at each meal)
DAY 2: Monitor your symptoms
DAY 3: Monitor your symptoms
DAY 4: Reintroduce Big Four category #1 (2 servings at each meal)
DAY 5: Monitor your symptoms
DAY 6: Monitor your symptoms
DAY 7: Monitor your symptoms

If you didn't have any reactions to the foods you introduced during week 1 and you're *certain* they don't cause any problems for you, you can include those foods intermittently (if you want to) throughout the rest of the reintroduction phase. However, if a food feels problematic at all, or if you are uncertain, it's best to remove it for the rest of the reintroduction phase so you can accurately gauge your reaction to the other Big Four categories.

If you react negatively to a specific food or your symptoms return after the first reintroduction day, *you are not required to eat it again on day 4.* You have just learned what its effect is on you—there's no need to subject yourself to more unless you think it could be helpful for gathering more information. To let your body heal and come back to the baseline you established during your 4x4, simply leave that Big Four category out for the rest of the week, and the following week, begin reintroducing the next category as planned.

Your second reintroduction day (on day 4) is meant to help you determine if you develop any symptoms with *a larger quantity* of that Big Four category. If this happens, you know your reactions are dose-dependent. If you develop symptoms, remove that category from your diet for the rest of your reintroduction phase. Begin reintroducing the next category the following week as planned.

When your reactions to a food or Big Four category are dose-dependent, we recommend eating it very selectively or removing it from your diet completely, because your body has clearly demonstrated an intolerance to it. While you may not feel the effects when you eat it in smaller doses, it could still cause inflammation. The good news is, you *can* handle that food in smaller doses without experiencing an immediate reaction. This is especially nice when you want a small indulgence or are exposed to a food unknowingly when dining out.

MONITORING YOUR SYMPTOMS

During the reintroduction phase, look for any negative physical, mental, or emotional reactions. These reactions can occur immediately after eating a food, but may take up to seventy-two hours to appear. A good place to start is the list you wrote down on your Reintroduction Worksheet of the symptoms that improved and those that completely resolved during the 4x4. If you didn't have any health conditions or symptoms to note prior to your 4x4, it is possible for new reactions to occur. This is because removing the Big Four allows chronic inflammation to subside, and your immune system is then able to react more strongly to what it perceives to be a problem. Possible negative reactions include:

- Anxiety
- Bloating
- Brain fog
- Congestion or sinus issues
- Diarrhea

- Fatigue
- Gas
- Headaches
- Joint pain
- Postnasal drip

Anything that is different from what you felt during your 4x4 could be a symptom. Use your Reintroduction Worksheet to keep track of any negative reactions you experience as you reintroduce the Big Four week by week.

Reintroduction Worksheet

Start of Reintroduction (Date):

During the 4x4

Symptoms that improved:	Symptoms that completely resolved:

Week #1: Dairy

Reintroduction Day #1	Reintroduction Day #2
Negative reactions?	Negative reactions?

Week #2: Grains

Reintroduction Day #1	Reintroduction Day#2
Negative reactions?	Negative reactions?

Week #3: Refined Sugar

Reintroduction Day #1	Reintroduction Day #2
Negative reactions?	Negative reactions?

Week #4: Vegetable Oils

Reintroduction Day #1	Reintroduction Day #2
Negative reactions?	Negative reactions?

WEEK 1: DAIRY

To kick off your reintroduction of the Big Four, you'll test your reaction to dairy. Dairy is the first category you'll reintroduce because it is the most complex of the Big Four. For some people, it can be a very healthful addition to their diet. For others, it can be harmful. The type and quality you consume can also greatly impact how your body reacts, and for this reason, it's important for you to experiment with different dairy products to make sure you are covering all your bases. On each reintroduction day, you should consume a few different types of dairy. We recommend starting with the most innocent of dairy products—butter, yogurt, and/or cream—during reintroduction day 1 and moving on to the more problematic ones, such as cheese and milk, on your second reintroduction day. Each type of dairy is listed in the following pages in order of most innocent to most problematic, along with more insight into each food.

Symptoms to look out for when reintroducing dairy include digestive problems such as bloating, gas, and diarrhea; acne; postnasal drip and other allergy-like symptoms; and joint pain. Of course, this is not an exhaustive list. In fact, since the proteins in dairy have been linked to inflammation and intestinal permeability, consuming dairy could cause *any symptom related to any autoimmune disease* to flare up. Be on the lookout for any symptom that arises or comes back.

BUTTER

When full-fat cream is churned or agitated, it separates into a solid (butterfat) and a liquid (buttermilk)—butter is the solid. It is about 80 percent fat, and the rest is mostly water. For this reason, it is typically well tolerated by most people because it contains only trace amounts of protein (the dairy proteins are casein and whey) and lactose (the dairy form of sugar). We recommend consuming grass-fed butter on reintroduction day 1, as it's great for testing the waters. If you notice any symptoms after consuming butter, it's best to back off and *not* move on to more problematic types of dairy.

FULL-FAT (HEAVY) CREAM

Much like butter, cream is composed of mostly fat and water, with small amounts of protein and lactose. We recommend including grass-fed unhomogenized heavy cream on reintroduction day 1, as many people can tolerate it well. If cream bothers you but butter does not, it may be either because of the higher lactose content (this would most likely cause only a digestive reaction) or the higher percentage of proteins (which could cause all kinds of symptoms, not just digestive distress).

FULL-FAT YOGURT

Yogurt can be an incredibly healthful food. Since it is bacteria-fermented milk, it contains live bacterial cultures, otherwise know as probiotics. Live bacterial cultures can be *great* for your gut health. The more probiotics you consume, the more "good" bacteria you have in your gut. These bacteria help protect your intestinal lining from damage, help break down food particles, and facilitate the absorption of nutrients into the bloodstream. Probiotic foods are incredibly healthy, so yogurt may merit some testing for you. It's another great option to try out on reintroduction day 1.

If you decide to reintroduce yogurt, go with a grass-fed, full-fat yogurt that doesn't have added sugar. Yogurt is much easier to digest than other dairy because its probiotics help to break down the lactose, so if you are sensitive to lactose, you may be able to tolerate small amounts of yogurt without issues. Yogurt contains a reasonably significant amount of dairy protein, as much as 10 grams in a typical 100-gram serving. If you struggle with yogurt, then dairy proteins are likely a problem for you.

If you happen to *not* tolerate yogurt, don't despair about the state of your gut bacteria. There are plenty of nondairy fermented alternatives you could consume instead. Any kind of fermented vegetable, coconut yogurt or kefir, and kombucha tea are all commonly available alternatives (read more about probiotic foods on page 76).

CHEESE

Cheese has lactose in it, but like yogurt, cheese, especially those aged for longer periods, doesn't have as much lactose as milk. Aged cheeses are generally handled quite well by people with lactose intolerance, though this varies from person to person and cheese to cheese. If you choose to reintroduce cheese, we recommend going with grass-fed, raw cheese. Cheese is a great food to bring back on your second reintroduction day (if you did fine with the foods you ate on reintroduction day 1).

If you can tolerate cheese but you can't tolerate milk, whey is likely the issue: While cheese is quite high in casein, the whey from the milk from which it's made is largely filtered or strained out during the cheesemaking process. If your symptoms are primarily digestive, the issue could be the lactose in the cheese.

FULL-FAT (WHOLE) MILK

Milk is the most potentially problematic of all dairy options, since it contains a whopping dose of both casein and whey, as well as lactose. For this reason, we recommend bringing milk back in on your second reintroduction day (if you choose to) and including only one serving of it. Quality can make a huge difference when it comes to how your body responds, so try to find grass-fed, nonhomogenized whole milk. This will be the most nutrient-dense option that has undergone the least amount of processing. You can often find high-quality milk from local farms and creameries at farmers' markets and natural grocery stores.

RAW MILK

If you have access to it, you can experiment with raw (unpasteurized) milk during your dairy reintroduction week to see how your body responds. Many people who suffer from lactose intolerance digest raw milk without any problems, as it contains probiotic bacteria and antimicrobial enzymes (which are removed with pasteurization). Pasteurization also destroys some of the nutrients in milk, so unpasteurized milk is much more nutrient-dense. Some people (including the FDA) deem raw milk unsafe. However, consider that while almost 10 million people are now consuming it regularly, there hasn't been a *single* death attributed to raw milk since the mid-1980s (peanuts, eggs, and cantaloupe—which are far more readily available—are the worst offenders when it comes to foodborne illnesses). Grass-fed raw milk can be purchased in stores in some states (check sites such as realmilk .com to see if your state is one of them), but you'll likely need to buy it directly from a local farm or at the farmers' market.

Noelle's Experience

*W*hile gluten generally makes me feel terrible, dairy is actually what triggers my IBS symptoms. This was a bit tricky to figure out, as I originally only reintroduced more innocent forms of dairy, including grass-fed butter and yogurt, which didn't cause me any issues in small doses. A few weeks later, I had some ice cream on vacation, thinking that it wouldn't be a big deal. Unfortunately, I had a *major* gut reaction that lasted all night and continued on the plane ride home. Needless to say, it's the last time I ever consumed ice cream or milk. To keep from making a similar mistake, make sure to follow our tips regarding how to reintroduce different types of dairy. Don't assume that dairy doesn't cause you any issue unless you've consumed all the different types during your reintroduction and observed the effects.

WEEK 2: GRAINS

Grains—specifically grains that contain gluten—are the most likely of the Big Four to cause negative reactions. For this reason, we recommend bringing back non-gluten-containing grains on reintroduction day 1, and including one or two servings of gluten-containing grains on your second reintroduction day if you didn't experience any negative reactions after the first day. If you experience negative reactions after the first day, remove grains from your diet for the rest of the week and continue with week 3 as planned.

NON-GLUTEN-CONTAINING GRAINS

Gluten-free grains include amaranth, buckwheat, corn, rice, millet, quinoa, sorghum, gluten-free oats, and teff. We suggest prioritizing whole, unrefined grains during your reintroduction. For example, you can make oatmeal (with rolled oats labeled "gluten-free") for breakfast, have some rice with lunch, and eat corn with dinner. While including grain products such as rice crackers or tortilla chips is fine, it can be hard to find brands that do not contain added refined sugar or vegetable oils, and those are the only ones that will work for your reintroduction. Some of our favorite brands (like Jackson's Honest, which makes tortilla chips with coconut oil) can be found on page 333.

GLUTEN-CONTAINING GRAINS

Gluten is the term used to refer to a combination of proteins—glutenin and gliadin—found in certain grains. Grains that are gluten-free have similar proteins, but they are made up of different amino acid chains that do not cause the same disruption as gluten does. Grains that contain gluten include wheat, barley, and rye, and related grains including spelt, Kamut, farro, durum, bulgur, semolina, triticale, and oats (unless labeled as gluten-free oats).

Until recently, doctors and scientists have thought of gluten consumption as a problem only for those suffering from celiac disease, an autoimmune condition. When people with celiac disease eat gluten, it triggers a cascade of inflammation both outside and inside the intestinal wall, and a loosening of the tight junctions that hold the cells of the gut together. When this loosening occurs, undigested gluten proteins "leak" through the gut barrier and interact with tissue transglutaminase (tTG), an enzyme the body releases in the gut to help repair damage. Because the invaders (gluten) are now crosslinked with the body's own tissue, the immune system creates antibodies to attack both gluten *and* gut cells. This can result in nutrient deficiencies, and a wide range of digestive problems.

In the past few years, research has shown that celiac disease is only one of many expressions of gluten intolerance. A general sensitivity to gluten, which many people experience, is now recognized as non-celiac gluten sensitivity (NCGS). Those with NCGS experience the same symptoms as those with celiac disease or a wheat allergy, but they don't produce antibodies to their body's own tissue, or have the same *severe* intestinal atrophy. Unfortunately, if you are sensitive to gluten, it can still trigger inflammation and leaky gut. Because inflammation and leaky gut are associated with a large number of diseases, symptoms to look out for when reintroducing grains include *just about all of them*. The most common symptoms of gluten sensitivity include IBS-like symptoms (abdominal pain, bloating, diarrhea, and constipation), brain fog, headaches, migraines, fatigue, joint and muscle pain, leg or arm numbness, dermatitis (eczema or skin rash), depression, anxiety, and anemia. Gluten sensitivity has also been associated with thyroid issues and hormonal imbalances.

If you already know you have celiac disease or NCGS, you should not reintroduce gluten-containing grains. However, you may want to exclusively test non-gluten-containing grains on both reintroduction days. Many people who have celiac disease or NCGS think that consuming grains without gluten is fine. Unfortunately, even relatively innocent grain proteins such as those found in amaranth or corn can trigger inflammation in those who suffer from celiac disease and NCGS, so it's important to test them.

Properly Preparing Grains

Most traditional cultures soak, sprout, or ferment grains prior to cooking and consuming them. These preparation methods break down the antinutrients in grains, which makes them much easier to digest. It also means the nutrients in the grains are better absorbed.

To soak grains—which is the easiest preparation method—all you need are filtered water, an acidic medium like apple cider vinegar, and time. This is a super-easy process! Simply place grains in a glass bowl and cover with warm filtered water. (The water needs to be slightly warmer than room temperature in order to break down the phytic acid.) Add 1 tablespoon apple cider vinegar for every 1 cup water. Then cover the bowl with a paper towel and let it sit in a warm area in your kitchen. Most grains should be soaked for 12 to 24 hours; buckwheat, brown rice, and millet have less phytic acid than other grains and only need to be soaked for 7 to 8 hours. Before cooking, drain the grains in a fine-mesh strainer and rinse them. (Note: Grains that were soaked will typically cook faster than grains that weren't.)

WEEK 3: REFINED SUGAR

If you consumed high quantities of sugar before, you probably noticed some huge changes during your 4x4. Once your blood sugar levels stabilized, your cravings may have decreased, your mental health improved, and your energy level increased (though sometimes this comes after a short period of fogginess, moodiness, and/or dizziness while the body adjusts). If you noticed significant changes and as a result have no interest in reintroducing refined sugar, that is A-OK! Simply skip this week and move right on to week 4. Long-term, you can continue to use natural sweeteners, such as those on page 30, to sweeten foods.

If you do choose to add sugar back into your diet, you may notice subtler symptoms during your reintroduction. Dairy and grains largely impact gut health and inflammation. Sugar can impact those, too, but its most potent effects are on your metabolism, mental health, and general feelings of energy and wellness.

There is no real need to distinguish between different kinds of sugar during your reintroduction. If it is "refined" or "processed" sugar, it's going to impact your body the same way. On reintroduction day 1, we recommend incorporating more isolated sources of sugar, such as adding coconut sugar to your morning coffee. On your second reintroduction day, you can include foods that contain added sugar, such as coconut milk ice cream or sweetened grass-fed yogurt (if you didn't react to dairy during week 1).

WEEK 4: VEGETABLE OILS

In order to test this last category, we don't invite you to bring a large container of soybean oil into your home. That would be unwise, to say the least. Instead, we want you to experiment with dining out however many times you want to on both reintroduction days. Go to a restaurant and get whatever you feel comfortable ordering, including foods that you've already reintroduced (but not ones you've decided are problematic). Or if you'd rather, get a premade meal at the supermarket. The point here isn't necessarily to pinpoint the effects of vegetable oils, but rather for you to experience the difference between days that include dining out and days that don't. We also want you to do your vegetable oil introduction at a restaurant because we really do *not* recommend bringing vegetable oils into your home. If you tolerate them, vegetable oils can be included in your diet sporadically but should never be reintroduced for use on a regular basis.

While reactions to vegetable oils typically aren't pronounced, you may experience symptoms associated with inflammation, such as digestive distress, joint pain, acne, or anxiety. Long-term, we recommend cooking with and consuming stable, high-quality fats and oils, such as those listed on page 127.

KNOWLEDGE IS POWER

The purpose of reintroduction is to teach you about the effects different foods have on your body. That way, going forward, you can make educated decisions about how you want to engage with certain foods. When faced with the option of dessert while dining out, for example, you could ask for a sorbet, which is dairy-free, if you know that dairy is a problem. Or, if dairy doesn't bother you as much, you could go ahead and get the ice cream. You could also decide to abstain entirely, because you might hate how tired you feel after you eat a large dose of sugar. It is entirely up to you. Remember: All foods are available to you, and you get to make the choice about how and what you want to eat based on what you know works best for you.

After going through the 4x4 and reintroduction phase, you are equipped with knowledge about your body. Now you can go forth and utilize it as you see fit. We have provided you with the *empowerment* of *familiarity with your body.*

TROUBLESHOOTING

If you find that some of your symptoms still remain after the 4x4, there are a few other foods that may be at the root of your reactions. Depending on your symptoms, you may wish to experiment with eliminating the following:

SOY

Many different products are soy-based: tofu, soy milk, tempeh, edamame, and miso, to name a few, and soy is also a component in many prepared foods in the form of soybean oil. Soy may contribute to hormone imbalance in the body for both men and women. Men may experience low libido, mood swings, low energy, and even the development of breast tissue if they consume too much soy. Women may suffer from a wide variety of symptoms based on their personal physiology. Soy increases estrogenic activity in some tissues and decreases it in others. This can lead to menstrual cramps, ovarian cysts, fibroids, PMS, mood swings, acne, hot flashes, and disrupted sleep. (In some cases, if you have *low* estrogen, some soy may help. It's best to work with a functional medicine practitioner if you are interested in using soy or other estrogenic compounds medicinally.)

Importantly, flaxseeds also have a high amount of estrogen-like compounds in them. They should be handled as carefully as soy.

Stefani's Experience

$\mathcal{I}$ have a *super*-sensitive endocrine system. One of the results of this is that I am quite sensitive to the effects of soy and flax. One time I used a soy-based lotion and I became so depressed I cried for days. Now I regularly avoid soy and flax, and I have a much better grip on all the systems they affect in my body. My periods are so regular I can time them to the hour, my skin is so clear I often don't wear foundation, and my mental health is no longer subject to dramatic swings.

NIGHTSHADES

Nightshades are fruits and vegetables that belong to the botanical family Solanaceae. These include tomatoes, potatoes, eggplants, sweet and hot peppers (but not black pepper), and chile-based spices (including paprika). Nightshades contain compounds (specifically lectin, saponin, and/or capsaicin) that can cause problems for some people. Those who are suffering from an autoimmune disease typically are the most sensitive to nightshades. If you find removing nightshades improves your symptoms, you may wish to consider following a diet plan tailored to people with autoimmune disease. We highly recommend *The Paleo*

Approach by Dr. Sarah Ballantyne and *The Autoimmune Wellness Handbook* by Mickey Trescott and Angie Alt for managing autoimmunity.

FODMAPS

FODMAP stands for fermentable oligosaccharides, disaccharides, monosaccharides, and polyols. The first word, *fermentable*, simply means what follows has the ability to ferment (specifically, in the gut). The rest of the words in the acronym are names of specific types of short-chain carbohydrates that aren't completely digested in the small intestine. While that may sound like a bad thing, short-chain carbohydrates that aren't entirely absorbed act as food for our resident gut flora. For some people, however, these short-chain carbohydrates ferment in excess in both the small and large intestines, causing gas, bloating, and abdominal pain. They also draw water into the large intestine, producing symptoms like bloating and diarrhea.

Foods that are high in FODMAPs include onions, garlic, asparagus, cauliflower, apples, cherries, peaches, pears, watermelon, gluten-containing grains, and dairy (to name a few). For a complete list of foods that are high in FODMAPs, go to http://coconutsand kettlebells.com/what-are-fodmaps.

If removing foods that are high in FODMAPs drastically reduces your symptoms, you likely have a FODMAP intolerance. While the causes of FODMAP intolerance can vary, it's often because of dysbiosis (an imbalance of bacteria in the gut), or a condition known as SIBO (small intestinal bacterial overgrowth). Treating the root cause will often result in a reduction of symptoms.

EGGS

While eggs are an incredibly healthful food, egg whites are packed with allergenic proteins because they are responsible for protecting the yolk from pathogens while the embryo grows. This means that some people can develop an egg allergy, which can cause skin inflammation or hives, nasal congestion, and digestive symptoms such as cramps and diarrhea.

People with autoimmune conditions can also be sensitive to eggs. Egg whites contain a proteolytic enzyme called lysozyme, which has the unique ability to pass through the gut barrier. When this happens, lysozymes can "leak" other allergenic proteins found in egg whites into the bloodstream at the same time. For healthy individuals, lysozymes usually have little to no effect. Those with autoimmune conditions, however, tend to have exaggerated immune and inflammatory responses to eggs. This could mean a flare-up of *any* symptom associated with autoimmune diseases.

FREQUENTLY ASKED QUESTIONS

Naturally, many questions arise when you're following an elimination diet like the 4x4. In order to smooth your transition and get you up and running on our plan as joyfully as possible, we've covered the most popular questions below.

WHAT DO I DO IF I STILL HAVE SYMPTOMS AFTER THE 4X4?

It is entirely possible that you will go through the 4x4 and reintroduction and still have unexplained symptoms. That's okay—even normal. All it means is that you have an underlying condition that either needs more time or a more specific intervention to heal.

First, it may be that you simply need to eliminate the Big Four *beyond* four weeks. While four weeks is sufficient time for most people's symptoms to subside, if you are dealing with a more chronic condition, it may take longer. We recommend trying the 4x4 for an additional one to three months to see if things resolve.

Second, there could be other foods that are causing your symptoms. Begin with the foods mentioned in the Troubleshooting section starting on page 55. If you suspect one of those foods may be at the root of your symptoms, eliminate it for four weeks, then reintroduce it using the guidelines on page 44. If your symptoms are associated with an autoimmune disease, two great resources for understanding food sensitivities are *The Paleo Approach* by Dr. Sarah Ballantyne and *The Autoimmune Wellness Handbook* by Mickey Trescott and Angie Alt.

Lastly, we recommend talking to a trusted medical practitioner (we are partial to functional medicine doctors because of their emphasis on identifying the root cause of symptoms) about your symptoms. You might be dealing with a specific nutrient deficiency or gut infection that needs a more targeted approach. It may take time to learn what's happening in your body, but with careful research (and teaming up with a practitioner who is willing to help), you will be able to figure out what your body needs to be its healthiest.

WHAT DO I DO IF THE REINTRODUCTION PHASE IS INCONCLUSIVE?

If you have more questions after your reintroduction phase, the first thing to do is reset: Go back to what you knew felt good and right. Stay there, eating foods that you are certain feel good for you (or as good as you can manage), for at least two weeks.

Then try reintroduction again. But this time, depending on where things started to become inconclusive, reintroduce each food from a Big Four category one at a time. For example, if you reintroduced a few different types of dairy on reintroduction day 1 during week 1, only test one dairy product (for example, butter) on day 1, and eat one serving at each meal. Monitor your symptoms for two days, then try another dairy product (such as yogurt), and monitor your symptoms for two days again. Keep doing this until you are able to pinpoint exactly which type of dairy (or grain) bothers you.

During this time, hold as many variables as possible constant, from how many hours you sleep each night to how many grains of rice you have with dinner (a *slight* exaggeration)—everything counts. The steadier you hold the rest of your life, the better your results will be.

WHAT HAPPENS IF I EAT ONE OF THE BIG FOUR DURING MY 4X4?

Whether it was an accidental exposure or a decision made out of desperation, if you end up eating one of the Big Four during your 4x4, we have one very specific recommendation for you: keep going. The whole experiment hasn't been derailed, we promise. Take this as a learning experience. Ask yourself, what caused you to deviate from the plan? Are there ways you can change your environment or your mind-set to help prevent that from happening in the future?

Also, take note of how you feel. Did you experience any symptoms after your slip? If so, that may feel unfortunate, but it also provides you with good information! This information could be so good and motivating that it could help you avoid the food you ate even more in the future (like if eating dairy gave you horrible diarrhea, for example).

While traveling and dining out may require some additional preparation, they're not nearly as intimidating as they may seem at first glance.

When you travel, there are two things you can do: pack your own food in advance, or try to get food when you arrive at your destination. Which you choose depends a lot upon where you are going. If you're going to be somewhere where a large grocery store will be hard to find, then it might be wise to pack your own nonperishable snacks beforehand. If you're going to be traveling to a major U.S. city, however, you will probably have access to some great options once you get there.

If you're traveling by car, you can simply pack a bag with nonperishable items (dried fruit, jerky, nut butters, canned wild salmon, Cinnamon-Toasted Coconut "Chips" [page 173], and nuts and seeds are all great options), and pack a cooler with whatever foods you'd like to eat for meals. If you are traveling by plane, you can pack non-perishable items in your suitcase and take a cooler bag with meals to eat on the plane as a carry-on (gel ice packs are allowed through security in the United States). Bring fresh fruit, some peeled hard-boiled eggs, or a salad with some meat on top, depending on how long your flight is. (Note: Food that is packaged with liquid (like canned salmon) will *not* be allowed through security.) Once you get to your destination, you can swing by the grocery store to get some additional snacks or food for meals before going to your hotel. Make sure your hotel room comes equipped with a small fridge to store any perishable food you purchase.

When traveling, don't be shy about bringing things that make you feel your best. Bring a small jar of olive oil or travel packets of coconut oil. Bring your own salt. Bring your own treats, such as Almond Shortbread Cookies (page 258). Pack enough dried fruit to last you a week. We like to pack enough snacks to get us through our trip. Then, when we arrive at our destination, we find the nearest grocery store and stock up on nonperishables. (For packaged snack and meal bars that we love, check out the list on page 333.) It's pretty much like eating at home, but in a hotel room without a stove.

For dining out, you have two options: First, if you have control over where you will be going, do a quick Internet search for "farm-to-table restaurants" or "gluten-free friendly restaurants" plus the name of the city you are in. These buzzwords will typically yield search results that include restaurants that have high-quality food and offer options for those with food sensitivities. Once you're at the restaurant, work with your server to figure out what the best option is for you. Second, you can't go wrong with vegetables and meat. Sides like salads (ask for olive oil for dressing) and steamed vegetables, and entrées that are broiled or baked are a great place to start.

CAN I DRINK ALCOHOL DURING MY 4X4?

During your 4x4 *and* your reintroduction phase, it's best to completely avoid alcohol. Alcohol can cause inflammation and disrupt gut flora, which can interfere with your reintroduction results. After your 4x4 and reintroduction period, reintroduce alcohol carefully and intentionally, as many forms of alcohol are made from grains. For example, beer is made from gluten-containing grains, so if you find you are sensitive to gluten, beer will also cause negative reactions. Some liquors, such as vodka and whiskey, are also typically made from grains (including gluten-containing grains). You may want to start with a gluten-free beer or a vodka made from grapes or potatoes.

WHAT IF I'M FEEDING A FAMILY?

Stefani lives alone, but Noelle's got a husband and a child to feed. This makes Noelle's situation more complicated than Stefani's. While Noelle's husband is completely on board with their food choices as a family, if he wants to eat something that Noelle is sensitive to (like dairy), he simply purchases enough for himself and eats it at his own will. Your family can operate the same way.

Before beginning the 4x4, we recommend proposing your plan to your family members—spouse and children alike. Tell them what you're going to be doing and ask if they want to join. It's possible they may want to try it too. Then all you have to do is start stocking your pantry for a full house and help whoever is responsible for the cooking (including you!) get the support they need.

If your family doesn't want to get on board, that's okay. It's important to communicate why you are doing it, and to let them know you need their support. The better you feel, the better you will operate as a family. Many of the meals in this book are *so* good, your family won't care whether they are free of the Big Four or not. So get them involved in choosing meals, snacks, and treats to cook while you're doing your 4x4.

If you're on a limited budget, you first need to figure out what your priorities are. We personally believe it's best to prioritize eating high-quality animal products. This is important not just for the environment but also for the sake of your health. The most affordable way to do this is to buy meat directly from local farms or at farmers' markets (see page 130 for detailed information and resources regarding purchasing from local farmers). There are unique health benefits that come from consuming grass-fed meat as opposed to industrialized meat, such as a preponderance of vitamin K, which we discuss at length on page 27.

If farmers' market prices are still out of your budget, that's okay. You can put local meat on a future wishlist, and in the meantime, simply buy conventional meat that has a very low percentage of fat. Toxins are stored in the animal's fat, which can be problematic if the meat comes from animals raised in concentrated animal feeding operations (CAFOs).

If you can afford it, purchase organic produce—and if you can't go *all* organic, try to buy a few fruits and vegetables from the organic section. When prioritizing which fruits and vegetables to purchase organic, use the Environmental Working Group's "Dirty Dozen" list as a guide (see page 131). In general, buying organic becomes more important when you eat the peel or skin of a fruit or vegetable. It is worth noting, too, that frozen fruits and vegetables tend to be less expensive than fresh, and also have a greater nutrient content since they are flash frozen right after harvest. Frozen organic produce can be a great way to maximize savings while choosing healthful foods.

It also helps to buy produce and other plant-based products in bulk. Purchasing large containers of spinach, big bags of apples and onions, coconut oils and butters, and nuts and nut flours, for example, in bulk from wholesale clubs is astoundingly cheaper than purchasing individual items at the grocery store. Larger containers of oils and spices tend to be more cost-effective than smaller ones, no matter what kind of store you purchase them from.

More recently, online-based retailers like Thrive Market (thrivemarket.com) and Vitacost (vitacost.com) have exploded because they offer many natural products at reduced costs. Purchasing from these sites in bulk when additional discounts are offered (during holidays, for example) can get you all kinds of different products, such as sauces, nuts and seeds, nut butters and flours, and snack and meal bars, for relatively cheap.

CAN I FOLLOW THE 4X4 IF I AM PREGNANT OR BREASTFEEDING?

It is perfectly safe to do the 4x4 if you are pregnant or breastfeeding. Removing the Big Four only cuts potentially problematic foods from your diet for a set period of time. As long as you are eating sufficient calories and maintaining a macronutrient ratio that works for you during your 4x4 (see page 12 for more information on this), your body will be well nourished. During your 4x4, we encourage you to track your calories and macronutrients to make sure you are eating enough. It's easy to unintentionally eat less—especially when you are busy—because you are no longer consuming hyperpalatable foods. Of course, because pregnancy and breastfeeding often make life more stressful and complicated, we encourage you to always prioritize your mental and emotional health. If at any time during your 4x4 you start to feel fatigued or drained (outside of the norm), discontinue the 4x4 and go back to eating however is most convenient for you.

IS IT OKAY TO EAT DESSERTS AND TREATS?

In short: absolutely. As long as a food is free of the Big Four, you can incorporate it into your 4x4. We are both fans of treats—and have no intention of depriving you of them. While you may be able to find some "paleo" treats at natural grocery stores, we recommend making your own treats using the recipes starting on page 244. We've included everything from Salted Dark Chocolate Almond Butter Cups (page 246) to Watermelon-Lime Gummies (page 266). All the recipes include nourishing ingredients and are free of the Big Four.

WHAT IF I AM A VEGETARIAN?

If you are a vegetarian, you can still do the 4x4. All the vegetarian recipes in this book are labeled as such; however, there are only a few main dishes that do not include meat. For this reason, we recommend having a few other vegetarian dinner recipes on hand when completing your 4x4. The best way to find vegetarian recipes that are 4x4-friendly is to search "paleo + vegetarian recipes" online.

Both of us spent many years (almost twenty between the two of us) as vegetarians because we believed it was healthier. But when looking at the research, we realized almost *all* the research that shows red meat is "bad" comes from observational studies, which do *not* prove causation. Additionally, these studies have absolutely no regard for the quality of the meat, and almost all the people who participate in these studies are consuming red meat sourced from CAFOs. (See page 70 for more information about meat quality.)

We believe the most healthful way to eat is to include high-quality animal products such as meat, fish, and eggs in your diet. Important nutrients, such as EPA and DHA, found in fatty fish; heme iron (which is more absorbable than the iron found in plants), found in beef and other ruminants; choline, an important B vitamin found mostly in eggs; and notably vitamin B_{12}, which is crucial for survival, are *not* found in plant products.

If you are passionate about the environment, sustainability, and the humane treatment of animals, as we are, consider getting involved in the world of what esteemed sustainability farmer Joel Salatin calls "grass farming." While CAFOs absolutely have a negative impact on the environment, grass farming has the *opposite* effect. Grass farming is based on the tenet that the diet of all the animals on a farm should be based on grass. When a farm is run as a grass farm, cows eat the grass, then the herd is rotated. Chickens come in behind the cows and peck through the manure, eating the fly larva, sanitizing the manure, and spreading it around. The grass is then able to rest, rejuvenate, and grow strong again. This type of farming not only results in the animals living a protected and productive life exactly how they were supposed to (birds follow omnivores in nature); it also doubles and triples the amount of biomass that grows. The more biomass that grows, the more carbon is moved from the atmosphere safely into the earth, since plants consume carbon dioxide as food. (For more information on this process, we recommend visiting Joel Salatin's website, polyfacefarms.com, and our friend Diana Rodgers's website, sustainabledish.com, where you can listen to her podcast.)

If you do choose to be vegetarian, we completely respect that. Long-term, in order to make sure you do not develop nutrient deficiencies, we suggest you supplement with vitamin B_{12} or a high-quality B-complex vitamin, as well as algal DHA (or better yet, if you are willing, a high-quality extra-virgin cod liver oil supplement). Be sure to also get enough protein. You can do so by consuming eggs, dairy (if you tolerate it well post-4x4), and/or high quantities of legumes.

WHAT IF I FEEL TOO FULL ON 2,000 CALORIES A DAY?

For most women, 2,000 calories a day is a great place to start. But if it's not right for you, that's okay. We understand that all bodies are different, and you may need fewer calories due to your build, height, and current lifestyle, for example. If you feel overfed or overstuffed eating 2,000 calories a day, you can slowly ramp down your caloric intake until you no longer feel too full, but also don't feel hungry. When doing this, we invite you to err on the side of eating *more* rather than less. Your caloric need may shift down and up at different points in your life according to your individual needs, so don't get hung up on the idea that you need "only" 1,800 or 1,500 calories a day because that's what you've always eaten or that's what some diet said to do. If you find that your appetite and needs are definitely for fewer than 2,000 calories a day—and *not* because you are lying to yourself and actually just trying to get lean the quick and unsustainable way—then listen to your body and give it what you think it needs.

WHAT ABOUT MEAL TIMING?

Eating three square meals, six small meals, or most of your calories in the morning are all ways you can eat food and be healthy.

That's right—there is literally no research that shows you cannot eat at whatever time you like and still be healthy. In fact, while many experts say to eat less at night or stop eating by a certain time, there are no studies that show eating at night is more likely to make you gain weight when compared to eating the exact same food earlier in the day.

Yes, we know that studies have demonstrated, for example, that people who eat breakfast are leaner and have more robust circadian rhythms. But there are *so* many confounding variables: people who eat breakfast may be leaner simply because they are more conscientious eaters, or because they get more sleep, or because they eat more calories (and nutrients) overall. There is not much reason to really believe that you *must* eat breakfast in order to be healthy. It may help, but you can be healthy with alternative eating patterns, too.

The key to being healthy is taking care of your own needs. Everybody's "cure" is different. Many people's "cures" are complete opposites. Some people may be helped by cutting back on carbohydrates, but other people might really need to add them to their diet. The same thing goes for the way in which you eat. Some people might feel really great and suffer no adverse symptoms when they fast intermittently. Others *really* suffer. Women who are recovering from hypothalamic amenorrhea (a condition that occurs when the body feels over-stressed or under-fed) or who are trying to get pregnant are great examples of those who should never regiment their meal times and should simply eat when they want to.

Personally, we both have tried various eating schedules. These days, Noelle is a big-time snacker. She carries snacks with her literally wherever she goes. She refuses to be hungry and therefore always keeps good fuel on hand. Stefani likes to work long hours, so she'll often eat two to three square meals a day or go a long time without eating (though not always).

So go ahead and eat on the schedule that works for you. Three meals with an occasional snack is a good place to start. But don't worry at all about deviating—you know what's best for your body.

5

LIVING WITH HEALTH, HAPPINESS, AND FREEDOM

Now that you've made it through the 4x4 and the reintroduction phase, the big question is—what's next? You've most likely discovered that some foods don't make you feel good, while others are just fine. Or maybe you didn't have any negative reactions, but you'd like to reduce your overall intake of certain foods for health reasons. While it would be easy to tell you to just eliminate those foods and leave it at that, we know how challenging it can be to make changes long-term without feeling deprived or getting stuck in the shame cycle (because yes, we've been there).

No strict elimination diet is successful in the long run, and you don't need to always be "on" the 4x4 to be healthy. Temptations, situations, and priorities come and go. This is perfectly fine. In fact, we actively embrace the messiness of life. Health is not about perfection; it's about being well—physically, mentally, and emotionally.

To help you facilitate the appropriate mind-set and live with health, happiness, and freedom beyond the 4x4, we've put together a list of the most important factors in supporting your physical and mental health. These principles will help you see how the 4x4 fits into the bigger picture, and protect you from living out the rest of your days trapped in the diet mentality.

SUPPORTING YOUR PHYSICAL HEALTH

When it comes to supporting your physical health long-term, there are three key principles to follow: (1) remain flexible, (2) eat nutrient-dense foods, and (3) optimize digestion and gut health. By focusing on these three things, you will create an incredibly solid foundation to operate from.

1. REMAIN FLEXIBLE

Now that you know which foods work best for your body, the number one thing you can do for your health is remain flexible. Your body doesn't have the exact same needs from day to day because it is dynamic and ever-changing. This means the number of calories and quantities of macronutrients you need will change, too. By staying in tune with what your body needs, you give yourself the freedom to fluctuate. You allow yourself to work *with* your body instead of against it.

Many people get stuck because they believe that if something works now, it will work forever. Or they think they need to always limit their calories to a set amount each day. This mind-set can be disastrous long-term, as it can lead to calorie and nutrient deficiencies that can stress your body. A body that is under chronic stress is unable to function optimally, especially when it comes to metabolizing food.

So remember this: there is nothing more important than eating enough and providing your body with all the nutrients it needs. Focus on meeting your minimums (as described in chapter 1) and add more food as you see fit. Some days, 2,000 calories may be just right. On others, you may need much more. The same goes for the amount of protein, carbs, and fats you consume. While you may feel best eating more fat right now, in a year or two you may feel better eating more carbs. There is no set number of calories (or carbs) you must limit yourself to in order to be healthy long-term. Simply focus on eating the foods that make you feel good, and eating enough of them.

2. EAT NUTRIENT-DENSE FOODS

Western culture tends to classify a food as "good" or "bad" based on the number of calories it contains. While calories—the energy a food provides—do play a part in how a food affects the body, they don't actually say anything about the food's nutritional value. For example, a single serving of Froot Loops cereal has 150 calories, while two fried eggs have about 180 calories. Some conventional advice would say that the better choice would be the cereal because it has fewer calories and less fat, although its nutritional value is much less overall. This thinking led to the explosion of cereals, breads, and bagels as breakfast foods in place of traditional, nutrient-dense foods such as eggs.

Focusing on nutrient density often means you're much more satisfied with less food. Studies have found that consuming eggs not only increases satiation, but also results in eating up to 400 calories less throughout the day when compared to an equal-calorie breakfast of a bagel.[1, 2]

When you stop restricting calories and instead focus on food quality, your body functions better. You have more energy, you feel more satiated after meals, and you are better able to trust your body to tell you how much to eat and when to stop. This is what it's like to have a healthy relationship with food. You eat when you are hungry, and you eat the things that make you feel good—both physically and emotionally.

In chapter 2, we talked about the Big Four—foods that tend to cause negative reactions and can actively *deplete* the body of nutrients. These foods are not inherently bad, but a diet high in these foods can absolutely lead to nutrient deficiencies. In contrast, there are many foods that *enrich* the body's nutrient status. Here we've included a list of the big hitters when it comes to nutrient density. As a general rule, we recommend consuming each of these at least two or three times a week.

DARK LEAFY GREENS

It's no secret—vegetables are good for you. They're anti-inflammatory and rich in antioxidants, which protect the body from damage caused by harmful molecules like free radicals. Vegetable-rich diets have repeatedly been linked to lower incidences of disease and better immune system function, as well as reduced risks for heart disease and cancer. In short, there is almost no such thing as eating too many vegetables.

Some of the most nutrient-dense vegetables are dark leafy greens. These include spinach, kale, chard, lettuce, collard greens, beet greens, endive, arugula, and mustard greens. Dark leafy greens are rich in vitamins A, C, E, and K; B vitamins; folate; and calcium. They're particularly important for women who are pregnant or trying to get pregnant, as folate is crucial for the development of the baby's brain and spinal cord.

GRASS-FED BEEF AND OTHER RUMINANT MEAT

Meat, particularly red meat, has been unfairly blamed as the root cause of many health issues, particularly heart disease. Every year or two, a new study comes out, is turned into a sensational headline, and is shared on social media, and the myth continues. But you can rest assured that almost all of the research that shows that red meat is "bad" comes from observational studies, which only demonstrate that there's a statistical relationship between reported red meat intake and health, and not that red meat intake is the cause of poor health. The people in these studies are eating red meat mostly from fast food, which is sourced from concentrated animal feeding operations (CAFOs). There is no regard for quality or source.

Additionally, these studies are flawed because of the "healthy user bias"—that is, because red meat has been vilified for years, the people who eat less of it are healthier because they are also likely to participate in other healthy behaviors such as exercising regularly and eating less sugar and fast food. The reality is that traditional cultures consumed greater amounts of red meat and still remained free of the chronic and degenerative diseases that plague our modern culture. We might have ninety-nine health problems, but meat (especially grass-fed meat) in our diet isn't one.

Beef, lamb, bison, game, and other ruminant (grazing) animals are incredibly nutrient-dense sources of essential amino acids, as well as important vitamins such as B vitamins (including B_{12}), vitamin D, iron, zinc, and more. When it comes to how an animal was treated as it lived on the earth, it's often said that "you are what they eat." For this reason, it's best to prioritize grass-fed meat, ideally from local farms and producers. (See page 26 for more information on the differences between grass-fed and grain-fed beef.)

LIVER AND OTHER ORGAN MEATS

Liver is possibly *the* most nutrient-dense food, packed with enough vitamin A in one pound to nourish a family of five for a month. It is also the best source of all the B vitamins and contains copper, iron, and fat-soluble vitamins, including A, D, E, and K. Liver from nearly any animal will pack a nutrient-dense punch, but liver from grass-fed cows is especially powerful because it contains vitamin K_2, which is essential for a healthy metabolism, heart, bones, and skin.

Liver is the most nutrient-dense organ meat, though hearts and kidneys are also great options.

EGGS

Contrary to popular belief, studies show that a diet rich in eggs will *not* cause heart disease or lead to unwanted weight gain. In fact, eggs contain *tons* of vitamins (we often call eggs "nature's multivitamins"). One of these is choline, a very rare but very important nutrient that prevents fatty liver disease and supports the body's natural detox mechanisms.

Importantly, the vast majority of an egg's nutrients are contained in the yolk. This means you'll want to eat the *whole* egg in order to get all the wonderful benefits.

WILD-CAUGHT FISH AND OTHER SEAFOOD

Salmon and other fatty fish contain high levels of vitamins D and A, as well as omega-3 fats. This supports the immune system, enhances cardiovascular health, strengthens the metabolism, and is key for having a healthy, happy brain. Examples of wild-caught fish dense in omega-3 fats include salmon, trout, and sardines. Examples of nutrient-rich shellfish include scallops and oysters, both of which are high in zinc.

BONE BROTH

Bone broth (or stock) is a nutritional powerhouse rich in collagen, amino acids, and the minerals necessary for strong bones, teeth, and skin, especially as you age. It also has a rare and important effect of helping to heal the gut lining. It's easy to make (see page 222) and you can use it in soup and stew recipes, or sip it from a mug in the morning.

3. OPTIMIZE DIGESTION AND GUT HEALTH

The evidence is clear. In order to have a healthy body, you must also have a healthy gut. The gut, also known as the gastrointestinal tract, is the long tube that's responsible for digesting the food you eat. In order to have a healthy gut, all the digestive processes must be supported and working properly.

THE PROCESS OF DIGESTION

When you sit down to a meal, the sight and smell of food triggers both saliva and stomach acid production, which prepare your body to eat food. Studies show that merely *talking* about food can stimulate digestive fluids, which is why commercials that talk about how wonderful a food tastes while showing you beautiful, appetizing images make you immediately want to eat the screen.

Once food is in the mouth, chewing mechanically breaks it down and mixes it with saliva. Saliva is much more than a mouth-moistening system: it actually contains electrolytes, antimicrobial agents, and enzymes that begin the chemical breakdown of food. This is why chewing food thoroughly before sending it downstream to be further digested is incredibly important.

Swallowing the chewed food (now called a *bolus*) sends it down the esophagus, and the cardiac sphincter at the bottom of the esophagus opens to allow the bolus to pass into the stomach. The stomach then secretes gastric juices to help "churn and burn"

The Organs Involved in Digestion

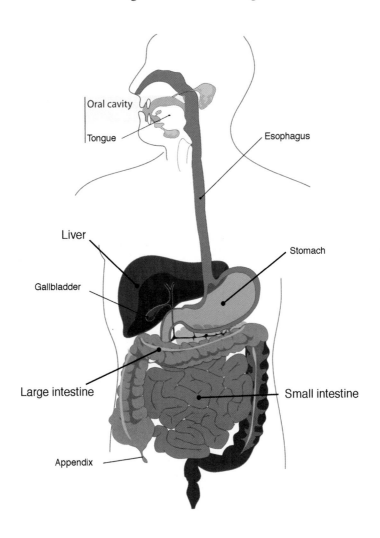

food. Both stomach acid and pepsinogen (a proenzyme that turns into the enzyme pepsin when it comes in contact with stomach acid) help to break down proteins into smaller strings of amino acids. Once the gastric juices have done their duty, the partially digested food (now called *chyme*) is released into the small intestine through the pyloric sphincter.

The small intestine is the star of the show when it comes to digestion. Essentially, it's a twenty-foot-long muscular tube that is responsible for the absorption of nutrients from food. When chyme enters the first part of the small intestine, the acidity triggers the secretion of two hormones into the bloodstream, *secretin* and *cholecystokinin (CCK)*. These two hormones communicate to other organs in the body that nutrients have entered the small intestine. Secretin stimulates the pancreas to release pancreatic juices into the small intestine, which raises the pH of the chyme and further breaks down the nutrients it contains, and CCK stimulates the gallbladder to release bile, which helps to emulsify fats so they can be absorbed into the body.

As the chyme travels through the small intestine, it becomes almost completely digested. Millions of villi and macrovilli (those tiny, finger-like projections lining the walls of the small intestine) absorb the nutrient molecules and pass them into the bloodstream.

Anything that is left over, including indigestible (insoluble) fiber, bile, water, and sloughed-off cells, then passes through the ileocecal valve into the large intestine. Here the water and nutrients are absorbed, and gut bacteria ferment indigestible materials and produce vitamins such as vitamins K and B_{12} and butyric acid. These nutrients are crucial for helping the digestive system function properly, as they nourish the gut lining and have even been shown to protect against colon cancer.

Any remaining undigested material ends its travels in the rectum and is eventually excreted.

In the Brain

When the body perceives stress, digestive functions are down-regulated in order to divert resources to the "fight or flight" response. Eating food in a stressed, or *sympathetic,* state can lead to issues such as gas, bloating, and diarrhea and disrupt the gut microbiome long-term. The body needs to be in "rest and digest" mode—or a *parasympathetic* state—for digestive processes to work properly. To help your body transition into a parasympathetic state before you eat, take 1 to 3 minutes to breathe deeply, or take a moment to pray or feel thankful for your food. It's also important to avoid eating in a stressful environment, such as at your desk at work or when driving, and to proactively seek out places that allow you to eat in a calm state.

In the Stomach

Stomach acid is a digestive fluid secreted in the stomach. It's responsible for breaking down food, killing any pathogenic bacteria that may have come along for the ride, and maintaining an acidic pH (1.5 to 3.0) in the stomach. It's estimated that 90 percent of people have chronically low stomach acid due to eating too fast, not chewing their food well enough, stress, nutrient deficiencies, and diets high in refined foods. When stomach acid isn't sufficient, large, undigested food particles and pathogens make it into the intestines, which can cause bloating, gas, diarrhea, constipation, and dysbiosis. To support stomach acid production, always chew your food thoroughly and prioritize eating in a parasympathetic state. If you suspect you have low stomach acid, drink 1 teaspoon apple cider vinegar in 1 cup water prior to meals.

In the Gallbladder

The gallbladder is a small organ located just beneath the liver that stores and releases bile. Though small in size, the gallbladder is a big player in digestion. When gallbladder function is impaired, which can be caused by, among other things, a diet high in vegetable oils, the body is unable to break down fats or absorb fat-soluble vitamins like A, D, E, and K. Common symptoms of a sluggish gallbladder include bloating, indigestion, fatigue after meals, light-colored stools, and diarrhea. If you suspect you aren't digesting fats properly, consuming beets regularly can help stimulate bile flow from the gallbladder. If your gallbladder has been removed entirely, it's important to take an ox bile supplement when eating a meal that contains fat; the ox bile will break down the fat in place of the bile from the gallbladder.

TAKING CARE OF YOUR GUT

While *all* the organs involved in digestion are important, much of the focus in the last decade has been on the health and integrity of the small and large intestines. This is because they are the primary surface of the body where an exchange happens between us and the exterior world. As a result, more than 70 percent of the immune system resides in the intestines.

That's big news, so it's worth repeating: your gut is inextricably linked with your immune system.

There are two parts to consider when talking about gut health: the microbiome, which is essentially all the bacteria that live in the gut, and the lining of the intestines. There are *trillions* of microorganisms in the gut—three to four pounds of bacteria, to be exact—and the health of your microbiome directly impacts the lining of your gut. Research shows that the health of the gut microbes and the integrity of the gut wall both have a profound effect on the body's ability to fight disease. Because of this connection, research surrounding some of the most complex diseases is now focused on the health of the gut and its relations to those diseases.

Unfortunately, many aspects of Western civilization have drastically decreased our exposure to beneficial microorganisms. Since the industrialization of food began in the late nineteenth century, consumption of traditional cultured and fermented foods, which are packed with probiotics, has taken a nosedive. Western children also spend more time inside and less time outdoors in nature, which helps inoculate the gut with microbes early in life.

The many other factors that can negatively impact gut health include:

- Antibiotics
- Medications such as NSAIDs and birth control
- Processed foods high in refined sugars and vegetable oils
- Exposure to foods the body is intolerant to
- Chlorine (typically found in tap water)
- Meat from animals exposed to antibiotics
- Chronic stress
- Nutrient deficiencies
- Lack of sleep
- Recurring gut infections

While the best way to maintain a healthy gut is to remove each one of these stressors, for most of us, that's unrealistic. This is why it's incredibly important to incorporate intentional gut-health strategies long-term.

Gut-Healing Strategy #1: Consume Probiotic Foods

Probiotics are live microorganisms that have beneficial qualities. While probiotics are everywhere, they're mainly found in soil and food and can be cultivated through preservation techniques such as fermentation. Popular fermented foods include raw (unpasteurized) sauerkraut, kombucha, kimchi, pickles, kvass, and grass-fed kefir and yogurt.

Regularly consuming probiotic-rich foods helps maintain a healthy balance of bacteria in the gut. When gut bacteria are healthy and flourishing, digestion functions appropriately and the immune system is balanced and able to fight disease.

To help gut microbes flourish, you also need prebiotics, which are nondigestible carbohydrates that act as food for probiotics in the gut. Prebiotics are found naturally in certain foods, including onions, garlic, asparagus, bananas, and leeks.

It's important to note that while probiotic supplements definitely have their place, building a healthy, robust, diverse colony of gut microbes is best done with a coordinated effort that includes both fermented foods and supplements.

If you're new to fermented foods, consume a small amount (1 to 2 tablespoons) each day for one to two weeks. After that, slowly increase your consumption until you're eating at least one serving (for example, ¼ cup sauerkraut or 1 cup kombucha) daily. Experiment with different kinds of probiotic foods, and consider switching up the types of foods you're consuming each week, as different probiotic-rich foods contain different probiotic strains.

Keep probiotic supplements on hand for times when you can't consume fermented foods, such as when you're traveling. Supplements are also good when digestive issues strike (constipation, diarrhea, and so on) that could disrupt gut microbes, and when you're taking antibiotics, which wipe out good *and* bad bacteria indiscriminately. Stick with high-quality probiotic supplements that have at least 10 billion CFU per capsule, and switch brands occasionally to diversify your exposure to probiotic strains.

Gut-Healing Strategy #2: Drink Bone Broth

After a long period of simmering in water, the bones, bone marrow, tendons, cartilage, and ligaments of pasture-raised animals release healing compounds, including collagen, proline, glycine, glucosamine, chondroitin sulphates, and glutamine. While all these nutrients are incredibly beneficial for the body, glutamine and collagen have specific gut-healing qualities.

Glutamine is an amino acid that is the primary fuel source for gut cells, and has been shown to enhance gut barrier function. *Collagen* is vital for the body and lends strength and structure to tendons, muscles, skin, hair, bones, and joints. The breakdown of animal collagen in bone broth produces gelatin, which soothes the gut lining, improves gut integrity and digestive function, and can increase gastric acid secretion. Bone broth is also packed with minerals, including calcium, magnesium, phosphorus, silicon, sulfur, and other trace minerals, in forms the body can easily absorb.

Bone broth is easy to make (you'll find our recipe on page 222), and we recommend drinking 4 to 6 ounces of bone broth daily (or using it in soups and stews). You can of course adjust the amount you consume depending on your body's needs. You can add collagen to your diet by supplementing with grass-fed beef gelatin or collagen peptides, which are both available in powder form. Beef gelatin will gel when added to liquids, making it great for homemade gummies, like the Watermelon-Lime Gummies on page 266. Collagen peptides do not gel and can be stirred into hot or cold liquids, smoothies, soups, or stews without adding any noticeable flavor.

Gut-Healing Strategy #3: Manage Stress

It's highly likely that, as an individual living in the twenty-first century, you're familiar with stress and experience it on a regular basis. Stress—put simply—is the body's response to a specific physiological or psychological demand, or *stimulus*. While the majority of stress is negative, stress can also be positive and lead to beneficial adaptations.

Despite being well aware of the harmful effects chronic stress can have on health, most people aren't proactively doing anything to mitigate their stress level. Managing stress often means changing or modifying established behaviors, and, well—that can be *stressful*. Unfortunately, without stress management, the body is much more susceptible to disease.

When we are under stress, whether from driving in traffic, sleep deprivation, working in a high-stress environment, or eating foods that create an inflammatory reaction, the body must divert resources to respond to that stress. If stress isn't managed appropriately and becomes chronic, many of these resources become depleted, and a chronic elevation of hormones involved in the stress response, such as cortisol, can create major imbalances in the body.

Studies show that chronic stress is linked to a number of conditions, including blood sugar dysregulation, weight gain, depression and anxiety, hormonal imbalances, a weakened immune system, cardiovascular disease, and damage to gut wall integrity. In short, if you aren't managing stress, all efforts to improve gut health will be ineffective.

While all the typical recommended stress-relieving activities can help, perhaps the best way to manage stress is to be *mindful* of it. Simply taking one to three minutes to breathe deeply and clear your mind when you feel anxious or stressed will help your body shift from a *sympathetic* state into a *parasympathetic* state. Incorporating intentional parasympathetic shifts into your day will help you have more control over your inner response to stress and prevent the "flight or fight" response from dominating everyday life. Other activities that can effectively facilitate this shift include spending time outdoors, listening to music, massage, acupuncture, going for a short walk, and meditating.

SUPPORTING YOUR MENTAL HEALTH

We firmly believe your mental health is just as important as your physical health. Unfortunately, many people become overly focused on controlling the things that impact their physical appearance—like food and exercise—and sacrifice their mental health in the process. This is largely because of the messaging we receive starting at a young age: *It is better to be smaller, and your worth as a human being is directly linked to what you look like.*

The underlying tone of *you aren't good enough* is pervasive in our culture. Shame sells, and if you feel like you need to be something else in order to be worthy, valued, and happy, you'll buy whatever is being sold that promises to help you get there. Constant exposure to this kind of messaging—which is pervasive in the diet and weight-loss industry—has resulted in most women feeling incredibly dissatisfied with their bodies. And oddly enough, the more women engage with diets or special fitness challenges that promise to "fix" them, the worse it gets.

We do not want that life for you. We both lived it for years—constantly chasing after a "better" body, hoping to finally find happiness in the next diet plan or fitness protocol. It's an endless road, and it almost never leads to health or a happier life. What *does* is pursuing health from a place of self-love, and knowing there is absolutely nothing "wrong" with you. You don't need to change your physical appearance to be worthy of love and attention: you are worthy of it *right now.*

Approaching health with this mind-set can change everything. It can change how you feel about your body and the actions you take to care for it. To help you facilitate this mind-set, we've compiled five important truths to live by. Understanding these truths will allow you to break down many of the lies you've been told and rebuild new conversations around your body, food, and health.

I. SELF-LOVE IS UNCONDITIONAL

Here is an incredibly important fact, perhaps the most important of all: You are supremely lovable, no matter what you eat, how you look, or the status of your health. You do not have to be a certain weight, shape, or size to love your body. You are worthy, right now—in this moment. There is no correlation between changing your outward appearance—like becoming leaner or gaining a six-pack—and becoming more lovable. Your worth is valid because you are human. There are no conditions to this.

The diet and weight-loss industry is masterful at getting us to believe that if we achieve a specific body weight or shape, we'll become more desirable, attractive, and happy. When you believe this—and see your worth as conditional upon it—behavior change is driven by negativity. When your actions are rooted in negativity, you prioritize choices that provide short-term solutions. You eat less even though you feel hungry. You work out longer even though you feel overly fatigued. You judge yourself—and others—more harshly and start comparing yourself to every person you come in contact with.

While this might come as a surprise, operating from a place of self-hate doesn't actually lead to health, happiness, or more satisfaction with your body. In fact, it results in exactly the opposite. It puts you in a position to constantly fight your body to make it become something else. In contrast, when you pursue health from a place of self-love, you make decisions according to what is going to be right for your body. You know that you are not more or less of a person because of the foods you choose to eat or your ability to maintain a six-pack. You are free to make the choices that are right for you—even if they are "off plan."

The truth that forever remains is this: Your body is always on your side, always trying to be healthy. You have a body that is strong, alive, and capable of amazing things, and the number of things it does right outweighs everything else. There is no wrong way to have a body, and you can be healthy at a variety of weights, sizes, and shapes. Pursuing health with this understanding will allow you to see health—and your body—in an entirely different light.

2. FOOD DOES NOT HAVE MORALITY

If you've ever eaten a food that is unhealthy, or deemed "bad" by all the health gurus, you haven't done *anything* wrong. There is no need to feel guilt or shame or beat yourself about it. You aren't lazy, worthless, or less than. You don't need to be punished. And you certainly aren't a bad person. Furthermore, no one is better than you because they do or don't eat certain foods—and vice versa. If someone chooses to eat differently from you, that doesn't make them "good" and you "bad"—it just means you made a different decision.

Food does *not* have morality, and therefore it is neither "good" nor "bad," so your food choices have no bearing on *your* morality. Of course, some foods are more nutrient-dense than others, and there may be foods that are detrimental to your health and don't make you feel well. But this does not mean those foods are inherently bad. Food is simply stuff you eat. Food is *neutral*.

Giving food morality means giving the power to *the food*, and when food has the power, your interactions with food will be accompanied by fear, anxiety, and judgment. This makes it virtually impossible to have any sort of balance or consistency when pursuing health. Punishing behaviors such as negative self-talk, overexercising, and caloric restriction are used to balance the scorecard and make "wrong" actions "right" again. Choices aren't made from a place of self-love; they are made to eliminate shame.

We invite you to remember that you are human and vulnerable. It is normal to want to be loved, respected, and desired. This yearning creates in you—in all of us—the fear of being rejected. It creates a fear of inferiority. It creates a fear of failure, a fear of being unacceptable. We both know this very, very well. We have suffered through years of self-tortured, self-defeating agony. After years of dieting, the number of times we've beaten ourselves up by going to the gym or starving ourselves after eating like we "shouldn't" is more than we can count. In the end, it never led us to a place of greater physical—and certainly never psychological—health. It always made us more entrenched, more self-critical, and more prone to uncertainty and doubt.

To overcome this mentality, we encourage you to dig into your psyche and expose your insecurities. If you do experience shame or guilt when you eat certain foods, ask yourself why. Dig deep into your attitude, your beliefs, and your history. Grab a pen and paper, and explore your feelings. Figure out what fears and motivations live deep inside you. Are you afraid of losing perceived authority? Are you afraid of not being in control? Or are you afraid of gaining weight? If you are, ask yourself why. Is it because society has made you believe you are unlovable or unworthy if you gain weight? If this is true—as it is for many people—it is important to convince yourself that you are wrong (which, to be clear, you are). If you feel the need to meet a certain arbitrary standard of beauty set by, for example, a particular group of your friends or acquaintances, it might be time to find new ones. Life is short, and yours shouldn't be wasted on people who are quick to judge or don't share your values.

3. THERE IS NO WAGON

Virtually everyone who has been on a diet or adopted a new way of eating has eventually broken the rules and made a mistake. This occurrence is commonly known as "falling off the wagon," and represents failure, inadequacy, and lack of willpower. While people tend to put an enormous amount of pressure on themselves to stay *on* the wagon, the truth is, *there is no wagon.* In fact, the wagon mentality is often why many people struggle to remain consistent.

The wagon we all refer to is really just a strict set of rules we hope will give us more control over our health, body, or other people's perception of us. When you're following the rules, you're in the wagon, and when you break a rule—you're out. This mentality can be incredibly ineffective at creating long-term behavior changes because it turns the pursuit of health into an all-or-nothing gambit: instead of enjoying a cookie, then going back to eating the foods that make you feel your best, breaking a rule results in working your way through an entire tub of cookie dough in a matter of hours.

Worst of all, the wagon mentality keeps you stuck in the shame cycle (see page 5). Falling off the wagon results in feelings of guilt and shame, and that shame often drives people straight into the arms of punishing behaviors such as more restriction and more rules, which become the new wagon. Each time perfection isn't maintained, it results in defeat, self-criticism, and desperation, and the only way to rectify these feelings is to get back on the wagon, which starts the process over again. This never-ending cycle is incredibly physically, mentally, and emotionally taxing, and can drain all the enjoyment from experiences involving food.

To stop the cycle, you must get out of the imaginary wagon. This does not mean throwing in the towel on pursuing health. It simply means understanding that the pursuit of health is a journey. There is no "on" or "off"—there is life, and your experiences help you learn what is going to serve you best in the long run. This allows you to nourish your body throughout all seasons of life without having to muster up the motivation to start over or wait until the conditions are *just* right.

It also means recognizing that health is the result of a number of different factors, including your mental, emotional, and social well-being. It's not just about what you eat, and eating perfectly is not a requirement of health. Often the mental banter that accompanies stressing about food is more detrimental than the food you are worried about. You can eat a cupcake in good company, enjoy it, and *move on*. You get to live with more flexibility and mindfulness as you pursue becoming more capable and experiencing all that life has to offer.

This does not mean that abstaining from something that is not serving you is wrong or ineffective. Not being "on the wagon" gives you the freedom to make choices that are right for your body without fear or judgment, or the obsession that often occurs when you categorize a food as "bad" or perceive you can't have something. All foods are available to you, and you get to make the choice about what you want to eat. There is no such thing as where you "should" be. Not with your body, and not with the food you eat. There is simply where you are and where you are going.

4. YOU DON'T NEED "MORE" WILLPOWER

A lot of people think *willpower* is the key to health. Eating healthfully is a chore, and you must rise to the occasion. You must set an alarm for five a.m. You must also make sure you work out on a daily basis. Then you must have a protein smoothie for breakfast and an organic kale salad for lunch. If you don't do these things, you are lazy and less than. You don't have enough willpower. The people who *do* work harder at it. They are the ones who make good decisions and deserve praise.

While this is generally accepted as how it all works, willpower is *not* an inherent quality of the morally superior. It isn't something you can have "more" or "less" of. Willpower is a skill that is shaped by how you set up your environment. Studies show willpower is a learned behavior. Like strengthening a muscle, the more you use it, the better you get at it. When people are successful at enacting willpower in their lives, it's largely because they have learned how to *minimize* the need for it.

You can think of willpower like a glass of water. You pour more water into your glass with positive inputs such as sleeping, eating nutrient-dense food, and using stress-management techniques. Each time you need to use willpower, you "drink" from the glass. Making yourself stay focused at work, resisting the urge to go out for lunch, and holding back from buying a pair of shoes you love all tap into your available water. By the end of the day, you're dehydrated and running on empty—without any willpower to your name.

To minimize the need for willpower, you must first eliminate fatiguing decisions. This is perhaps the most powerful way to support your mental and emotional health when making changes or following a protocol like the 4x4. If you'd like to stop eating a specific food because it doesn't make you feel well, removing that food from your home eliminates the need to continually choose not to eat it. Instead of waiting until the morning to decide whether you are going to go for a walk, make the decision the night before. When you get up, move right into it.

Second, prepare and have a plan. If your goal is to cook dinner at home during the week, plan out your meals a few days in advance and prep food for those meals if possible. This will allow you to move right into making dinner when the time comes. It's also important to plan for the unexpected. If you end up having only twenty minutes to work out instead of an hour, having shorter workouts that you can shift to makes the decision to still work out quick and easy. (Lucky you—this book can help with both of those things!)

Lastly, make the action you want to take the path of least resistance. Small, simple steps can make a huge difference when it comes to deciding whether to take action. By laying out your workout clothes the night before and having your workout space already prepared, you have very little resistance to actually getting up and working out. When you set up these practices, they become habit. When they become routine, they stop being hard. They become easy, normal things about your life that you do every day. This is how you make it sustainable in the long run.

You can also support your mental health by facilitating a mind-set that recognizes your success. Some ways to do this are by positively reinforcing yourself and confidently acknowledging your skills. When you have a "win," celebrate it! Don't put pressure on yourself to perform or to be perfect. That isn't necessary for health, and health and happiness aren't destinations to be achieved. They are part of the journey. Find ways to feel gratitude for the opportunity to move your body and make healthy choices. Get excited about the potential impact the 4x4 is going to have on your life. If progress feels slow, remind yourself that these things can take time. Anything you can do to give yourself a sense of patience, a sense of gratitude, a sense of excitement, and love for yourself and your new approach to health and wellness will make your journey easier and more joyful.

5. HAVING BODY FAT DOES NOT MAKE YOU UNHEALTHY

The science is now clear: people can be healthy and live long lives at a variety of weights and shapes. It remains true that there is an association between obesity and certain health conditions such as heart disease, but the correlation is much looser than scientists previously thought. In fact, current research has found that body fat does not necessarily create negative health consequences. Instead, weight gain is often a *symptom* of a disease state in the body. When looking at the validity of how we assess someone's body fatness—and health—there are also huge inconsistencies. A recent study out of UCLA looked at 40,420 individuals and found that nearly half of "overweight" people and 29 percent of "obese" people (according to the BMI scale) were quite healthy. On the flip side, more than 30 percent of people who were at a "normal" weight were metabolically unhealthy.[3] In short, being overweight doesn't mean being unhealthy, and being thin is no guarantee of good health.

The only way to truly tell if someone is healthy is to know exactly how their body is functioning. Blood tests that look at insulin sensitivity, inflammatory markers, immune function, nutrient status, and hormonal secretions are all great indicators of health status and longevity. These numbers do not necessarily correlate with weight. And in some cases, having more fat on your body is *healthier*. For example, people who suffer from certain cancers appear to benefit from having more body fat. The basic idea here is that body fat can protect you. Body fat is a rich source of energy. It is also where the body stores all the fat-soluble vitamins you need for good health. Women who have higher body fat percentages also tend to live longer than those who do not. This isn't the case 100 percent of the time, but it *is* good reason to refrain from being judgmental about anyone's size, including your own.

In sum, you do not need to fear your body or your body size. Western society puts significant pressure on people—especially women—to adhere to a specific body type: small, lean, with little body fat. We see no problem with this body type, but we also see no problem with larger ones, too. These high-pressure norms come from media outlets that do their best to make you feel bad about yourself; they actually have very little to do with your health. If anything, they are attempting to worsen your health by making you feel self-conscious and unhappy and driving you to do things like go on crash diets over and over again.

If you do wish to lose weight, that is also totally okay. We have absolutely no problem with the desire to change your body, as long as that desire comes from a place of self-love, and as long as you know you do not need to become something else to be worthy. By eating 2,000 calories a day and setting minimums instead of maximums, it is totally possible and likely that weight loss will happen, especially if your health improves. Changes in body fat percentages that are sustainable and *real* happen over the long-term when the body feels safe, fed, and healed. There is no way to *force* weight loss using quick fixes and have the body stay that way. Weight loss must start with healing, first and foremost in your body and mind. Then it simply takes place as a downstream effect.

When approaching health, we encourage you to embrace your body and enjoy all that it is capable of. True happiness doesn't come from what your body *is*—what size, what shape—it comes from what your body *does*. When your happiness is contingent on a specific state of being, happiness is fleeting and fluctuating because bodies fluctuate and change, which is totally normal. Thinking these fluctuations are wrong or bad or make your body unacceptable is the number one way to derail yourself from a healthy way of eating and fall into despair. But how amazing and wonderful would life be if all of us could stop judging ourselves and one another and simply appreciate our bodies for their abilities to sustain life? While this may seem easier said than done, we *know* it is possible. If we were both able to break free of our judgment of, shame about, and anxiety around our bodies, food, and health, anyone can. All it takes is some time; some good, hard introspection; and a heaping dose of commitment to overcoming what society tries to make you feel about yourself. We hope this book facilitates that journey for you.

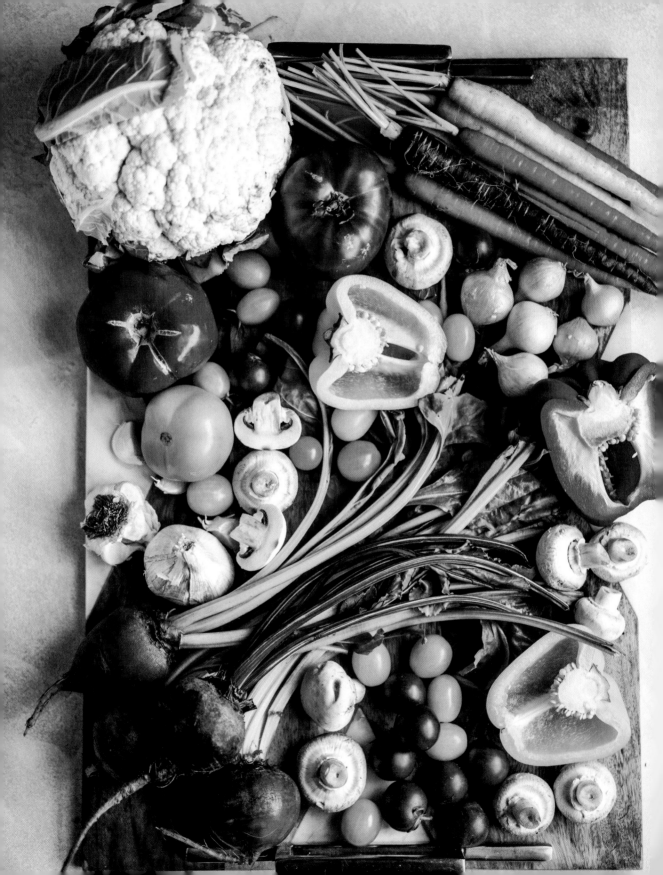

PART II

The PLAN in ACTION: MEAL PLANS, RECIPES, and FITNESS PLAN

6

THE COCONUTS AND KETTLEBELLS MEAL PLANS

Planning and preparation are an absolute *must* when it comes to carrying out a successful 4x4. Because—like most people—you've probably got a lot on your plate, we've done all the work for you and created two separate meal plans: one for bread lovers and one for butter lovers (see page 15 if you haven't yet figured out if you're a bread or butter lover). The bread lover's plan is great for people who do better with more carbs, while the butter lover's plan is great for those who do better with more fat. With each meal plan, we've included everything you need to get started—a weekly shopping list, a guide to kitchen tools and equipment, and a detailed pantry guide. And best of all, batch cooking and meal-prep days are built in, which keeps your time in the kitchen to a minimum.

When following one of the meal plans, remember to listen to your body. While each meal plan provides you with more than enough food to meet your minimums, your individual needs may vary. You may need more carbs, more fat, more protein, or more calories on certain days. To help you customize each plan, we've included tips on how to boost calories, plus quick and easy 4x4-friendly snacks you can add if you need to. These meal plans aren't here to limit you or your choices, and they certainly aren't the only way you can be successful on the 4x4. If you'd like to make small adjustments and swap out a meal with one you're more familiar with—go for it!

As a special reminder—a serving size is whatever is going to serve *your* body. The recipes in this book contain serving sizes that are consistent with conventional standards. But this doesn't mean you should eat only one serving for a meal. For most meals, you'll likely eat two or three servings. The meal plans are made up so that you'll have plenty to eat at meals with room to spare. If you have leftovers, you can eat them as snacks or throw them in the freezer to eat at a later date.

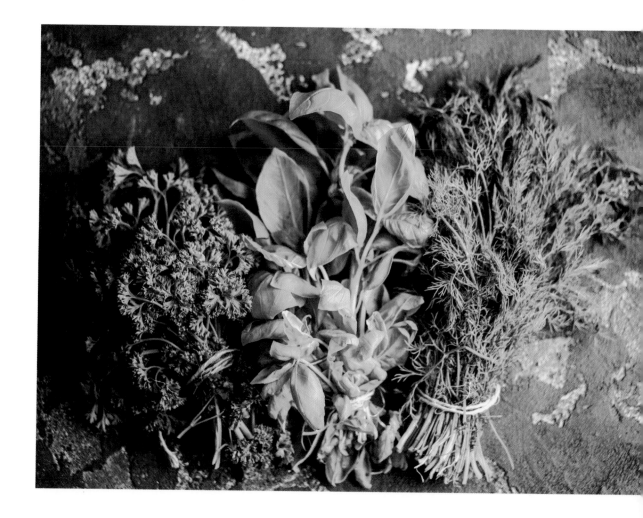

Here are some special notes about how to shop and plan out your meals when using the meal plans:

Food Quantity

- Each meal plan feeds one person for four weeks. If your family is on board for the 4x4, you'll need to increase the amount of food you make depending on the number of mouths you have to feed.

- After cooking food on meal-prep days, separate the food you've cooked into individual containers. Certain items, such as Homemade Bone Broth (see page 222), should be frozen in individual portions, then transferred to the refrigerator the night before to thaw.

- When a meal has "(double)" after it, you'll need to make a double portion of the meal. The shopping list provided for each week accounts for this.

Leftovers

- When leftovers are to be eaten for a meal, the meal will have "(leftover)" after it.

- If the meal is in italics in the meal plan, it indicates that the food has already been made during your meal-prep days or is a leftover meal. Meals that are not in italics will have to be made that day.

- Each meal plan is made up so that you'll have plenty to eat at meals with room to spare. Take note of when a meal is going to be eaten as leftovers and for how many meals. Then separate the leftovers into individual containers so you can easily grab the meal when it's time to eat. If you have extra leftovers, you can eat them as snacks or throw them in the freezer to eat later.

Time Management

- Each week, you are given two meal-prep days. We recommend making these the Saturday and Sunday before your week starts. If you have different days off or your week starts on a different day, you can shift your meal-prep days around. You can also make all the food on one day, depending on your schedule. Just make sure your meal-prep day(s) occur just prior to the start of your week.

- When following each meal plan, we recommend shopping at the grocery store once a week. It's best to do this on the weekend just prior to beginning your meal prep.

- While there is plenty of variety, we've added the perfect amount of repetition so you can get into a groove and benefit from familiarity with some of the recipes.

Shopping List

- Each shopping list provides you with all the food you'll need to make your meals for the week. The list provides quantities that are as specific as possible. However, if you need only half an item (such as a red onion), the shopping list includes 1 red onion to keep it simple.

- Fresh herbs are used throughout the recipes in small quantities. If you see it on the shopping list, simply purchase a single bunch.

- A guide to all the pantry items can be found on page 124, "Stocking the Pantry." In the shopping list, we've included what items from the pantry will be needed. Make sure you are well stocked with the pantry items listed for the week (including spices). If you need a special amount (more than normal), we've called attention to it.

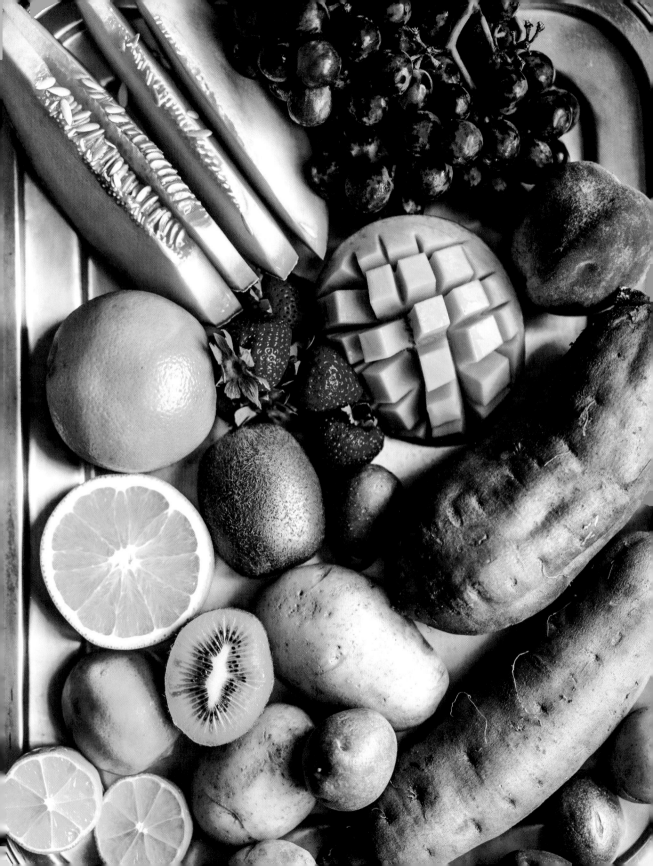

BREAD LOVER'S MEAL PLAN

Our Bread Lover's Meal Plan is specifically for people who feel better eating more carbs. It's packed with nutrient-dense foods and incorporates snacks and sides that have a good dose of carbohydrates.

Ways to Boost Calories

- Add fresh fruit to breakfast: apples, bananas, and berries are great options.

- Roast whole sweet potatoes and add them to lunch or dinner: Pierce each sweet potato several times with a fork and bake at 400°F until tender, about 45 minutes.

- Add a treat after dinner, such as Avocado Chocolate Mousse (page 264) or Dark Chocolate Mug Cake (page 250).

Quick Snack Ideas

- Apple, banana, or carrot sticks with almond butter

- Dates

- Fruit and nut bars (see our favorite brands on page 333)

- Dried fruit (unsweetened)

BREAD LOVER'S WEEK I

MEAL PREP

Day 1
- Make Bacon-Wrapped Eggs, page 146 (freeze)
- Make Chocolate-Cherry Energy Bites, page 172 (freeze)

Day 2
- Make Pumpkin Breakfast Muffins, page 154 (freeze for week 1 and week 2)
- Make Strawberry Cobb Salad, page 182 (toss the salad without the dressing and refrigerate)
    - Hard-boil 3 eggs
    - Make Dairy-Free Ranch Dressing, page 192
- Cook 2 chicken breasts (freeze)

Notes
- Put frozen breakfast foods (Bacon-Wrapped Eggs and Pumpkin Breakfast Muffins) in the refrigerator the night before to thaw.
- Put 2 chicken breasts in the refrigerator to thaw the night before you make the Apple, Avocado, and Chicken Salad, page 177.
- Add the dressing to the Strawberry Cobb Salad just before eating.

BREAD LOVER'S WEEK I SHORTCUTS

- Use store-bought mayonnaise to make the Dairy-Free Ranch Dressing, or use store-bought dairy-free ranch dressing. We recommend the brand Primal Kitchen.

SHOPPING LIST

Meat/Poultry/Fish/Eggs

1 large (4-pound) whole chicken

2 pounds ground turkey

1½ pounds wild-caught salmon fillet

1½ pounds bacon (26 slices)

1 pound ground beef

2 chicken breasts

24 large eggs

Produce

2 large heads romaine lettuce

2½ cups baby spinach

1 head cauliflower

1½ pounds small white potatoes

2 large sweet potatoes

5 medium red potatoes

5 sweet onions

1 red onion

2 scallions

3 carrots

1 pound broccoli florets

1 bell pepper

1 small zucchini

1 medium tomato

1 celery stalk

1¼ cups cherry tomatoes

1 cup white mushrooms

4 sweet apples (such as Fuji or Pink Lady)

3 large avocados

1½ cups strawberries

10 Medjool dates

1 cup unsweetened dried cherries

1 lemon (for juice)

4 heads garlic

Fresh chives

Fresh parsley

Fresh basil

Fresh cilantro

Fresh rosemary

Pantry

Coconut oil (or ghee)

Extra-virgin olive oil

Cold-pressed avocado oil (or macadamia nut oil)

Coconut flour

Almond flour

Almond butter

Raw honey

Pure maple syrup

Baking soda

Pure vanilla extract

Cacao powder (or unsweetened cocoa powder)

Coconut aminos

Balsamic vinegar

Apple cider vinegar

Dijon mustard

Canned full-fat coconut milk (one 13.5-ounce can)

Canned pumpkin (one 15-ounce can)

Canned crushed tomatoes (two 28-ounce cans)

Sriracha sauce

Tomato paste

Chai tea

Grass-fed collagen peptides

Unsweetened coconut flakes

Unsweetened baking chocolate (optional)

Raw almonds

Raw pecans

Spices

Sea salt

Black pepper

Garlic powder

Ground cinnamon

Ground nutmeg

Dried dill

Onion powder

Dried oregano

Dried thyme

Smoked paprika

Paprika

Ground sage

Ground turmeric

Chili powder

Ground cumin

Ground ginger

Red pepper flakes

Bread Lover's Week I Menu

	BREAKFAST	LUNCH	DINNER	SNACK
MONDAY	*Bacon-Wrapped Eggs*	*Strawberry Cobb Salad*	Classic Italian Turkey Meatballs (double) + Rosemary Roasted Potatoes	*Chocolate-Cherry Energy Bites*
TUESDAY	*Bacon-Wrapped Eggs*	*Strawberry Cobb Salad*	*Classic Italian Turkey Meatballs + Rosemary Roasted Potatoes (leftover)*	*Chocolate-Cherry Energy Bites*
WEDNESDAY	*Bacon-Wrapped Eggs*	*Classic Italian Turkey Meatballs (leftover) + Strawberry Cobb Salad*	Slow Cooker Chicken + Creamy Mashed Cauliflower	Easy Apple "Cookies"
THURSDAY	*Pumpkin Breakfast Muffins + Superfood Coconut Chai Latte*	*Slow Cooker Chicken (leftover)*	Zucchini-Beef Taco Skillet	*Easy Apple "Cookies" (leftover)*
FRIDAY	*Pumpkin Breakfast Muffins + Superfood Coconut Chai Latte*	*Zucchini-Beef Taco Skillet (leftover)*	*Slow Cooker Chicken + Creamy Mashed Cauliflower (leftover)*	*Easy Apple "Cookies" (leftover)*
SATURDAY	Apple Bacon Sweet Potato Hash	Apple, Avocado, and Chicken Salad	Firecracker Salmon + Lemon-Garlic Roasted Broccoli	*Chocolate-Cherry Energy Bites*
SUNDAY	*Apple Bacon Sweet Potato Hash (leftover)*	*Apple, Avocado, and Chicken Salad (leftover)*	*Firecracker Salmon + Lemon-Garlic Roasted Broccoli (leftover)*	*Chocolate-Cherry Energy Bites*

Italics indicate that food is already made or is a leftover meal.

BREAD LOVER'S WEEK 2

MEAL PREP

Day 1

- Make Homemade Bone Broth, page 222 (separate into three or four small containers and freeze for week 2 and week 4)
- Make Cinnamon-Toasted Coconut "Chips," page 173 (store in an airtight container)

Day 2

- Make Raspberry Apple Cider Vinaigrette, page 191 (refrigerate)
- Make Chicken-Sage Meatballs, page 206 (refrigerate)

Notes

- Put frozen breakfast foods (Pumpkin Breakfast Muffins, made during week 1) in the refrigerator the night before to thaw.
- Thaw Homemade Bone Broth for the Slow Cooker Garlic-Thyme Pot Roast, page 216, and Slow Cooker Bison Chili, page 226, in the refrigerator the night before.

BREAD LOVER'S WEEK 2 SHORTCUTS

- Use olive oil and balsamic vinegar as dressing for the Roasted Beets and Berries Salad, page 180, instead of making Raspberry Apple Cider Vinaigrette.
- Purchase store-bought bone broth for recipes. We recommend the brand Kettle & Fire.

SHOPPING LIST

Meat/Poultry/Fish/Eggs

3 to 4 pounds mixed
  beef bones
1 (3- to 4-pound)
  chuck roast
4 (6-ounce)
  mahimahi fillets

2 pounds ground
  chicken
2 pounds ground
  bison
5 large eggs

Produce

3 large sweet
  potatoes
5 medium red
  potatoes
6½ cups baby
  arugula
3 sweet onions
3 carrots
2 medium beets
1 red bell pepper
1 bell pepper
  (any color)
1 medium tomato
3 jalapeños
2 large mangoes
2 bananas

1¼ cups fresh
  raspberries
¾ cup fresh
  blueberries
2 large sweet apples
  (such as Fuji or
  Pink Lady)
1 bag frozen
  strawberries
  (at least 2 cups)
2 avocados
2 limes (for juice)
2 heads garlic
Fresh cilantro
Fresh bay leaves
  (optional)

Pantry

Coconut oil
  (or ghee)
Extra-virgin olive oil
Almond flour
Coconut flour
Almond butter
Pure vanilla extract
Raw honey
Pure maple syrup
Apple cider vinegar
Baking soda
Canned full-fat
  coconut milk
  (four 13.5-ounce
  cans)
Canned crushed
  tomatoes (one
  28-ounce can)

Grass-fed collagen
  peptides
Chai tea
Unsweetened
  coconut flakes
  (at least 4 cups)
Unsweetened
  shredded coconut
Unsweetened
  baking chocolate
  (optional)
Macadamia nuts
  (at least 1½ cups)
Raw pecans
Raw walnuts

Spices

Sea salt
Black pepper
Ground cinnamon
Black peppercorns
Dried basil
Ground sage
Dried parsley
Garlic powder
Ground chipotle
  chile

Ground cumin
Dried thyme
Paprika
Dried oregano
Chili powder
Cayenne pepper
  (optional)

Bread Lover's Week 2 Menu

	BREAKFAST	LUNCH	DINNER	SNACK
MONDAY	Breakfast Smoothie Trio (Strawberry-Banana Smoothie)	*Chicken-Sage Meatballs*	Coconut Macadamia Nut-Crusted Mahimahi + Mango-Jalapeño Salsa	*Cinnamon-Toasted Coconut "Chips"*
TUESDAY	Breakfast Smoothie Trio (Strawberry-Banana Smoothie)	*Chicken-Sage Meatballs*	Sweet Potato Chipotle Bison Sliders	*Cinnamon-Toasted Coconut "Chips"*
WEDNESDAY	*Pumpkin Breakfast Muffins* + Superfood Coconut Chai Latte	*Coconut Macadamia Nut-Crusted Mahimahi + Mango-Jalapeño Salsa (leftover)*	*Sweet Potato Chipotle Bison Sliders (leftover)*	Easy Apple "Cookies"
THURSDAY	*Pumpkin Breakfast Muffins* + Superfood Coconut Chai Latte	*Chicken-Sage Meatballs*	Slow Cooker Garlic-Thyme Pot Roast	*Easy Apple "Cookies" (leftover)*
FRIDAY	*Pumpkin Breakfast Muffins* + Superfood Coconut Chai Latte	*Slow Cooker Garlic-Thyme Pot Roast (leftover)*	Slow Cooker Bison Chili	*Easy Apple "Cookies" (leftover)*
SATURDAY	Fluffy Coconut Pancakes	Roasted Beets and Berries Salad	*Slow Cooker Garlic-Thyme Pot Roast (leftover)*	*Cinnamon-Toasted Coconut "Chips"*
SUNDAY	*Fluffy Coconut Pancakes (leftover)*	*Roasted Beets and Berries Salad (leftover)*	*Slow Cooker Bison Chili (leftover)*	*Cinnamon-Toasted Coconut "Chips"*

Italics indicate that food is already made or is a leftover meal.

BREAD LOVER'S WEEK 3

MEAL PREP

Day 1
- Make Bacon-Wrapped Eggs, page 146 (freeze)
- Make Chocolate-Cherry Energy Bites, page 172 (freeze)

Day 2
- Make Pumpkin Breakfast Muffins, page 154 (freeze for week 3 and week 4)
- Make Strawberry Cobb Salad, page 182 (toss the salad without the dressing and refrigerate)
  - Hard-boil 3 eggs
  - Make Dairy-Free Ranch Dressing, page 192
- Cook 2 chicken breasts (freeze)

Notes
- Put frozen breakfast foods (Bacon-Wrapped Eggs and Pumpkin Breakfast Muffins) in the refrigerator the night before to thaw.
- Put 2 chicken breasts in the refrigerator to thaw the night before you make the Apple, Avocado, and Chicken Salad, page 177.
- Add the dressing to the Strawberry Cobb Salad just before consuming.

BREAD LOVER'S WEEK 3 SHORTCUTS
- Use store-bought mayonnaise to make the Dairy-Free Ranch Dressing, or use store-bought dairy-free ranch dressing. We recommend the brand Primal Kitchen.

SHOPPING LIST

Meat/Poultry/Fish/Eggs

1 large (4-pound) whole chicken

1½ pounds wild-caught salmon fillet

1½ pounds bacon (24 slices)

1 pound ground turkey

1 pound ground beef

2 chicken breasts

4 ounces beef liver

24 large eggs

Produce

3 large sweet potatoes

5 medium red potatoes

2 large heads romaine lettuce

2½ cups baby spinach

2 pounds carrots

1 pound parsnips

1 pound broccoli florets

2 sweet onions

1 red onion

1 cup white mushrooms

1 medium tomato

1¼ cup cherry tomatoes

2 scallions

1 celery stalk

3 sweet apples (such as Fuji or Pink Lady)

1½ cups strawberries

10 pitted Medjool dates

1 cup unsweetened dried cherries

2 large avocados

1 lime (for juice)

1 medium lemon (for juice)

2 heads garlic

Fresh chives

Fresh parsley

Fresh cilantro

Pantry

Coconut oil (or ghee)

Extra-virgin olive oil

Avocado oil (or macadamia nut oil)

Coconut flour

Almond butter

Raw honey

Pure maple syrup

Pure vanilla extract

Cacao powder (or unsweetened cocoa powder)

Baking soda

Apple cider vinegar

Coconut aminos

Balsamic vinegar

Sriracha sauce

Dijon mustard

Chai tea

Grass-fed collagen peptides

Canned pumpkin (one 15-ounce can)

Canned full-fat coconut milk (two 13.5-ounce cans)

Unsweetened coconut flakes

Unsweetened baking chocolate (optional)

Raw almonds

Raw pecan

Raw walnuts

Raw pumpkin seeds

Spices

Sea salt

Black pepper

Garlic powder

Ground cinnamon

Ground nutmeg

Dried dill

Onion powder

Smoked paprika

Paprika

Dried oregano

Dried thyme

Ground sage

Turmeric powder

Ground cumin

Chili powder

Ground ginger

Red pepper flakes

Bread Lover's Week 3 Menu

	BREAKFAST	LUNCH	DINNER	SNACK
MONDAY	*Bacon-Wrapped Eggs*	*Strawberry Cobb Salad*	Slow Cooker Chicken	*Chocolate-Cherry Energy Bites*
TUESDAY	*Bacon-Wrapped Eggs*	*Strawberry Cobb Salad*	*Slow Cooker Chicken (leftover)*	*Chocolate-Cherry Energy Bites*
WEDNESDAY	*Bacon-Wrapped Eggs*	*Slow Cooker Chicken (leftover) + Strawberry Cobb Salad (leftover)*	Bacon-Liver Meatballs + Parsnip and Carrot Fries	Easy Apple "Cookies"
THURSDAY	Pumpkin Breakfast Muffins + Superfood Coconut Chai Latte	*Bacon-Liver Meatballs (leftover)*	Cilantro-Lime Turkey Burgers + Sweet Potato Wedges	*Easy Apple "Cookies" (leftover)*
FRIDAY	Pumpkin Breakfast Muffins + Superfood Coconut Chai Latte	*Cilantro-Lime Turkey Burgers + Sweet Potato Wedges (leftover)*	Firecracker Salmon + Lemon-Garlic Roasted Broccoli	*Easy Apple "Cookies" (leftover)*
SATURDAY	Cinnamon Vanilla N'Oatmeal	Apple, Avocado, and Chicken Salad	*Bacon-Liver Meatballs + Parsnip and Carrot Fries (leftover)*	*Chocolate-Cherry Energy Bites*
SUNDAY	*Cinnamon Vanilla N'Oatmeal (leftover)*	*Apple, Avocado, and Chicken Salad (leftover)*	*Firecracker Salmon + Lemon-Garlic Roasted Broccoli (leftover)*	*Chocolate-Cherry Energy Bites*

Italics indicate that food is already made or is a leftover meal.

BREAD LOVER'S WEEK 4

MEAL PREP

Day 1

- Make Cinnamon-Toasted Coconut "Chips," page 173 (freeze)
- Make Watermelon-Lime Gummies, page 266 (refrigerate)

Day 2

- Make Chicken-Sage Meatballs, page 206 (refrigerate)
- Make Raspberry Apple Cider Vinaigrette, page 191 (refrigerate)
- Prepare Japanese sweet potatoes for Shepherd's Pie, page 218 (refrigerate)

Notes

- Put frozen breakfast foods (Pumpkin Breakfast Muffins, made during week 3) in the refrigerator the night before to thaw.
- Thaw enough Homemade Bone Broth (made during week 2) for the Shepherd's Pie and Slow Cooker Bison Chili, page 226, in the refrigerator the night before.

BREAD LOVER'S WEEK 4 SHORTCUTS

- Use olive oil and balsamic vinegar as dressing for the Roasted Beets and Berries Salad instead of making Raspberry Apple Cider Vinaigrette.
- Purchase store-bought bone broth for recipes. We recommend the brand Kettle & Fire.

SHOPPING LIST

Meat/Poultry/Eggs

2 pounds ground chicken

1 (1½-pound) sirloin steak

1½ pounds ground beef (or lamb)

1 pound ground bison

1 pound bacon (10 slices)

1 large egg

Produce

6 cups arugula

2 large Japanese sweet potatoes

3 large sweet potatoes

1½ pounds small white potatoes

5 cups sliced white mushrooms (about 12 ounces)

2 medium beets

1 small eggplant, such as Japanese or Italian

2 zucchini

4 sweet onions

2 carrots

1 medium yellow squash

1 red bell pepper

1 bell pepper (any color)

2 celery stalks

1 jalapeño

3 Roma (plum) tomatoes

2 scallions

1 small watermelon (or 2 cups 100% watermelon juice)

2 bananas

3 sweet apples (such as Fuji or Pink Lady)

1¼ cups raspberries

¾ cup blueberries

1 avocado

1 lime (for juice)

2 heads garlic

Fresh basil

Fresh rosemary

Fresh cilantro

Pantry

Coconut oil (or ghee)

Extra-virgin olive oil

Pure toasted sesame oil

Almond flour

Almond butter

Raw honey

Pure maple syrup

Apple cider vinegar

Coconut aminos

Sriracha sauce

Grass-fed gelatin

Grass-fed collagen peptides

Tomato paste

Marinara sauce

Canned crushed tomatoes (one 28-ounce can)

Canned full-fat coconut milk (three 13.5-ounce cans)

Chai tea

Unsweetened coconut flakes (at least 3 cups)

Raw walnuts

Sesame seeds

Spices

Sea salt

Black pepper

Ground cinnamon

Ground nutmeg

Ground sage

Dried parsley

Garlic powder

Dried basil

Paprika

Dried thyme

Dried oregano

Red pepper flakes

Chili powder

Ground cumin

Ground ginger

Cayenne pepper (optional)

Bread Lover's Week 4 Menu

	BREAKFAST	LUNCH	DINNER	SNACK
MONDAY	Breakfast Smoothie Trio (Apple Pie Smoothie)	*Chicken-Sage Meatballs*	Shepherd's Pie	*Cinnamon-Toasted Coconut "Chips"*
TUESDAY	Breakfast Smoothie Trio (Apple Pie Smoothie)	*Chicken-Sage Meatballs*	*Shepherd's Pie (leftover)*	*Cinnamon-Toasted Coconut "Chips"*
WEDNESDAY	*Pumpkin Breakfast Muffins* + Superfood Coconut Chai Latte	*Shepherd's Pie (leftover)*	Baked Ratatouille + Rosemary Roasted Potatoes	*Watermelon-Lime Gummies*
THURSDAY	*Pumpkin Breakfast Muffins* + Superfood Coconut Chai Latte	*Chicken-Sage Meatballs*	Slow Cooker Bison Chili	*Watermelon-Lime Gummies*
FRIDAY	*Pumpkin Breakfast Muffins* + Superfood Coconut Chai Latte	*Baked Ratatouille + Rosemary Roasted Potatoes (leftover)*	Asian Beef Stir-Fry	*Watermelon-Lime Gummies*
SATURDAY	Apple Bacon Sweet Potato Hash	Roasted Beets and Berries Salad	*Slow Cooker Bison Chili (leftover)*	*Cinnamon-Toasted Coconut "Chips"*
SUNDAY	*Apple Bacon Sweet Potato Hash (leftover)*	*Roasted Beets and Berries Salad (leftover)*	*Asian Beef Stir-Fry (leftover)*	*Cinnamon-Toasted Coconut "Chips"*

Italics indicate that food is already made or is a leftover meal.

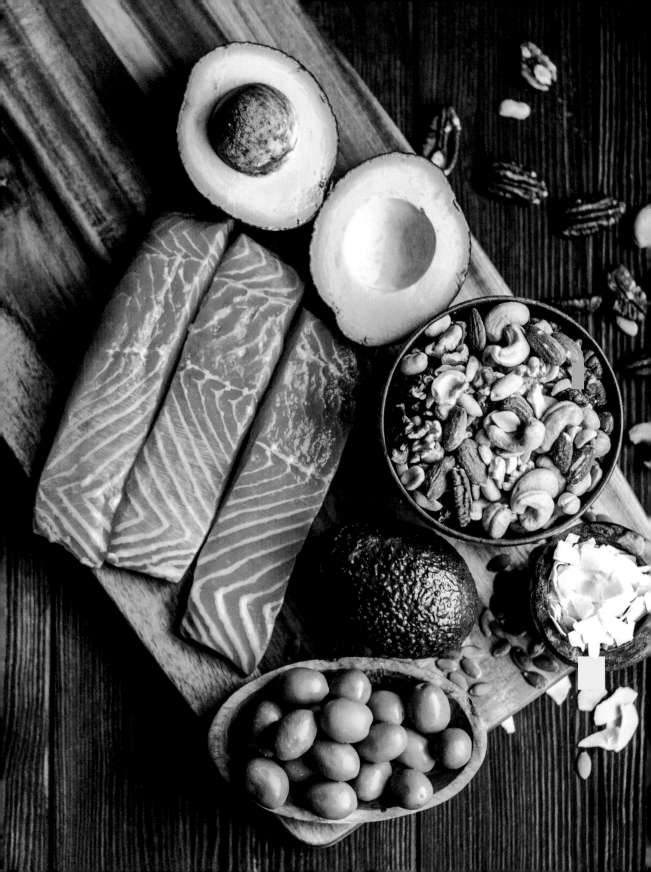

BUTTER LOVER'S MEAL PLAN

Our Butter Lover's Meal Plan is specifically for people who feel better eating more fat. It's packed with nutrient-dense foods and incorporates snacks and sides that are lower in carbohydrates.

Ways to Boost Calories

- Add sliced avocado or fresh berries to breakfast.

- Make a batch of Dairy-Free Ranch Dressing (page 192) and use it as a dip for sliced veggies.

- Add a treat after dinner, such as Whipped Coconut Cream (page 248) or Chocolate Coconut Bombs (page 245). You can also make a berries-and-cream bowl: Place frozen berries in a bowl and pour coconut milk on top, then top with Homemade Chocolate Shell (page 252).

Quick Snack Ideas

- Macadamia nuts

- Hard-boiled eggs

- Carrot sticks with nut butter

- Jerky or collagen protein bars (see our favorite brands on page 333)

BUTTER LOVER'S WEEK I

MEAL PREP

Day 1
- Make Bacon-Wrapped Eggs, page 146 (freeze)
- Make Spiced Rosemary Roasted Nuts, page 174 (store in an airtight container)

Day 2
- Make Pumpkin Breakfast Muffins, page 154 (freeze for week 1 and week 2)
- Make Strawberry Cobb Salad, page 182 (toss the salad without the dressing and refrigerate)
  - Hard-boil 3 eggs
  - Make Dairy-Free Ranch Dressing, page 192
- Cook 2 chicken breasts (freeze)

Notes
- Put frozen breakfast foods (Bacon-Wrapped Eggs and Pumpkin Breakfast Muffins) in the refrigerator the night before to thaw.
- Put 2 chicken breasts in the refrigerator to thaw the night before you make the Apple, Avocado, and Chicken Salad, page 177.
- Add the dressing to the Strawberry Cobb Salad just before consuming.

WEEK I SHORTCUT
- Use store-bought mayonnaise to make the Dairy-Free Ranch Dressing, or use store-bought dairy-free ranch dressing. We recommend the brand Primal Kitchen.

SHOPPING LIST

Meat/Poultry/Fish/Eggs

2 pounds ground turkey

1 (1½- to 2-pound) flank steak

1½ pounds wild-caught salmon fillet

1½ pounds bacon (26 slices)

1 pound ground beef

2 chicken breasts

30 large eggs

Produce

2 large heads romaine lettuce

2½ cups baby spinach

1 head cauliflower

1 pound asparagus

1 pound broccoli florets

1 bell pepper

1 small zucchini

1 medium tomato

1¼ cup cherry tomatoes

1 cup white mushrooms

1 red onion

3 sweet onions

2 scallions

1 celery stalk

3 avocados

3 sweet apples (such as Fuji or Pink Lady)

1½ cups strawberries

1 medium lemon (for juice)

3 heads garlic

Fresh chives

Fresh rosemary

Fresh parsley

Fresh basil

Fresh cilantro

Pantry

Coconut oil (or ghee)

Extra-virgin olive oil

Avocado oil (or macadamia nut oil)

Coconut flour

Almond flour

Almond butter

Raw honey

Pure maple syrup

Pure vanilla extract

Apple cider vinegar

Coconut aminos

Balsamic vinegar

Sriracha sauce

Baking soda

Dijon mustard

Tomato paste

Grass-fed collagen peptides

Chai tea

Canned pumpkin (one 15-ounce can)

Canned crushed tomatoes (two 28-ounce cans)

Canned full-fat coconut milk (two 13.5-ounce cans)

Unsweetened coconut flakes

Unsweetened baking chocolate (optional)

Raw almonds (at least 2 cups)

Raw walnuts (at least 1½ cups)

Raw cashews

Raw pecans

Raw pumpkin seeds

Spices

Sea salt

Black pepper

Garlic powder

Cayenne pepper

Ground cinnamon

Ground nutmeg

Dried dill

Onion powder

Dried oregano

Ground ginger

Red pepper flakes

Chili powder

Ground cumin

Paprika

Dried thyme

Butter Lover's Week I Menu

	BREAKFAST	LUNCH	DINNER	SNACK
MONDAY	*Bacon-Wrapped Eggs*	*Strawberry Cobb Salad*	Classic Italian Turkey Meatballs (double) + Creamy Mashed Cauliflower	*Spiced Rosemary Roasted Nuts*
TUESDAY	*Bacon-Wrapped Eggs*	*Strawberry Cobb Salad*	*Classic Italian Turkey Meatballs + Creamy Mashed Cauliflower (leftover)*	*Spiced Rosemary Roasted Nuts*
WEDNESDAY	*Bacon-Wrapped Eggs*	*Classic Italian Turkey Meatballs + Strawberry Cobb Salad (leftover)*	Firecracker Salmon + Bacon-Wrapped Asparagus Bundles	Easy Apple "Cookies"
THURSDAY	Pumpkin Breakfast Muffins + Superfood Coconut Chai Latte	*Firecracker Salmon + Bacon-Wrapped Asparagus Bundles (leftover)*	Zucchini-Beef Taco Skillet	*Easy Apple "Cookies" (leftover)*
FRIDAY	Pumpkin Breakfast Muffins + Superfood Coconut Chai Latte	*Zucchini-Beef Taco Skillet (leftover)*	*Firecracker Salmon + Bacon-Wrapped Asparagus Bundles (leftover)*	*Easy Apple "Cookies" (leftover)*
SATURDAY	Fluffy Coconut Pancakes	Apple, Avocado, and Chicken Salad	Grilled Balsamic Flank Steak + Lemon-Garlic Roasted Broccoli	*Spiced Rosemary Roasted Nuts*
SUNDAY	*Fluffy Coconut Pancakes (leftover)*	*Apple, Avocado, and Chicken Salad (leftover)*	*Grilled Balsamic Flank Steak + Lemon-Garlic Roasted Broccoli (leftover)*	*Spiced Rosemary Roasted Nuts*

Italics indicate that food is already made or is a leftover meal.

BUTTER LOVER'S WEEK 2

MEAL PREP

Day 1

- Make Homemade Bone Broth, page 222 (separate into three or four small containers and freeze for week 2 and week 4)
- Make Cinnamon-Toasted Coconut "Chips," page 173 (store in an airtight container)

Day 2

- Make Honey-Lime Dressing, page 193 (refrigerate)
- Make Chicken-Sage Meatballs, page 206 (refrigerate)

Notes

- Put frozen breakfast foods (Pumpkin Breakfast Muffins, made during week 1) in the refrigerator the night before to thaw.
- Thaw Homemade Bone Broth for the Slow Cooker Garlic-Thyme Pot Roast, page 216, and Balsamic Wine Pork Chops, page 234, in the refrigerator the night before.

BUTTER LOVER'S WEEK 2 SHORTCUTS

- Use olive oil and balsamic vinegar as dressing for the Chili-Lime Shrimp Salad, page 178, instead of making Honey-Lime Dressing.
- Purchase store-bought bone broth for recipes. We recommend the brand Kettle & Fire.

SHOPPING LIST

Meat/Poultry/Seafood/Eggs

3 to 4 pounds mixed beef bones

1 (3- to 4-pound) chuck roast

2 pounds ground chicken

1 (1½-pound) sirloin steak

1 pound ground turkey

4 boneless pork chops

1 pound large shrimp

½ pound bacon (6 slices)

1 large egg

Produce

1 head romaine lettuce

1 large bunch kale

6 cups mixed baby greens

5 medium red potatoes

2 cups spinach

1½ pounds white mushrooms (about 20 ounces)

1 jicama

2 pounds carrots

1 pound parsnips

1 red bell pepper

1 small zucchini

1 medium tomato

10 cherry tomatoes (about 1 cup)

4 sweet onions

1 red onion

2 scallions

1 large avocado

2 bananas

2 large sweet apples (such as Fuji or Pink Lady)

1 bag frozen cherries (2 cups), pitted

5 limes (for juice)

Red wine or 100 percent red grape juice (½ cup)

3 heads garlic

Fresh cilantro

Fresh parsley

Fresh bay leaves (optional)

Pantry

Coconut oil (or ghee)

Extra-virgin olive oil

Pure toasted sesame oil

Almond flour

Almond butter

Raw honey

Pure maple syrup

Apple cider vinegar

Balsamic vinegar

Grass-fed collagen peptides

Coconut aminos

Sriracha sauce

Sesame seeds

Chai tea

Canned full-fat coconut milk (three 13.5-ounce cans)

Unsweetened coconut flakes (at least 3½ cups)

Unsweetened baking chocolate (optional)

Raw pecans

Spices

Sea salt

Black peppercorns

Ground cinnamon

Garlic powder

Ground sage

Dried parsley

Ground ginger

Ground cumin

Chili powder

Dried thyme

Paprika

Dried oregano

Butter Lover's Week 2 Menu

	BREAKFAST	LUNCH	DINNER	SNACK
MONDAY	Breakfast Smoothie Trio (Cherry-Spinach Smoothie)	*Chicken-Sage Meatballs*	Asian Beef Stir-Fry	*Cinnamon-Toasted Coconut "Chips"*
TUESDAY	Breakfast Smoothie Trio (Cherry-Spinach Smoothie)	*Chicken-Sage Meatballs*	Cilantro-Lime Turkey Burgers + Parsnip and Carrot Fries	*Cinnamon-Toasted Coconut "Chips"*
WEDNESDAY	*Pumpkin Breakfast Muffins + Superfood Coconut Chai Latte*	*Asian Beef Stir-Fry (leftover)*	*Cilantro-Lime Turkey Burgers + Parsnip and Carrot Fries (leftover)*	Easy Apple "Cookies"
THURSDAY	*Pumpkin Breakfast Muffins + Superfood Coconut Chai Latte*	*Chicken-Sage Meatballs*	Slow Cooker Garlic-Thyme Pot Roast	*Easy Apple "Cookies" (leftover)*
FRIDAY	*Pumpkin Breakfast Muffins + Superfood Coconut Chai Latte*	*Slow Cooker Garlic-Thyme Pot Roast (leftover)*	Balsamic Wine Pork Chops	*Easy Apple "Cookies" (leftover)*
SATURDAY	Kale and Bacon Breakfast Skillet	Chili Lime Shrimp Salad	*Slow Cooker Garlic-Thyme Pot Roast (leftover)*	*Cinnamon-Toasted Coconut "Chips"*
SUNDAY	*Kale and Bacon Breakfast Skillet (leftover)*	*Chili Lime Shrimp Salad (leftover)*	*Balsamic Wine Pork Chops (leftover)*	*Cinnamon-Toasted Coconut "Chips"*

Italics indicate that food is already made or is a leftover meal.

BUTTER LOVER'S WEEK 3

MEAL PREP

Day 1
- Make Bacon-Wrapped Eggs, page 146 (freeze)
- Make Spiced Rosemary Roasted Nuts, page 174 (store in an airtight container)

Day 2
- Make Pumpkin Breakfast Muffins, page 154 (freeze for week 3 and week 4)
- Make Strawberry Cobb Salad, page 182 (toss the salad without the dressing and place in the refrigerator)
  - Hard-boil 3 eggs
  - Make Dairy-Free Ranch Dressing, page 192
- Cook 2 chicken breasts (freeze)

Notes
- Put frozen breakfast foods (Bacon-Wrapped Eggs and Pumpkin Breakfast Muffins) in the refrigerator the night before to thaw.
- Put 2 chicken breasts in the refrigerator to thaw the night before you make the Apple, Avocado, and Chicken Salad, page 177.
- Add the dressing to the Strawberry Cobb Salad just before consuming.

BUTTER LOVER'S WEEK 3 SHORTCUTS
- Use store-bought mayonnaise to make the Dairy-Free Ranch Dressing, or use store-bought dairy-free ranch dressing. We recommend the brand Primal Kitchen.

SHOPPING LIST

Meat/Poultry/Fish/Eggs

1 large (4-pound) whole chicken
4 (6-ounce) mahimahi fillets
1½ pounds bacon (24 slices)
1 pound large shrimp
1 pound ground beef
2 chicken breasts
4 ounces beef liver
30 large eggs

Produce

1 head cabbage
1 large head romaine lettuce
4½ cups baby spinach (more optional)
5 medium red potatoes
1 pound broccoli florets
2 pounds carrots
1 pound parsnips
1 red bell pepper
1 medium tomato
1¼ cup cherry tomatoes
3 cups white mushrooms
3 sweet onions
1 red onion
1 celery stalk
3 sweet apples (such as Fuji or Pink Lady)
2 large avocados
1½ cups strawberries
1 medium lemon (for juice)
1 lime (for juice)
2 head garlic
Fresh chives
Fresh rosemary
Fresh parsley
Fresh cilantro
Fresh basil

Pantry

Coconut oil (or ghee)
Extra-virgin olive oil
Avocado oil (or macadamia nut oil)
Coconut flour
Almond flour
Almond butter
Raw honey
Pure maple syrup
Pure vanilla extract
Baking soda
Apple cider vinegar
Coconut aminos
Sriracha sauce
Canned pumpkin (one 15-ounce can)
Grass-fed collagen peptides
Dijon mustard
Chai tea
Canned full-fat coconut milk (two 13.5-ounce cans)
Unsweetened coconut flakes
Unsweetened shredded coconut
Unsweetened baking chocolate (optional)
Raw almonds (at least 2 cups)
Raw walnuts (at least 1½ cups)
Macadamia nuts (at least 1½ cups)
Raw pecans
Raw cashews
Raw pumpkin seeds

Spices

Sea salt
Black pepper
Garlic powder
Cayenne pepper
Ground cinnamon
Ground nutmeg
Dried dill
Onion powder
Smoked paprika
Paprika
Dried oregano
Dried thyme
Ground sage
Ground turmeric
Ground ginger

Butter Lover's Week 3 Menu

	BREAKFAST	LUNCH	DINNER	SNACK
MONDAY	*Bacon-Wrapped Eggs*	*Strawberry Cobb Salad*	*Slow Cooker Chicken*	*Spiced Rosemary Roasted Nuts*
TUESDAY	*Bacon-Wrapped Eggs*	*Strawberry Cobb Salad*	*Slow Cooker Chicken (leftover)*	*Spiced Rosemary Roasted Nuts*
WEDNESDAY	*Bacon-Wrapped Eggs*	*Slow Cooker Chicken (leftover) + Strawberry Cobb Salad (leftover)*	Bacon-Liver Meatballs + Parsnip and Carrot Fries	Easy Apple "Cookies"
THURSDAY	Pumpkin Breakfast Muffins + Superfood Coconut Chai Latte	Bacon-Liver Meatballs *(leftover)*	Shrimp and Cabbage Stir-Fry	*Easy Apple "Cookies" (leftover)*
FRIDAY	Pumpkin Breakfast Muffins + Superfood Coconut Chai Latte	*Shrimp and Cabbage Stir-Fry (leftover)*	Coconut Macadamia Nut–Crusted Mahimahi + Lemon-Garlic Roasted Broccoli	*Easy Apple "Cookies" (leftover)*
SATURDAY	Spinach, Tomato, and Mushroom Frittata	Apple, Avocado, and Chicken Salad	*Bacon-Liver Meatballs + Parsnip and Carrot Fries (leftover)*	*Spiced Rosemary Roasted Nuts*
SUNDAY	Spinach, Tomato, and Mushroom Frittata *(leftover)*	Apple, Avocado, and Chicken Salad *(leftover)*	Coconut Macadamia Nut–Crusted Mahimahi + Lemon-Garlic Roasted Broccoli *(leftover)*	*Spiced Rosemary Roasted Nuts*

Italics indicate that food is already made or is a leftover meal.

BUTTER LOVER'S WEEK 4

MEAL PREP

Day 1

- Make Raspberry Apple Cider Vinaigrette, page 191 (refrigerate)
- Make Cinnamon-Toasted Coconut Chips, page 173 (store in an airtight container)

Day 2

- Make Everyone's Favorite Guacamole, page 184 (refrigerate)
- Make Chicken-Sage Meatballs, page 206 (refrigerate)

Notes

- Put frozen breakfast foods (Pumpkin Breakfast Muffins, made during week 3) in the refrigerator the night before to thaw.
- Thaw Homemade Bone Broth (made during week 2) for the Slow Cooker Garlic-Thyme Pot Roast, page 216, and Slow Cooker Bison Chili, page 226, in the refrigerator the night before.

BUTTER LOVER'S WEEK 4 SHORTCUTS

- Use olive oil and balsamic vinegar as dressing for the Roasted Beets and Berries Salad, page 180, instead of making Raspberry Apple Cider Vinaigrette.
- Purchase store-bought bone broth for recipes. We recommend the brand Kettle & Fire.

SHOPPING LIST

Meat/Poultry/Eggs

1 (3- to 4-pound) chuck roast

2 pounds ground chicken

4 boneless, skinless chicken breasts

1 pound ground beef

1 pound ground bison

½ pound bacon (8 slices)

1 large egg

Produce

5 medium red potatoes

1 large sweet potato

6 cups baby arugula

2 cups spinach

1 head romaine lettuce

1 head cauliflower

3 carrots

3 sweet onions

2 bell peppers

2 jalapeños

1 zucchini

2 medium beets

1 medium tomato

1 vine-ripened tomato

5 avocados

2 bananas

2 large sweet apples (such as Fuji or Pink Lady)

1 bag frozen cherries (2 cups), pitted

1¼ cups raspberries

¾ cup blueberries

1 lime (for juice)

2 heads garlic

Fresh chives

Fresh cilantro

Pantry

Coconut oil (or ghee)

Extra-virgin olive oil

Almond flour

Almond butter

Raw honey

Pure maple syrup

Pure vanilla extract

Apple cider vinegar

Grass-fed collagen peptides

Chai tea

Canned full-fat coconut milk (three 13.5-ounce cans)

Canned crushed tomatoes (one 28-ounce can)

Unsweetened coconut flakes (4 cups)

Unsweetened baking chocolate (optional)

Raw pecans

Raw walnuts

Raw almonds

Raw pumpkin seeds

Spices

Sea salt

Black pepper

Ground cumin

Cayenne pepper

Ground sage

Dried parsley

Garlic powder

Onion powder

Dried basil

Ground cinnamon

Dried thyme

Paprika

Dried oregano

Chili powder

Butter Lover's Week 4 Menu

	BREAKFAST	LUNCH	DINNER	SNACK
MONDAY	Breakfast Smoothie Trio (Cherry-Spinach Smoothie)	*Chicken-Sage Meatballs*	Bacon-Guacamole Chicken Rolls + Creamy Mashed Cauliflower	*Cinnamon-Toasted Coconut "Chips"*
TUESDAY	Breakfast Smoothie Trio (Cherry-Spinach Smoothie)	*Chicken-Sage Meatballs*	Slow Cooker Garlic-Thyme Pot Roast	*Cinnamon-Toasted Coconut "Chips"*
WEDNESDAY	*Pumpkin Breakfast Muffins + Superfood Coconut Chai Latte*	*Bacon-Guacamole Chicken Rolls + Creamy Mashed Cauliflower (leftover)*	*Slow Cooker Garlic-Thyme Pot Roast (leftover)*	Easy Apple "Cookies"
THURSDAY	*Pumpkin Breakfast Muffins + Superfood Coconut Chai Latte*	*Chicken-Sage Meatballs*	Zucchini-Beef Taco Skillet	*Easy Apple "Cookies" (leftover)*
FRIDAY	*Pumpkin Breakfast Muffins + Superfood Coconut Chai Latte*	*Slow Cooker Garlic-Thyme Pot Roast (leftover)*	Slow Cooker Bison Chili	*Easy Apple "Cookies" (leftover)*
SATURDAY	Cinnamon Vanilla N'Oatmeal	Roasted Beets and Berries Salad	*Zucchini-Beef Taco Skillet (leftover)*	*Cinnamon-Toasted Coconut "Chips"*
SUNDAY	*Cinnamon Vanilla N'Oatmeal (leftover)*	*Roasted Beets and Berries Salad (leftover)*	*Slow Cooker Bison Chili (leftover)*	*Cinnamon-Toasted Coconut "Chips"*

Italics indicate that food is already made or is a leftover meal.

KITCHEN TOOLS AND EQUIPMENT

While there may be a few items on this list that are new to you, the tools and equipment needed to make the recipes in this book are very common. In fact, there's a good chance you already own most of them. Each item makes preparing and cooking meals easier and faster, saving you time and effort in the kitchen.

KITCHEN TOOLS

Airtight glass containers: Great for storing both dry and liquid ingredients. The two most popular brands are Weck and Le Parfait.

Apple corer: Quickly removes the core and seeds while keeping the rest of the apple intact. A corer is a must-have tool when slicing apples crosswise, as for Easy Apple "Cookies" (page 168).

Bamboo cooking spoon: Great for stirring and incorporating foods in stainless-steel cookware.

Box grater: A four-sided stainless-steel box that allows for slicing, and grating to a coarse, medium, or fine consistency. You'll find this most useful when thinly slicing vegetables and fruits like zucchini or plantains.

Chef's knife: A good-quality chef's knife will make chopping, slicing, and dicing much faster and easier. This all-purpose knife is usually about 8 inches long and will become your go-to knife for the majority of kitchen tasks.

Cutting boards: A set of three wooden or bamboo cutting boards will serve you well for slicing, dicing, and serving. Smaller cutting boards can be used to cut up vegetables or fresh herbs and larger cutting boards are useful for resting or carving cooked meats.

Dry measuring cups: Used for dry ingredients, such as coconut flour or cacao powder. Get a set that includes at least five separate measuring cups, including 1 cup, ½ cup, ⅓ cup, ¼ cup, and ⅛ cup (which is the equivalent of 2 tablespoons).

Fine-mesh strainer: Great for straining bone broth and freshly blended fruit juices or sifting coconut flour into an even consistency.

Food scale: Helps make sure you've got the right ratio of ingredients to spices. A digital scale that allows you to measure both ounces and grams will be the most useful.

Garlic press: An undervalued time-saving tool, but keep in mind that pressed garlic will release slightly more flavor than minced garlic.

Glass measuring cup: For liquid ingredients, such as water or fresh lime juice. Because it's heat safe, it's also great for melting and combining ingredients that need to be poured.

Kitchen shears: Shears have a variety of uses in the kitchen, including opening food packaging, snipping herbs, and trimming meats.

Ladle: A large, long-handled, deep spoon for serving soups, stews, and chilis.

Lemon/lime squeezer: A sturdy squeezer will help you extract every last drop of juice from halved lemons and limes.

Mandoline slicer: Makes quick work of cutting tasks. By running food along the inclined plane, you can make perfectly even and uniform slices. The blades on a mandoline slicer are extremely sharp, so *always* use the hand guard.

Measuring spoons: Used for both wet and dry ingredients, these will likely be the most-used tools in your kitchen. Invest in a set of six measuring spoons, including 1 tablespoon, 1 teaspoon, ¾ teaspoon, ½ teaspoon, ¼ teaspoon, and ⅛ teaspoon. Look for ones with a narrow head that can easily fit into spice jars.

Mixing bowl set: A basic set of three mixing bowls can be used for a variety of cooking and baking tasks. A durable stainless-steel set with lids will hold up for the long haul and let you prep, store, and transport ingredients with ease.

Paring knife: Another all-purpose knife that allows for small or intricate work, such as mincing garlic cloves or removing the seeds from a jalapeño. When you need more precision than a chef's knife can provide, this knife will take on the task.

Silicone spatulas: Flexible silicone spatulas are great for stirring, mixing, folding, and scraping down both hot and cold foods. A set of three spatulas in small, medium, and large will fit a variety of pans and bowls.

Stainless-steel spatula: When cooking with cast iron, a stainless-steel spatula with flat edges and round corners will help keep the surface smooth, seasoned, and slick. Sometimes called a pancake turner, a Dexter-Russell 5-inch all-purpose stainless-steel spatula is great for most cooking tasks, including sautéing vegetables and crumbling ground meat.

Silicone turner-spatula: Perfect for lifting cookies from the pan or flipping eggs or burgers in stainless-steel and nonstick cookware.

Tongs: Stainless-steel tongs are great for browning meats in the skillet. A pair of 12-inch tongs that lock closed will provide the most versatility and be easy to clean and store.

Vegetable peeler: A good-quality vegetable peeler will let you easily remove the skin from vegetables such as carrots and potatoes, or fruits such as apples. A basic swivel peeler with a solid handle is good for all-around use.

Whisk: Essential for properly incorporating eggs and blending both liquid and dry ingredients. A standard 10-inch stainless-steel balloon whisk will serve you well for the recipes in this book.

Wooden skewers: Skewers about 4 inches long are great for securing food that has been rolled up or stacked, such as Sweet Potato Chipotle Bison Sliders (page 224).

KITCHEN EQUIPMENT

Baking cups: A must when using metal muffin tins. Both parchment paper and silicone baking cups do a great job at preventing sticking, especially when baking batter made with coconut flour.

Baking sheet: A flat metal pan with a rim on one or two sides. This makes it easy to hold and lets cookies slide right off. They're also useful when placing no-bake treats in the fridge or freezer to chill.

Blender: Essential for blending smoothies, dressings, dips, and batters. A 6-cup (or larger) blender with at least 600 watts of power will get food to the proper consistency with ease.

Broiler pan: A heavy-duty two-part pan specifically designed for broiling food in the oven. It has a slotted upper pan and a deeper lower pan to catch drips, and can withstand high temperatures and direct heat from above.

Cast-iron skillet: Durable, inexpensive, and great at heat retention. A new cast-iron pan will likely come preseasoned. Cast-iron cookware requires different care than your other pots and pans, but once you see how easy it is to cook with and clean, it will likely become your go-to pan.

Food processor: Makes food prepping tasks astonishingly easy. While they come in a variety of sizes, go for a 9-cup (or larger) food processor that has blades or attachments for chopping, slicing, shredding, and blending, as you'll likely end up using it on a regular basis.

Glass baking dish: Used for marinating, baking, roasting, and storing. For everyday cooking, go for set of three baking dishes with lids, including an 8-inch square dish and medium and large rectangular dishes.

Handheld mixer or stand mixer: Lets you easily stir, beat, and whip ingredients to an even consistency. While a standard handheld mixer will meet most of your needs, a larger stand mixer comes in handy for bigger, more involved mixing tasks.

Ice pop molds: Ice pop molds come in many shapes and sizes. To make your life easy, get a set of six 3- to 4-ounce molds that stand upright in the freezer and have reusable sticks that snap onto each mold. This will eliminate spills and keep the sticks secured in place as the ice pops freeze.

Ice pop sticks: Natural (untreated) wooden sticks that are 4½ inches long can be used as skewers for freshly cut fruit, or with ice pop molds that don't have reusable sticks.

Loaf pan: A standard 8½ x 4½-inch glass or metal loaf pan can be used to set no-bake snacks and treats or to bake bread or meat loaf.

Muffin pans: A standard 12-cup metal muffin tin and a 24-cup metal mini-muffin tin are kitchen staples if you love baking muffins and other treats.

Rimmed baking sheet (sheet pan): A flat metal pan with rimmed sides. Great for roasting vegetables and meats because it keeps juices from spilling. Use a 13 x 18-inch baking sheet unless otherwise noted in the recipe.

Saucepan: A pot with tall, straight sides, great for cooking sauces and soups. You'll get plenty of use out of 1½- and 3-quart saucepans.

Silicone candy molds: These flexible molds come in fun shapes and sizes and let treats like homemade gummies and candies pop right out with a little push from the bottom. Always make sure to place silicone molds on a baking sheet so they remain level when you transfer them to the fridge or freezer to set.

Silicone muffin pans: A standard 12-cup silicone muffin pan and a 24-cup silicone mini-muffin pan are great for preparing smooth and uniform treats, such as Salted Dark Chocolate Almond Butter Cups (page 246). They're also safe to use in the oven, and baked goods will pop right out of the molds once they've cooled. Always make sure to place silicone molds on a baking sheet so they remain level when you transfer them to the oven, fridge, or freezer.

Skillet and sauté pan: You can accomplish most kitchen tasks with a basic 8-or 10-inch skillet, a larger 12-inch skillet, and a deep 4-quart sauté pan (if you're not sure what the difference is, a skillet has sloping sides, while a sauté pan has relatively tall, straight sides). While there are a variety of materials to chose from, stainless-steel pans with an aluminum core (sometimes called "tri-ply" or "multiclad") heat evenly, and unlike nonstick cookware, they can withstand high heat and be transferred directly from the stovetop to the oven.

Slow cooker: This electric appliance is an absolutely must for anyone with a busy schedule. A slow cooker simmers food for an extended period of time at low temperatures, making it perfect for cooking whole chickens, roasts, stews, and chilis. Simply throw the ingredients in the pot in the morning, and you'll have a delicious, ready-for-you-meal at dinnertime. The recipes in this book require a 6-quart (or larger) slow cooker.

Soup pot: To make soups and stews, you'll need a large 8- or 10-quart soup pot. You can also use this pot to boil large quantities of food, such as eggs, chicken wings, or potatoes.

Wire rack: Lets air circulate freely to cool baked goods, such as cookies and muffins, which prevents them from becoming soggy.

STOCKING THE PANTRY

A well-stocked pantry is a must for maintaining balance and consistency throughout the week. To help you purchase the items you need, each pantry item included in the recipes in this book is listed here, along with some additional details and buying tips. Many of the pantry items are used in multiple recipes and can easily be incorporated into dishes you cook or create on the fly.

Almond flour: Although almond flour and almond meal are both made from ground almonds and are sometimes labeled interchangeably, almond flour is traditionally made from blanched (skinless) almonds. For all the recipes in this book that call for it, you'll get the best results by using a blanched almond flour versus almond meal, which is made from raw almonds with their skins still on. Almond flour, such as Bob's Red Mill Super-Fine Almond Flour, gives baked goods a buttery texture; you'll get a denser, grainy texture if you use almond meal instead.

Almond butter: A delicious, spreadable paste made from ground almonds. When purchasing almond butter, check the ingredients list to make sure the only ingredient is raw or dry-roasted almonds, as many brands have added refined oils and/or sugar. For most recipes, you can swap out almond butter for another nut butter.

Apple cider vinegar: Look for raw apple cider vinegar that still contains the "mother." A great option is Bragg Organic Raw Unfiltered Apple Cider Vinegar.

Balsamic vinegar: Great for dressings and marinades, true balsamic vinegar is a thick syrup produced in Italy from grape must (whole pressed grapes, including their stems, seeds, and skins). Local olive oil and vinegar taprooms are a great place to find high-quality aged balsamic vinegars, but you can also find them at most grocery stores.

Baking chocolate (unsweetened): This chocolate is 100 percent cacao, meaning no sweeteners, flavors, or other ingredients are added to it. For a smooth, rich texture, look for SunSpire's Organic Fair Trade 100% Cacao Unsweetened Baking Bar.

Dijon mustard: A condiment made from mustard seeds and a combination of vinegar, salt, and spices. Two great brands include Organicville and Annie's Naturals.

Cacao powder: A rich, chocolaty powder made from unheated and unprocessed cacao beans. Packed with antioxidants, fiber, and minerals like magnesium and calcium, it's become much more widely available recently and can be found at most local grocery stores and online. Three great brands are Navitas Naturals, Healthworks, and Divine Organics. If you don't have access to cacao powder, you can use unsweetened cocoa powder instead, which is made from roasted cacao.

Canned pumpkin: When choosing canned pumpkin, make sure it's 100 percent pumpkin puree and nothing else. Most grocery chains have store-brand canned pumpkin, but if not, look for Farmer's Market Foods Organic Pumpkin.

Coconut aminos: This soy-free seasoning sauce can add a lot of variety to your cooking. It's made from coconut sap and has a deep, sweet-savory flavor. You can use it for sauces and marinades or add it directly to the pan when sautéing vegetables. The most widely available brand is Coconut Secret Coconut Aminos.

Coconut butter: A spread made from the meat of coconuts that is typically used as a condiment or baking ingredient. Because it has a slightly dry texture, it needs to be gently heated before being mixed with other ingredients. A great product is Artisana Organics Raw Coconut Butter.

Coconut flour: A soft, fine flour made from ground dried coconut meat. Two great brands include Bob's Red Mill and Let's Do . . . Organic. Please note that coconut flour cannot be swapped equally in recipes for other flours such as almond flour because it is very dry and requires added moisture.

Coconut milk: For all the recipes in this book that call for it, use canned full-fat coconut milk. It has a thick, creamy texture and no added sweeteners or flavors. While different brands of canned coconut milk can be found at just about any grocery store, Native Forest Classic Organic Coconut Milk has the best texture. When you open the can, the milk will likely have separated somewhat into opaque coconut cream and a clear liquid. To recombine, simply pour the contents of the can into a bowl and whisk or use a handheld mixer to blend it for 5 to 10 seconds into an even consistency.

Coconut, shredded or flakes (unsweetened): Coconut flakes are larger pieces of dried coconut, whereas shredded coconut is shaved into smaller, finer strips. Both varieties can be purchased unsweetened from the brand Let's Do . . . Organic.

Coconut water: Great for cooking, adding to smoothies, and drinking as a refreshing beverage, coconut water is versatile and delicious. Look for 100 percent coconut water—no additives, not from concentrate.

Collagen peptides: These are short-chain amino acids derived from collagen protein. They are highly bioavailable, digestible, and soluble in cold water, meaning they can be easily added to smoothies or drinks. Look for collagen products from grass-fed beef. A high-quality product is Vital Proteins Collagen Peptides (blue canister).

Crushed tomatoes: A mixture of fresh crushed tomatoes and tomato puree or paste. The tomatoes have a slightly finer texture than diced tomatoes, making them great for sauces and stews. Choose crushed tomatoes that are organic and preserved in a BPA-free can or glass jar.

Diced tomatoes: Tomato chunks packed in tomato juice. Go for diced tomatoes that are organic, don't have added preservatives, and come in a BPA-free can or glass jar.

Gelatin: Derived from collagen, beef gelatin is very similar to collagen peptides in look and texture, but because of its structure, it must be dissolved in hot liquid. When cooled, gelatin will gel (like Jell-O), which is why it's used to make Watermelon-Lime Gummies (page 266). Look for gelatin from grass-fed beef. A high-quality product is Vital Proteins Beef Gelatin (green canister).

Hot sauce: Traditionally made from aged cayenne red peppers and a mixture of vinegar, water, and spices. Two great products include Tessemae's All-Natural Hot Buffalo Sauce and Frank's RedHot.

Marinara sauce: An Italian sauce usually made with tomatoes, garlic, herbs, and onions. You can also use a basic tomato-basil pasta sauce in its place. When purchasing tomato-based pasta sauces, watch out for added refined sugars and oils. Two great options are Organico Bello and Yellow Barn Biodynamic.

Pure vanilla extract: When purchasing vanilla extract, watch out for additives and "imitation" vanilla extract. A good vanilla extract will be in a dark glass bottle and contain only pure vanilla bean extractives, water, and alcohol. Two great brands are Simply Organic and Frontier Co-op.

Red Boat Fish Sauce: Red Boat Fish Sauce is a made from fresh wild-caught anchovies and salt and contains no added sugar, as other brands of fish sauce do. It gives marinades and sauces a unique, rich, and satisfying dimension.

Sriracha sauce: If you're a fan of heat, sriracha sauce is the perfect pantry staple. It can be used in marinades, sauces, and sautés, and you need only a small amount to add a kick of flavor. The best brand for the job is Organicville Sky Valley.

Thai red curry paste: A mixture of aromatic herbs and fresh red chiles that can be added to stir-fries, soups, or coconut milk to create delicious Thai curry. The recipes in this book use Thai Kitchen Red Curry Paste, which is available at most grocery stores.

Tomato paste: A thick paste made by cooking tomatoes for several hours to reduce the water content. Look for tomato paste that is organic and preserved in a BPA-free can, tube, or glass jar. The only ingredient listed should be tomatoes. A great option is Bionaturae Organic Tomato Paste.

CHOOSING THE RIGHT INGREDIENTS

COOKING OILS

Naturally occurring saturated fats are great to cook with because they are stable and can withstand exposure to medium to high heat without being damaged. In the recipes in this book, coconut oil and ghee (clarified butter) are the two recommend cooking fats, but you can use other saturated fats from the chart below depending on your preference. When purchasing cooking fats, look for products that are organic, unrefined, and/or from grass-fed or pasture-raised sources. When purchasing oils for low- to medium-heat cooking and cold uses, use only extra-virgin or cold-pressed oils.

Guide to Cooking Fats

FATS FOR MEDIUM- TO HIGH-HEAT COOKING

Beef tallow	Ghee (clarified butter)
Coconut oil	Lard
Duck fat	

FATS FOR LOW- TO MEDIUM-HEAT COOKING

Avocado oil	Macadamia nut oil
Extra-virgin olive oil	

FATS FOR COLD USES/FINISHING DISHES

Sesame oil
Walnut oil

SALT

All salt is *not* created equal. A quick glance at the ingredients list on most salts will reveal that they contain additives like dextrose (sugar) and anticaking agents. In addition, traditional table salt is heavily processed, bleached, and stripped of its naturally occurring minerals. Unrefined sea salt, on the other hand, is harvested directly from ancient sea beds or evaporated seawater and can contain up to sixty trace minerals, depending on the source. Essentially, unrefined sea salt is a synergistic package of minerals. Because the minerals remain in the salt, unrefined sea salt is often slightly pink or gray in color. For the recipes in this book, you'll get the best results using Redmond Real Salt (fine salt) or Selina Naturally Celtic Sea Salt (fine ground). Both are reputable brands that put a lot of care and attention into their sourcing.

SWEETENERS

While there are a variety of natural sweeteners to choose from (see the complete list on page 30), the two added sweeteners used throughout the recipes in this book are raw honey and pure maple syrup. Both contain naturally occurring beneficial compounds such as vitamins, minerals, and antioxidants. When purchasing honey and maple syrup, source and quality are important. Much of the conventional honey sold in grocery stores is not pure honey at all and has been cut with ingredients such as high-fructose corn syrup.[1] For this reason, always purchase raw, unfiltered honey, preferably from a local producer. Because raw honey often has a slightly thicker consistency, you may need to heat it for a few seconds before using it in recipes. When purchasing maple syrup, look for a dark maple syrup that is 100 percent pure. In general, honey and maple syrup can be used interchangeably in recipes, so feel free to experiment and use the one you prefer.

NUTS AND SEEDS

For the recipes in this book, always use raw nuts and seeds (unroasted and unsalted) unless otherwise noted. Packaged nuts and seeds often contain added refined oils and/or sugar, so make sure to check the ingredients. To save money, you can buy raw nuts and seeds in bulk and store them in airtight containers in the refrigerator or freezer until you're ready to use them.

MEAT AND FISH

When purchasing meat and fish, prioritize meat that is grass-fed and/or pastured-raised and fish that is wild. Today, 99 percent of all animal products sold in the United States originate in confined animal feed operations (CAFOs), where the goal is producing the highest possible output for the lowest possible cost. To accomplish this, animals are kept in tight quarters, often without access to sunlight or room to move, and fed grain- and soy-based feeds that include additives such as stale candy and bakery waste still wrapped in plastic.[2]

Unfortunately, this not only negatively impacts the animals and the environment, but also results in meat that is far less nutrient-dense. When animals are given the opportunity to eat their natural diet, live outside, and grow at a normal rate, they absorb more nutrients and rarely require antibiotics. As a result, grass-fed beef, for example, is higher in antioxidants, including in beta-carotene and vitamin E, B vitamins, and important minerals such as calcium, magnesium, and potassium in comparison to grain-fed meat. It's also leaner, is a significant source of conjugated linoleic acid (CLA), and has higher levels of omega-3 fatty acids.[3] Similarly, farm-raised fish have less vitamin D and higher levels of omega-6 fatty acids compared to wild fish, and are often treated with antibiotics and pesticides.

While grass-fed/pasture-raised meats and wild fish are becoming more readily available at grocery stores, the best place to purchase affordable, high-quality animal products is from farmers' markets or directly from local farms. According to the latest data from the USDA, the number of farmers' markets in the United States has grown by 76 percent in the last decade. This means there's a very good chance there are a few in your area. To find your local farmers' markets, you can search online directories such as Local Harvest (localharvest.org), the National Farmers Market Directory (nfmd.org), and the USDA Farmers Market Directory (search.ams.usda.gov/farmersmarkets). Because vendors get to sell directly to consumers, prices are often much cheaper. In fact, vendors are typically more flexible with their prices and do promotions or sales each week. When you visit your local farmers' market for the first time, ask vendors where their farms are located, how they raise their animals, and if they sell directly from the farm (which is often cheaper). Many farms produce weekly emails or newsletters with specials and will even do drops to deliver meats and other animal products throughout the winter when farmers' markets are closed. You may also have the option to purchase a cow share, where farmers will butcher a whole steer and sell it to a set number of people at a flat rate. The items you'll find at farmers' markets will largely depend on what's local to your area (this is especially the case when it comes to fish), so you may find you stock up on certain items at farmers' markets and others at the grocery store depending on what's available and your budget.

EGGS

Like meat and fish, the best place to purchase affordable, high-quality eggs is from farmers' markets or directly from local farms. Eggs from local farms will likely be from pasture-raised hens, meaning the hens have roamed outside in the sun and fed on grass and bugs.

Because of this, pasture-raised eggs have more folate and vitamin B$_{12}$ and substantially higher amounts of beta-carotene; vitamins A, E, and D; and omega-3 fatty acids in comparison to factory-farmed eggs.[4, 5] If you're purchasing eggs at the grocery store, watch out for labels that are tricky or deceptive. In general, eggs labeled with basic, nonspecific terms such as "natural" or "farm fresh" are from hens raised in battery cages. Eggs labeled "cage-free" come from hens that were kept in tight quarters in large indoor barns, and "free-range" means the hens were kept in large indoor barns with some sort of outdoor access, although typically just a small area. If eggs are labeled "organic," it means the hens were fed organic corn and soy feed and did not receive antibiotics. While chickens can receive antibiotics, it is illegal to give chickens hormones, so the term "hormone-free" is nothing more than a marketing ploy. Of course, if pasture-raised eggs aren't available to you or within your budget, that's okay. Purchase eggs from a brand you trust and make decisions based on what's important to you.

PRODUCE

Buying produce that is locally grown and in-season is the best way to get budget-friendly, high-quality fruits and vegetables. Produce grown locally has more vitamins and enzymes because it takes much less time to get to you, and more minerals because it is grown in nutrient-rich soil.[6] Local produce can be purchased at farmers' markets, directly from local farms or farm stands, or through a CSA (community-supported agriculture) cooperative, which allows you to receive a share of a local farm's produce for a specified number of weeks.

By definition, organic produce is free of synthetic fertilizers and almost all synthetic pesticides, genetic engineering, radiation, and sewage sludge. Pesticides have been linked to a variety of health problems, including brain and nervous system toxicity, cancer, hormone disruption, and skin, eye, and lung irritation, so reducing your overall exposure is recommended when possible. (It's important to note that many local farms do not use the USDA's "certified organic" label because certification is incredibly costly, but their pest-management techniques are still organic and much less invasive in comparison to industrial farming techniques.) If you can't afford to buy all organic produce, prioritize buying organic versions of the fruits and vegetables on the Environmental Working Group's (EWG) "Dirty Dozen" list (see opposite). In contrast, the items on the EWG's Clean Fifteen have a very low percentage of detectable pesticides, so buying organic isn't as important, especially when you're on a budget.

Dirty Dozen

1.	Strawberries	5.	Peaches	9.	Celery
2.	Spinach	6.	Pears	10.	Tomatoes
3.	Nectarines	7.	Cherries	11.	Sweet bell peppers
4.	Apples	8.	Grapes	12.	Potatoes

Clean Fifteen

1.	Sweet corn*	6.	Frozen sweet peas	11.	Honeydew melon
2.	Avocados	7.	Papayas	12.	Kiwi
3.	Pineapples	8.	Asparagus	13.	Cantaloupe
4.	Cabbage	9.	Mangoes	14.	Cauliflower
5.	Onions	10.	Eggplant	15.	Grapefruit

*Sweet corn is considered a grain, so it is not included in the 4x4.

SPICES

When your spice rack (or drawer) is full, the flavor possibilities are endless. For this reason, it's best to invest in some basic dried herbs and spices in glass jars and eventually transition to purchasing spices in bulk when you know what you like. If you're just getting started on your stash, begin with staples such as whole black peppercorns (with a pepper mill or in a grinder jar), basil, parsley, thyme, oregano, paprika, chili powder, ground sage, garlic powder, onion powder, and ground cinnamon. Then add a new herb or spice or two to your grocery list as you work your way through the recipes in this book. You can purchase affordable, high-quality dried herbs and spices in bulk from specialty grocery stores or online. For online purchases, two great retailers are Mountain Rose Herbs and Frontier Co-op. To make sure they retain their flavor, store dried herbs and spices in a cool, dark place, and swap out your stash every twelve to eighteen months. (Herbs and spices don't expire, but they lose their potency over time.)

THE RECIPES

All the recipes in this book are free of the Big Four—grains, dairy, refined sugars, and vegetable oils. This means that any recipe can be used while you are following the 4x4. Each recipe also has additional labels for further customization:

- *Egg-Free:* Does not contain eggs.

- *Nightshade-Free:* Contains no tomatoes, potatoes, peppers, or eggplant, or spices derived from these ingredients.

- *Nut-Free:* Does not contain nuts or seeds (but may include seed-based spices).

- *Vegetarian:* Does not include meat.

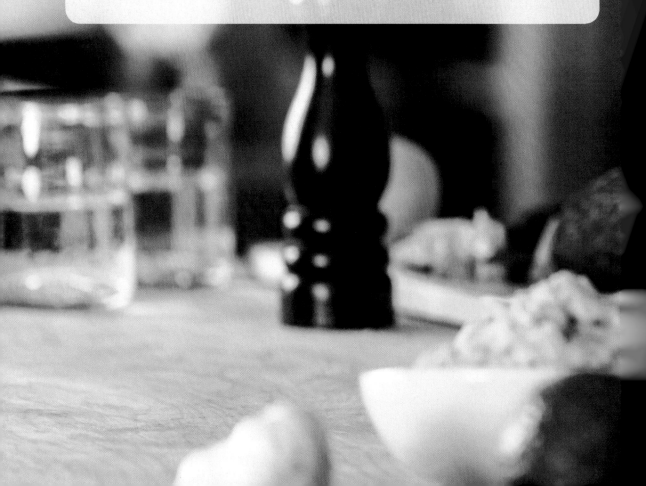

From Noelle's Kitchen

I created all the recipes in this book in my small home in South Philadelphia while balancing a full-time job and a newborn baby girl. So you can rest assured that you don't need a fancy kitchen or an endless amount of time to cook these recipes. Many of them are staples in my home, and I use them to get a nourishing, flavorful meal on the table in a short amount of time. With most of the recipes, I've included special tips and options for changing things up if you'd like to customize the recipe to your needs. My ultimate goal is to give you everything you need to cook each meal with confidence and make your time in the kitchen enjoyable, not stressful.

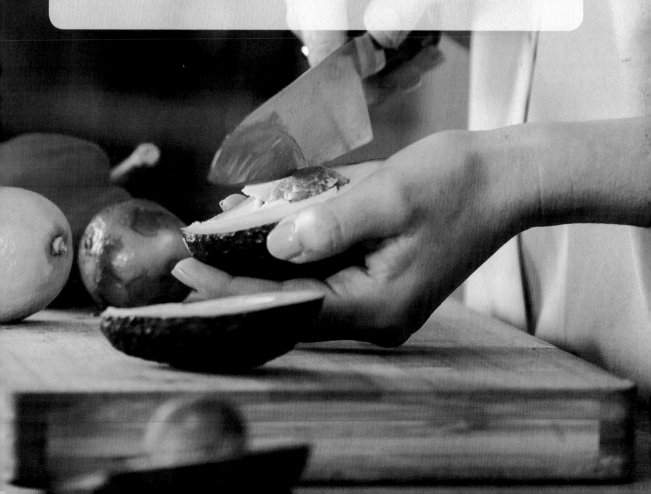

Breakfast Smoothie Trio

EGG-FREE, NIGHTSHADE-FREE, NUT-FREE
(CHERRY-SPINACH SMOOTHIE ONLY), VEGETARIAN

This smoothie triple threat will keep your mornings colorful and balanced with the perfect blend of carbohydrates and a kick of nutrient-dense fats.

Place all the ingredients in a blender and blend until smooth.

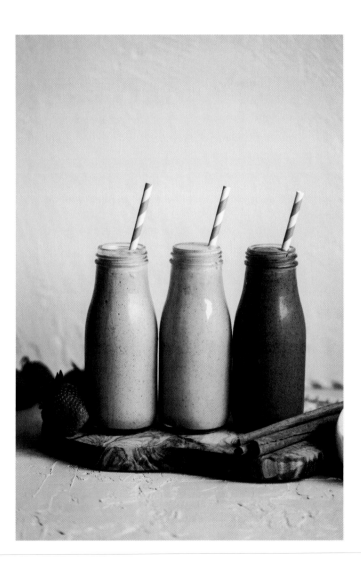

Each version makes one 16-ounce serving
Prep time: **5 minutes**
Cooking time: none

Strawberry-Banana Smoothie

1 cup frozen strawberries
1 banana, sliced
1 cup canned full-fat coconut milk
1 tablespoon almond butter
½ teaspoon pure vanilla extract

Apple Pie Smoothie

1 banana, peeled, frozen, and sliced
1 cup sliced apples
1 cup canned full-fat coconut milk
1 tablespoon almond butter
¼ teaspoon ground cinnamon
⅛ teaspoon ground nutmeg
1 teaspoon raw honey or pure maple syrup

Cherry-Spinach Smoothie

1 banana, peeled, frozen, and sliced
1 cup frozen pitted cherries
1 cup canned full-fat coconut milk
Large handful of spinach

Noelle's tip: Using some frozen fruit makes the smoothies slightly thick and creamy but still easy to blend. If you'd like to thin out the smoothie, simply add a little more coconut milk or coconut water.

Change it up: Add 1 scoop grass-fed collagen peptides to each smoothie to give it gut-healing properties.

Superfood Coconut Chai Latte

EGG-FREE, NIGHTSHADE-FREE, NUT-FREE

Give your breakfast or afternoon tea superpowers with this special-ingredient coconut chai latte. While a frothing wand may be a relatively new contraption for you, it's definitely worth the small investment. It's easy to use and makes the coconut milk silky and smooth.

Makes one 10-ounce latte (1 serving)

Prep time: less than 10 minutes

Cooking time: none

1. Boil ¾ cup water in a teapot. Place the tea bag in a mug (or place loose tea in a tea ball or strainer) and pour the water over the tea. Steep for 4 to 6 minutes.

2. While the tea is steeping, heat the coconut milk in a small saucepan until just warm. Do not let the coconut milk boil.

3. Pour the coconut milk into a glass measuring cup or tall glass and froth it with a frothing wand. You can also froth the milk in a bowl with a handheld mixer or in a blender. Set the milk aside.

4. Remove the tea bag or loose tea from the mug and stir in the maple syrup and collagen peptides.

5. Slowly pour the frothed milk into the mug. Top with the cinnamon and enjoy.

1 chai tea bag, or 1 teaspoon loose chai tea

½ cup canned full-fat coconut milk

1 teaspoon pure maple syrup or raw honey, or more to taste

1 tablespoon grass-fed collagen peptides

Pinch of ground cinnamon

Special equipment: Frothing wand (optional)

Change it up: Give the latte a stronger chai flavor by using 2 chai tea bags or 2 teaspoons loose chai tea and the same amount of water.

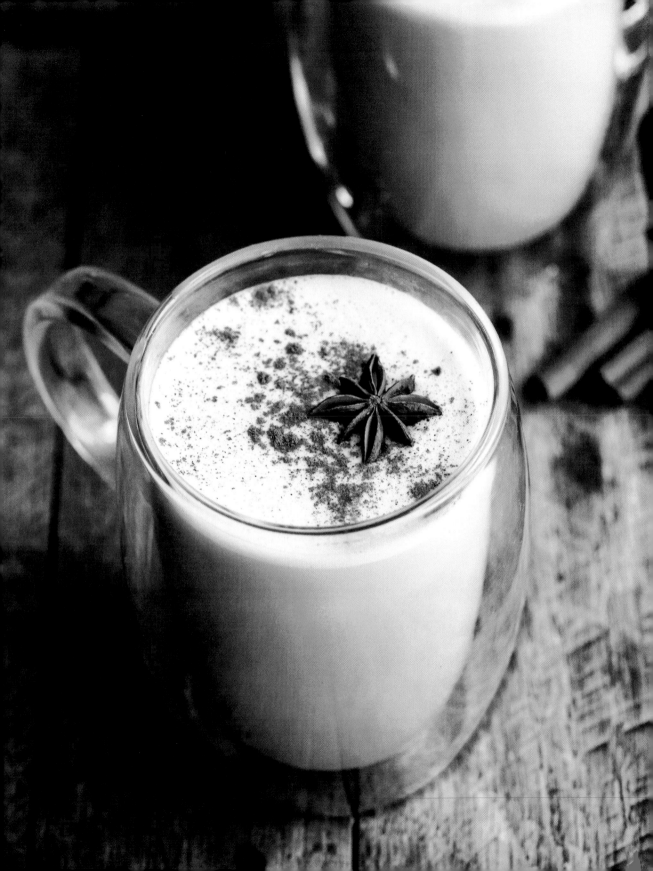

Raspberry-Coconut Smoothie Bowl

EGG-FREE, NIGHTSHADE-FREE, VEGETARIAN

This smoothie-in-a-bowl has a slightly thicker consistency, making it perfect for eating with a spoon. To add to the fun, you can jazz up the bowl with your favorite toppings, turning each breakfast into a new Instagram photo opportunity. #smoothiebowl

1. To make the smoothie base, place the banana, coconut milk, and coconut water in a blender and pulse until combined. Add the raspberries, almond butter, and vanilla and blend until smooth, scraping down the sides of the blender as necessary.

2. Pour the smoothie into a bowl, sprinkle with the desired toppings, and delight in eating a smoothie with a spoon.

Makes one 16-ounce serving
Prep time: **5 minutes**
Cooking time: **none**

Smoothie bowl base

1 banana, peeled, frozen, and sliced
1 cup canned full-fat coconut milk
2 tablespoons coconut water
1 cup frozen raspberries
1 tablespoon almond butter
½ teaspoon pure vanilla extract

Toppings

Fresh fruit, such as raspberries, sliced kiwi, or sliced dragon fruit
Chopped nuts, such as walnuts, or pecans, or pumpkin seeds
Unsweetened coconut flakes
Freeze-dried fruit chunks

Change it up: Add 1 scoop grass-fed collagen peptides to the smoothie (while blending) to give it gut-healing properties.

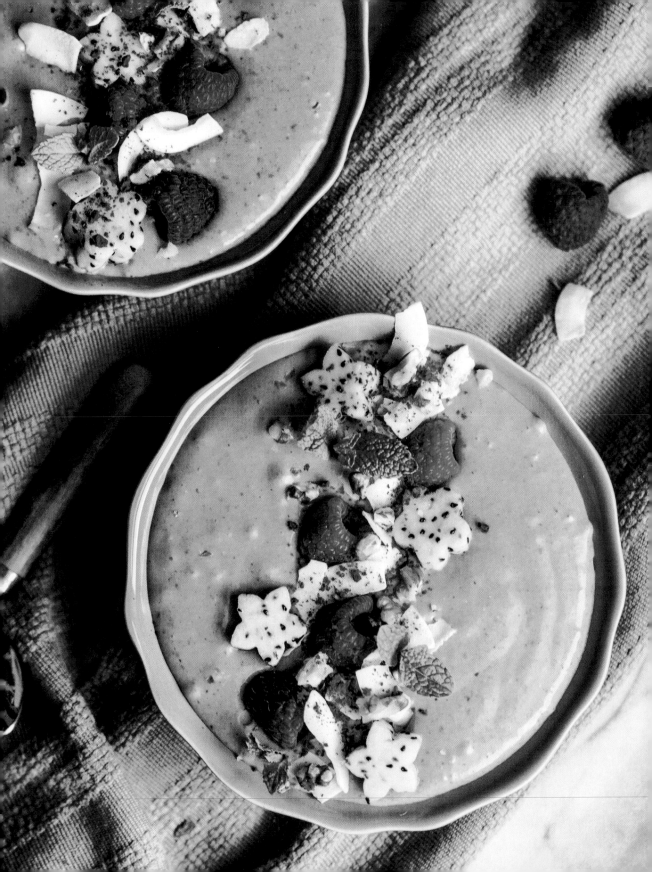

Apple Bacon Sweet Potato Hash

EGG-FREE, NIGHTSHADE-FREE, NUT-FREE

This hash is a great dish to prepare when serving breakfast or brunch to a group of friends or family. It pairs nicely with eggs cooked any style and brings the combination of sweet and savory to the scene.

Makes 4 to 6 servings
Prep time: **20 minutes**
Cooking time: **20 minutes**

1. Preheat the oven to 400°F. Line a baking sheet with parchment paper or aluminum foil.

2. In a large bowl, toss the sweet potatoes with 2 tablespoons of the coconut oil until all sides are coated. Arrange the potatoes in a single layer on the prepared baking sheet and sprinkle with ¼ teaspoon of the salt. Roast until just soft, 12 to 14 minutes.

3. Meanwhile, in a large skillet, melt the remaining ½ tablespoon coconut oil over medium heat. Add the bacon and cook until just crisp, 4 to 5 minutes. Add the onion, remaining ¼ teaspoon salt, and the pepper and cook until the onion is soft, 3 to 4 minutes.

4. Stir in the apple, cinnamon, and sage and cook for 1 to 2 minutes. Stir in the sweet potatoes and cook until they are lightly golden brown, 7 to 8 minutes.

5. Transfer to a platter and serve warm.

2 large sweet potatoes, peeled and diced
2½ tablespoons coconut oil or ghee, melted
½ teaspoon sea salt
6 bacon slices, chopped into small pieces
1 sweet onion, diced
¼ teaspoon freshly ground black pepper
1 apple, cored and diced
½ teaspoon ground cinnamon
¼ teaspoon ground sage

Noelle's tip: Use a 12-inch (or larger) skillet for this recipe so the sweet potatoes brown evenly when added at the end.

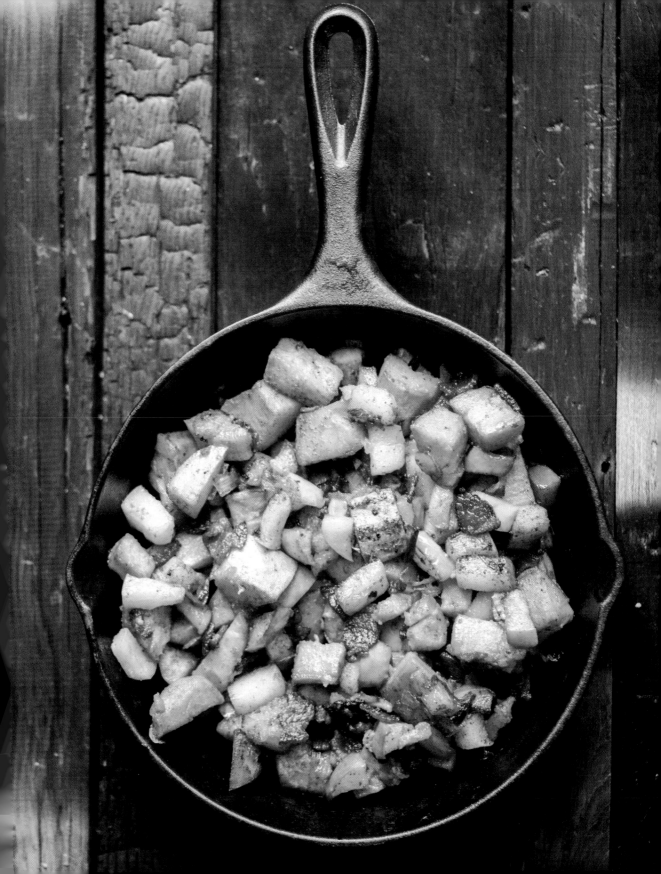

Twice-Baked Breakfast Sweet Potatoes

NIGHTSHADE-FREE, NUT-FREE

Twice-baked breakfast sweet potatoes are guaranteed to elevate your breakfast game to champion status. The second baking round makes the potatoes hearty and decadent, and melds all the flavors of breakfast together into one beautiful bite.

1. Preheat the oven to 400°F.

2. Pierce the sweet potatoes with fork and place them on a baking sheet. Roast until they can be pierced easily with a fork, about 1 hour. Set the sweet potatoes aside to cool but leave the oven on.

3. Meanwhile, in a large skillet, melt ½ tablespoon of the coconut oil over medium heat. Add the bacon and cook until just crisp, 4 to 5 minutes on each side. Set the bacon aside on a paper towel to cool, then crumble it into small pieces.

4. When the sweet potatoes are cool to the touch, slice them in half lengthwise and scoop out the flesh into a large bowl, leaving the potato skins intact with a thin layer of potato behind. Set the skins on the baking sheet.

5. Add the remaining 2 tablespoons coconut oil, the coconut milk, rosemary, salt, and pepper to the bowl with the sweet potato flesh and whip with a handheld mixer until smooth. Fold in half the bacon pieces. Divide the filling among the sweet potato skins, making a deep well in the center with a spoon to hold an egg. Crack 1 egg into the center of each sweet potato and sprinkle with salt and pepper.

6. Bake until the egg whites are cooked but the yolks are still slightly soft, 15 to 20 minutes. Garnish with the remaining bacon and the chives.

Makes 8 servings

Prep time: 20 minutes

Cooking time: 1 hour 20 minutes

4 large sweet potatoes
2½ tablespoons coconut oil or ghee
8 bacon slices
¼ cup canned full-fat coconut milk
½ teaspoon dried rosemary
½ teaspoon sea salt, plus more to taste
¼ teaspoon freshly ground black pepper, plus more to taste
8 large eggs
1 teaspoon minced fresh chives, for garnish

Noelle's tip: It's totally fine if the egg runs over the sweet potato a bit. Once cooked, it will give the potatoes a nice rustic look, making you look like a professional chef (because of course you are).

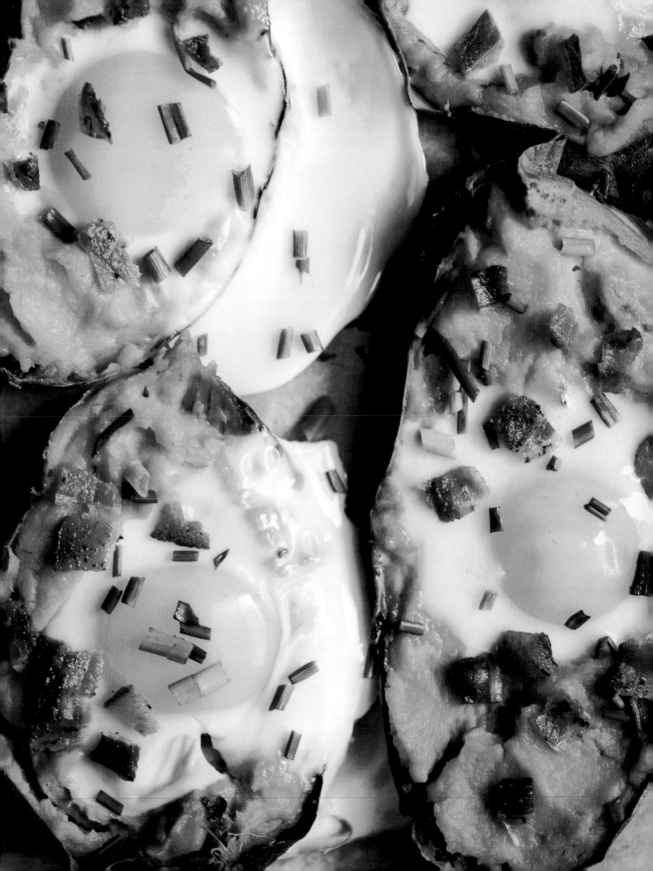

Spinach, Tomato, and Mushroom Frittata

NUT-FREE, VEGETARIAN

"Frittata" is not only fun to say, it also offers a nice change of pace from the typical preparation methods for eggs. Sticking true to its Italian roots, this frittata is sure to please all palates and preferences, thanks to the medley of spinach, tomato, and fresh basil.

Makes 3 servings

Prep time: **10 minutes**

Cooking time: **20 minutes**

1. Preheat the oven to 375°F.

2. In a large bowl, combine the eggs, ⅛ teaspoon of the salt, the pepper, and the basil. Set aside.

3. In a medium oven-safe skillet, melt the coconut oil over medium heat. Add the garlic and mushrooms and cook, stirring, until soft, 3 to 4 minutes. Add the spinach and remaining ⅛ teaspoon salt and cook until the spinach wilts, 2 to 3 minutes. Stir in the tomato.

4. Spread the vegetables so that they cover the bottom of the skillet. Pour the egg mixture over the top and cook until the edges set, about 1 minute.

5. Transfer the skillet to the oven and bake until the eggs are set in the center, 10 to 12 minutes.

6. Slide the frittata out of the skillet onto a cutting board. Slice into wedges, then serve.

6 large eggs, beaten
¼ teaspoon sea salt
⅛ teaspoon freshly ground black pepper
2 teaspoons chopped fresh basil
2 tablespoons coconut oil or ghee
2 garlic cloves, minced
1 cup coarsely chopped white mushrooms
2 cups baby spinach
1 medium tomato, diced

Noelle's tip: To easily slide the frittata out of the skillet, run a silicone spatula around the edge to gently loosen it from the pan.

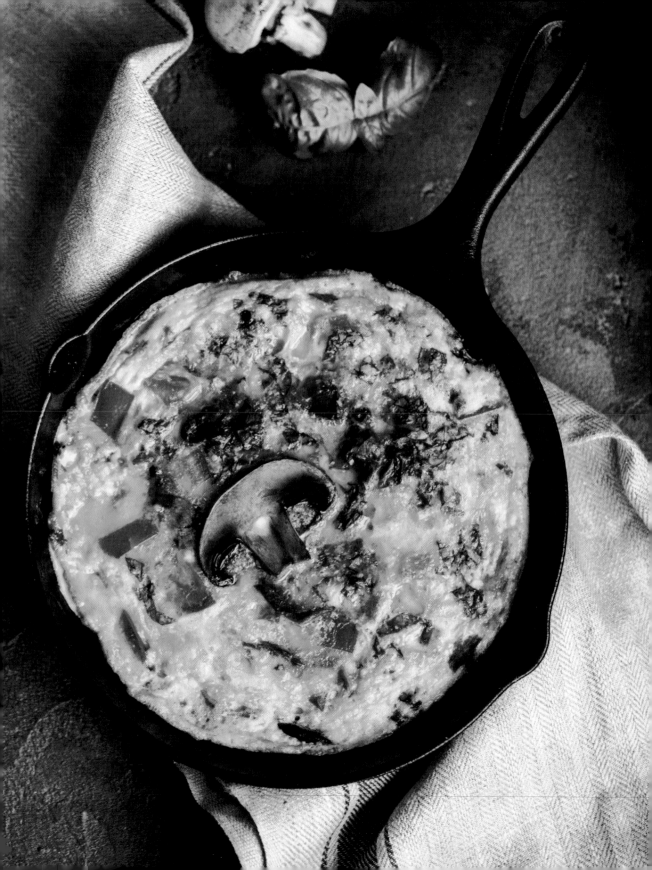

Bacon-Wrapped Eggs

NIGHTSHADE-FREE, NUT-FREE

These bacon-wrapped eggs are the perfect breakfast in a cup. If you're short on time in the mornings, you can make these in bulk and store them in the refrigerator or freezer for the week ahead. If you're storing them in the freezer, simply put them in the fridge to thaw the night before; the next morning, eat them chilled or warmed in the microwave for 10 to 15 seconds.

Makes 6 servings
  (2 eggs per serving)
Prep time: **15 minutes**
Cooking time: **less than**
  25 minutes

1 tablespoon coconut oil or
  ghee, plus more to grease
  the pan
12 bacon slices
2½ cups baby spinach
⅔ cup chopped white
  mushrooms
⅛ teaspoon garlic powder
12 large eggs
1 teaspoon minced fresh
  chives
Pinch of sea salt
Pinch of freshly ground black
  pepper

1. Preheat the oven to 400°F. Lightly grease a 12-cup muffin tin with coconut oil.

2. In a large skillet, melt the coconut oil over medium heat. Add the bacon and cook until the fat has just rendered but the bacon is still soft and pliable, 3 to 4 minutes on each side. Set the bacon aside on a paper towel.

3. Pour out all but 1 tablespoon of the rendered bacon fat from the skillet. Return the skillet to the heat, add the spinach, mushrooms, and garlic powder, and stir. Cook until the spinach becomes soft, 1 to 2 minutes. Transfer the mixture to a bowl and set aside.

4. Place 1 piece of bacon inside each well of the prepared muffin tin, wrapping it around the sides. Spoon about 2 teaspoons of the vegetable mixture into each well inside the bacon.

5. Crack 1 egg into each well on top of the vegetables. Sprinkle evenly with the chives, salt, and pepper.

6. Bake for 12 to 15 minutes, until the eggs are cooked to your desired doneness. Watch closely to prevent overcooking.

7. Gently run a spatula or small butter knife around the edge of each bacon-wrapped egg to release it from the pan. Serve warm.

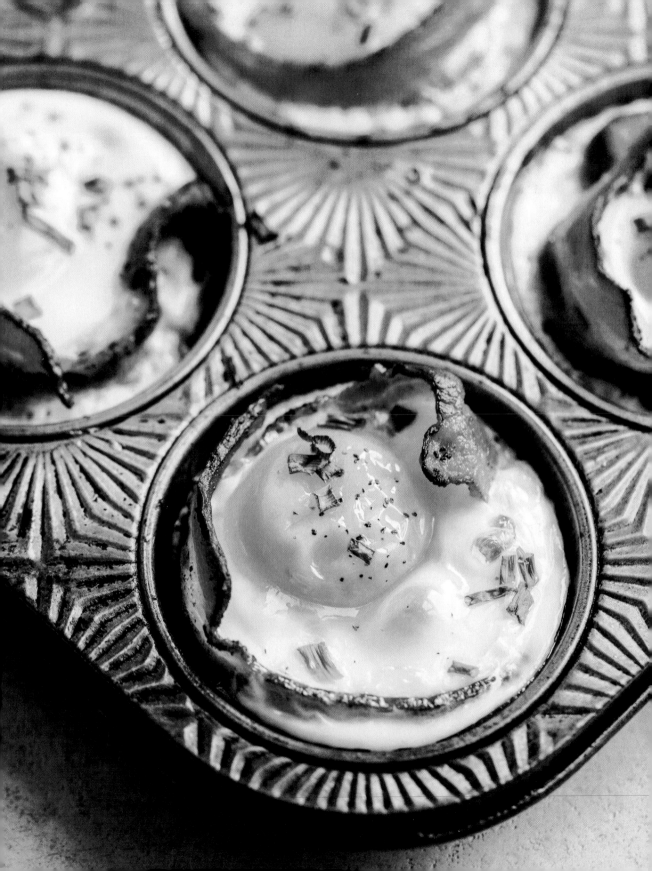

Kale and Bacon Breakfast Skillet

EGG-FREE, NIGHTSHADE-FREE, NUT-FREE

This breakfast skillet is a quick and simple dish that's pre-pared in a single pan. It's great to make during the week when you've had enough of eggs and want to power up your day in a new way.

1. In a large skillet, melt the coconut oil over medium heat. Add the bacon and cook until just crisp, 4 to 5 minutes.

2. Add the onion and garlic and cook until just soft, 3 to 4 minutes. Add the mushrooms and cook, stirring, for 2 minutes more.

3. Add the kale, salt, and pepper and cook until the kale wilts and turns dark green, 2 to 3 minutes. Serve warm.

Makes 3 or 4 servings

Prep time: 10 minutes

Cooking time: less than 15 minutes

1½ teaspoons coconut oil or ghee
6 bacon slices, chopped into small pieces
½ medium onion, diced
1 garlic clove, minced
1 cup chopped white mushrooms
5 large kale leaves, stemmed and chopped
Pinch of sea salt
Pinch of freshly ground black pepper

Change it up: Use another hearty green such as Swiss chard instead of kale.

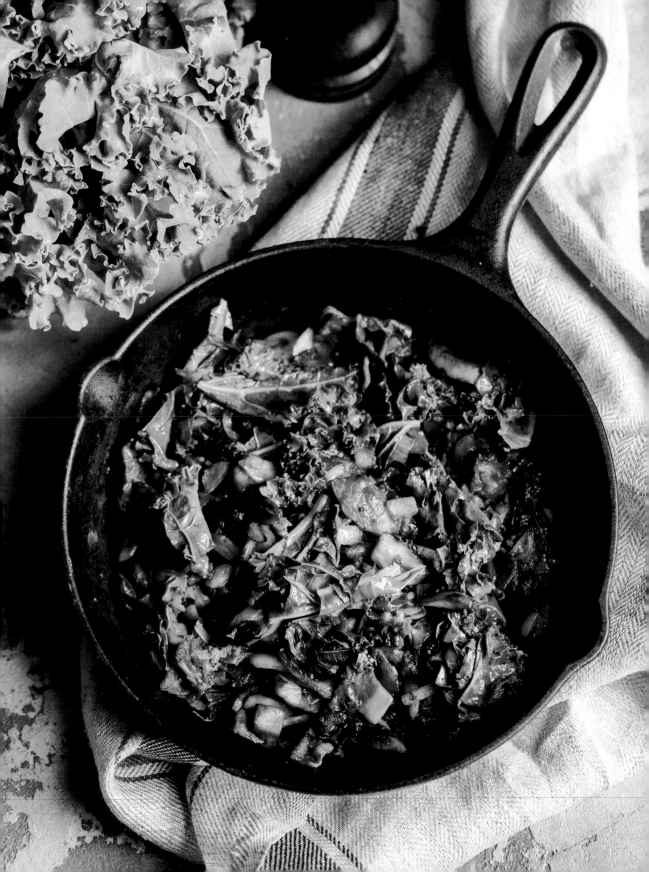

Fluffy Coconut Pancakes

NIGHTSHADE-FREE, VEGETARIAN

When I was growing up, my dad used to make pancakes for the family every Saturday morning. This is a version of his current recipe, which he still makes for us when we're visiting. According to Dad, the secret to fluffy pancakes is mixing the ingredients in the blender—so don't skip that step!

1. Place the eggs, almond flour, coconut flour, coconut milk, honey, vanilla, vinegar, baking soda, and cinnamon in a blender and blend on high speed for 30 to 45 seconds, until completely blended.

2. In a large skillet, melt about 1 teaspoon coconut oil over medium heat. Pour enough batter into the skillet to make 2 medium pancakes, spreading each pancake with the back of the ladle to smooth it evenly into a circle. When the pancakes start to bubble on top and the sides firm up, carefully flip them and cook until golden brown on the second side, 1 to 2 minutes. Remove the pancakes from the skillet and set aside.

3. Add more oil to the skillet and repeat with the remaining batter. Serve warm, garnished with your toppings of choice.

Makes 3 servings (about 10 medium pancakes)
Prep time: **10 minutes**
Cooking time: **less than 20 minutes**

4 medium eggs, lightly beaten
¾ cup almond flour
¼ cup coconut flour
½ cup canned full-fat coconut milk
2 tablespoons raw honey
1 teaspoon pure vanilla extract
½ teaspoon apple cider vinegar
¼ teaspoon baking soda
¼ teaspoon ground cinnamon
Coconut oil or ghee

Toppings (optional)

Fresh fruit
Ghee or coconut oil
Pure maple syrup
Whipped Coconut Cream (page 248)

Noelle's tip: These pancakes keep well in the refrigerator or freezer, so feel free to double the batch and add them to your grab-n-go breakfast stash.

Change it up: Just after pouring the batter into the pan, add a few fresh blueberries or slices of banana to each pancake.

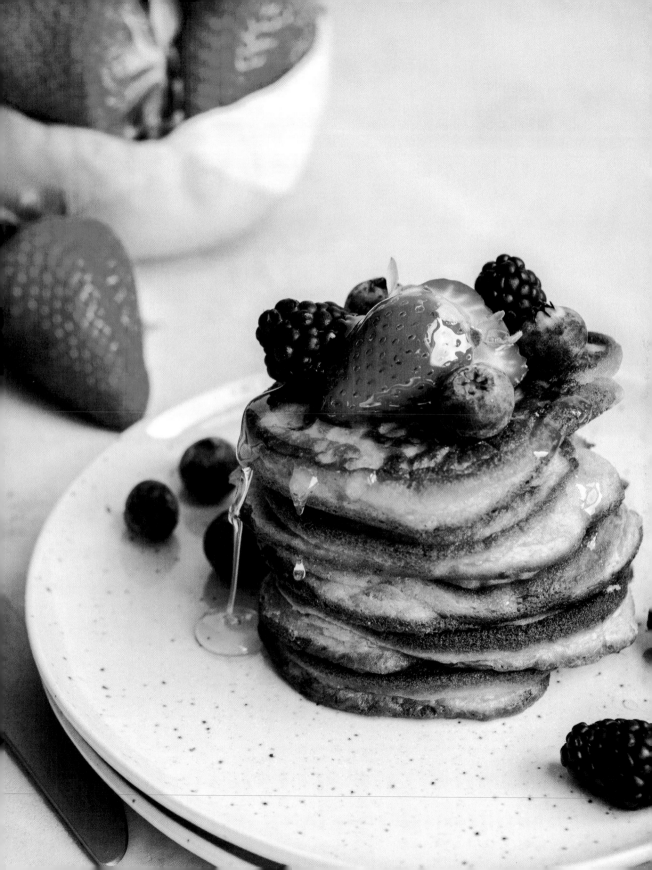

Cinnamon Vanilla N'Oatmeal

EGG-FREE, NIGHTSHADE-FREE, VEGETARIAN

When you're craving a warm and cozy breakfast, this (not) oatmeal is the perfect nutrient- and energy-packed meal. It's become a snow-day staple in my home that tends to get gobbled up after the sidewalk's been shoveled.

Makes 3 or 4 servings
Prep time: 10 minutes
Cooking time: less than 10 minutes

1. Place the coconut flakes, pecans, walnuts, almonds, and pumpkin seeds in a food processor and pulse until coarsely ground, stopping before the mixture breaks down into a powder.

2. Place a medium saucepan over medium heat and add the nut mixture. Slowly pour the coconut milk into the pan and stir. Cook, continuing to regularly stir as the mixture begins to bubble, until it starts to thicken, 4 to 5 minutes.

3. When the mixture has reached your desired consistency, add the honey, vanilla, and cinnamon and stir. Remove the pan from the heat.

4. Transfer the n'oatmeal to a bowl and serve warm with your toppings of choice.

½ cup unsweetened coconut flakes
¼ cup raw pecans
¼ cup raw walnuts
¼ cup raw almonds
¼ cup raw pumpkin seeds
1 cup canned full-fat coconut milk
2 teaspoons raw honey
½ teaspoon pure vanilla extract
¼ teaspoon ground cinnamon

Toppings (optional)

Fresh fruit
Dried fruit, such as raisins or unsweetened dried cherries
Canned full-fat coconut milk

Prep ahead: Make the ground nut mixture in bulk ahead of time and store it in an airtight container in the refrigerator.

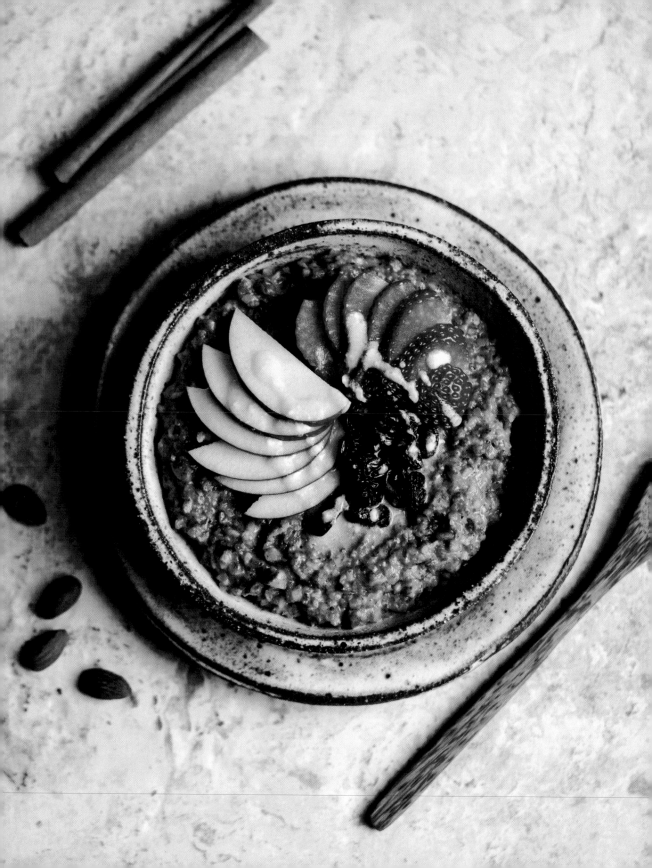

Pumpkin Breakfast Muffins

NIGHTSHADE-FREE, NUT-FREE, VEGETARIAN

These pumpkin muffins are a fan favorite because they're moist and flavorful, with the perfect amount of sweetness. They're also nut-free, which makes them great for kids or family members with nut allergies. If you're new to baking with coconut flour, do yourself a favor and purchase a set of reusable silicone baking cups. The muffins pop right out of the liners, cutting down on frustration and cleanup time.

1. Preheat the oven to 350°F. Line a 12-cup muffin tin with silicone or parchment paper baking cups.

2. In a medium bowl, combine the coconut flour, baking soda, cinnamon, nutmeg, and salt. In a large bowl, lightly whisk the eggs, honey, coconut oil, vanilla, and vinegar. Slowly add the dry ingredients to the wet ingredients and mix until there are no lumps. Fold in the canned pumpkin.

3. Scoop the batter evenly into the prepared muffin tin, filling each liner about three-quarters full. Sprinkle the coconut flakes on top, pressing them down gently into the batter to make them stick.

4. Bake for 25 to 30 minutes, until the edges are lightly golden brown. Let the muffins cool in the pan for 10 minutes, then transfer to a wire rack to cool completely.

5. Store in an airtight container in the refrigerator for up to 1 week or in the freezer for up to 3 months.

Makes 12 muffins (1 per serving)
Prep time: 15 minutes
Cooking time: 25 minutes

½ cup coconut flour
½ teaspoon baking soda
1½ teaspoons ground cinnamon
½ teaspoon ground nutmeg
¼ teaspoon sea salt
6 large eggs, lightly beaten
⅓ cup raw honey
¼ cup coconut oil or ghee, melted
1 teaspoon pure vanilla extract
1 teaspoon apple cider vinegar
⅔ cup canned pure pumpkin puree
Unsweetened coconut flakes, for garnish

Noelle's tip: To make blending the batter easier, pulse the dry ingredients in a food processor until relatively smooth, then add the wet ingredients and pulse until blended, scraping down the sides of the bowl as needed to make sure everything's incorporated.

Change it up: Top the muffins with raw pumpkin seeds, pecans, or walnuts.

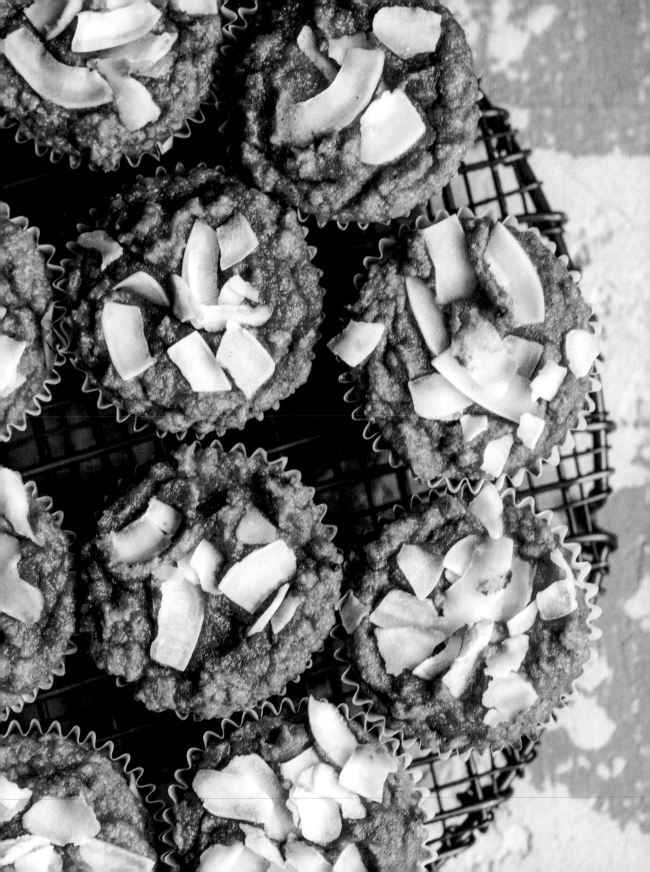

8

SIDES AND SNACKS

Creamy Mashed Cauliflower

EGG-FREE, NIGHTSHADE-FREE, NUT-FREE, VEGETARIAN

This creamy mashed cauliflower has become a holiday staple in our home because it can be served alongside a variety of dishes. It has a smooth and velvety consistency that everyone loves, and I always get requests to share the recipe—especially when people find out it's made from cauliflower.

Makes 4 servings

Prep time: 10 minutes

Cooking time: less than 10 minutes

1 head cauliflower, cut into small florets

2½ tablespoons coconut oil or ghee

2 garlic cloves, chopped

3 tablespoons canned full-fat coconut milk

½ teaspoon sea salt

⅛ teaspoon freshly ground black pepper

1 teaspoon chopped fresh chives, for garnish

1. Bring a large pot of water to a boil. Add the cauliflower and cook until soft, 6 to 8 minutes. Drain the cauliflower and pat it dry with a paper towel.

2. Meanwhile, in a small skillet, melt ½ tablespoon of the coconut oil over medium heat. Add the garlic and cook until fragrant, about 1 minute. Remove the skillet from the heat.

3. Place the cauliflower, garlic, remaining 2 tablespoons coconut oil, the coconut milk, salt, and pepper in a food processor and process until smooth.

4. Transfer to a serving dish and garnish with the chives. Serve warm.

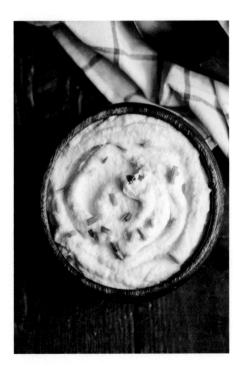

Savory Sweet Potato Wedges

EGG-FREE, NUT-FREE, VEGETARIAN

Sweet potato wedges are perfect for any occasion. They're simple, savory, and downright delicious, which means you'll likely be battling it out for the last wedge. Bring your A game!

Makes 3 or 4 servings
Prep time: **15 minutes**
Cooking time: **35 minutes**

1. Preheat the oven to 400°F. Line a baking sheet with parchment paper or aluminum foil.

2. In a large bowl, toss the sweet potatoes with the coconut oil until all sides are coated. Arrange the potatoes in a single layer on the prepared baking sheet and season them with the paprika, salt, pepper, and cinnamon. Toss gently to coat.

3. Roast for 30 to 35 minutes, until golden brown and tender, flipping once halfway through to ensure even cooking.

3 large sweet potatoes, scrubbed and cut lengthwise into 1-inch wedges
2 tablespoons coconut oil or ghee, melted
1 teaspoon paprika
1 teaspoon sea salt
¼ teaspoon freshly ground black pepper
¼ teaspoon ground cinnamon

Noelle's tip: To make the outside slightly crispier, finish the potatoes under the broiler for about 2 minutes on each side. In general, the thinner you cut the wedges, the quicker the outer shell will brown when roasting. Watch them carefully under the broiler!

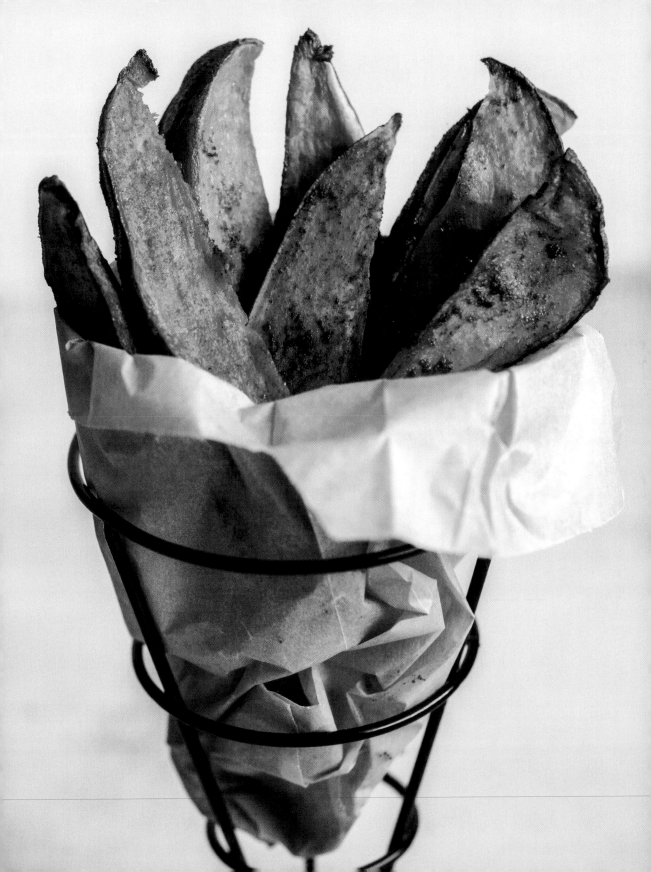

Parsnip and Carrot Fries

EGG-FREE, NIGHTSHADE-FREE, NUT-FREE, VEGETARIAN

These oven-roasted "fries" will completely change your perception of parsnips and carrots. Their mildly sweet flavor and slightly crisp exterior make eating your vegetables an irresistible task.

Makes 3 or 4 servings

Prep time: **20 minutes**

Cooking time: **35 minutes**

1 pound carrots, peeled
1 pound parsnips, peeled
3 tablespoons coconut oil or ghee, melted
1 teaspoon dried thyme
½ teaspoon garlic powder
½ teaspoon sea salt, or more to taste
¼ teaspoon freshly ground black pepper

1. Preheat the oven to 450°F. Line a baking sheet with parchment paper or aluminum foil.

2. Cut each carrot in half crosswise, then cut each half lengthwise into ½-inch-thick strips. Repeat with the parsnips.

3. In a large bowl, toss the carrots and parsnips with the coconut oil until all sides are coated. Arrange the fries in a single layer on the prepared baking sheet and season them with the thyme, garlic powder, salt, and pepper. Toss gently to coat.

4. Roast for 30 to 35 minutes, until the vegetables are golden brown, flipping once halfway through to ensure even cooking.

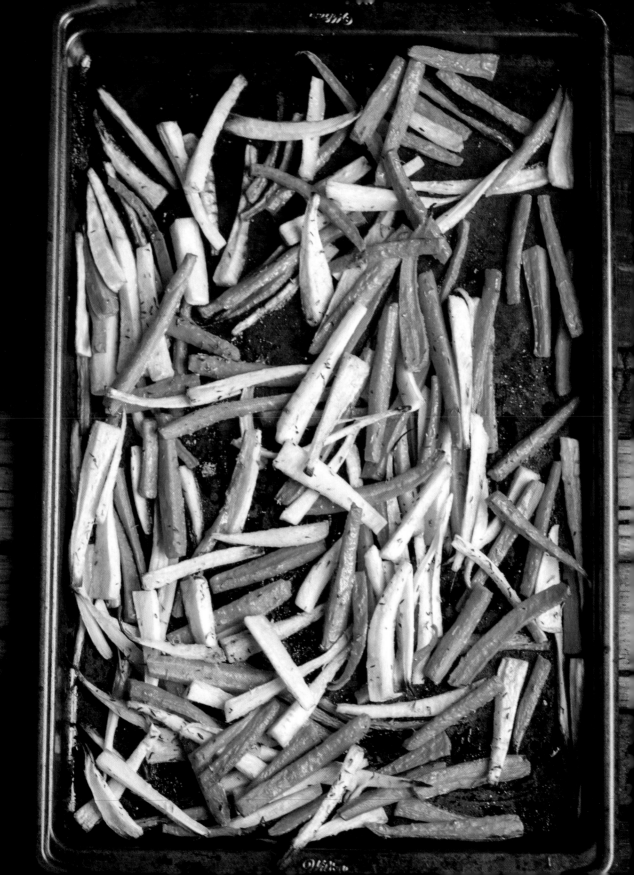

Bacon-Wrapped Asparagus Bundles

EGG-FREE, NIGHTSHADE-FREE, NUT-FREE

The first time I made this dish was for a Christmas party we hosted at our house for friends and family. Despite it being an incredibly simple dish, it was the first thing to go—and left everyone wishing they had grabbed an extra bundle or two when they had the chance. The next year, I doubled the recipe, and everyone was happy.

Makes 3 servings (2 bundles per serving)
Prep time: 10 minutes
Cooking time: 20 minutes

1 pound asparagus, tough ends trimmed
6 bacon slices
1 tablespoon coconut oil or ghee, melted
1 tablespoon balsamic vinegar
¼ teaspoon freshly ground black pepper
⅛ teaspoon garlic powder

1. Preheat the oven to 400°F. Line a baking sheet with parchment paper or aluminum foil.
2. Separate the asparagus into six even bundles. Wrap one piece of bacon tightly around each bundle, starting 1 inch from the bottom of the asparagus. Place the bundles on the prepared baking sheet.
3. In a small bowl, whisk together the coconut oil and vinegar and pour over the bundles. Sprinkle the bundles evenly with the pepper and garlic powder.
4. Roast for 20 minutes, until the asparagus is tender and the bacon is crisp.

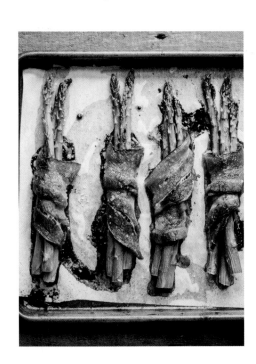

Lemon-Garlic Roasted Broccoli

EGG-FREE, NIGHTSHADE-FREE, NUT-FREE, VEGETARIAN

Even if all you have is 5 minutes to prep, you can have a pan full of crispy, caramelized roasted broccoli that even the pickiest of eaters will devour.

Makes 2 or 3 servings
Prep time: **5 minutes**
Cooking time: **20 minutes**

1. Preheat the oven to 400°F. Line a baking sheet with parchment paper or aluminum foil.
2. Arrange the broccoli florets in a single layer on the prepared baking sheet. Drizzle the broccoli with the coconut oil and season it with the garlic, salt, and pepper. Toss gently to coat.
3. Roast until golden brown in spots, 15 to 20 minutes. Drizzle with the lemon juice before serving.

1 pound broccoli florets
3 tablespoons coconut oil or ghee, melted
3 garlic cloves, minced
½ teaspoon sea salt
½ teaspoon freshly ground black pepper
1 teaspoon fresh lemon juice

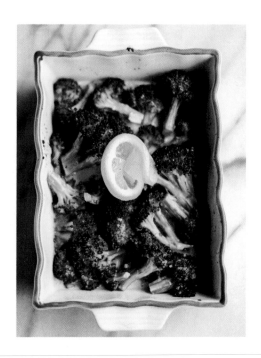

Rosemary Roasted Potatoes

EGG-FREE, NUT-FREE, VEGETARIAN

Roasted potatoes are one of my mom's specialties. According to her, the secret to irresistible potatoes is using sufficient oil and roasting the potatoes past mere tenderness to give them a nice golden brown color. Since adopting her technique, I've experimented with a variety of fresh herbs and spices, and nothing beats the combination of garlic and fresh rosemary.

Makes 3 or 4 servings

Prep time: **10 minutes**

Cooking time: **30 minutes**

1½ pounds small white
potatoes (such as fingerling
or new potatoes)
3 tablespoons coconut oil or
ghee, melted
2 garlic cloves, minced
1 tablespoon finely chopped
fresh rosemary
½ teaspoon sea salt
¼ teaspoon freshly ground
black pepper

1. Preheat the oven to 425°F. Line a baking sheet with parchment paper or aluminum foil.

2. Slice the potatoes in half crosswise or lengthwise, depending on the size of the potatoes.

3. In a large bowl, toss the potatoes with the coconut oil until all sides are coated. Arrange the potatoes in a single layer on the prepared baking sheet and season them with the garlic, rosemary, salt, and pepper. Toss gently to coat.

4. Roast for 25 to 30 minutes, until golden brown, stirring halfway through to ensure even cooking.

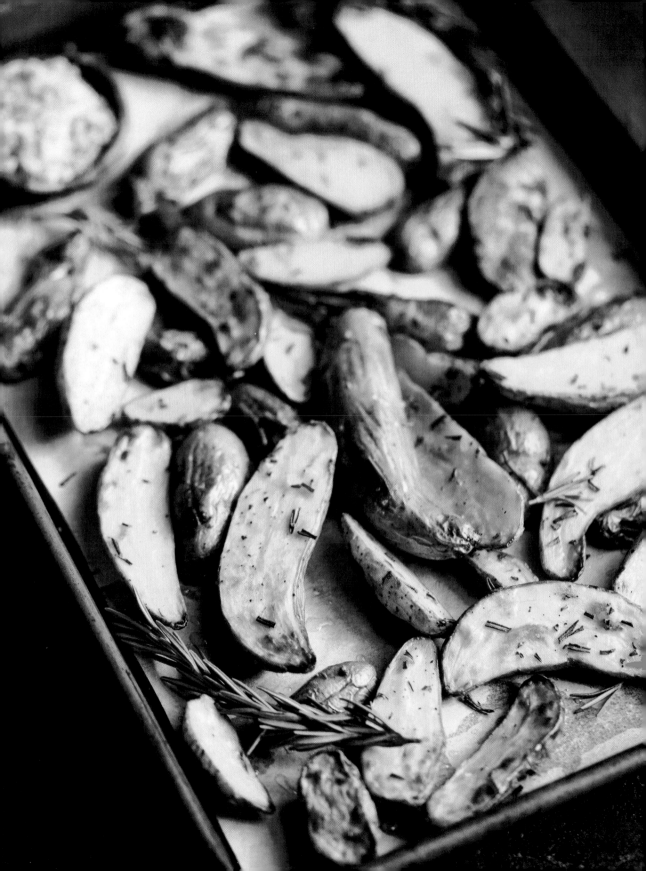

Zucchini-Tomato Sauté

EGG-FREE, NUT-FREE, VEGETARIAN

This sauté is one of the quick and simple side dishes I keep in my toolbox for busy weeknights. While the ingredients are minimal, the taste is anything but!

Makes 3 or 4 servings

Prep time: **10 minutes**

Cooking time: **less than 15 minutes**

1. In a large skillet, melt the coconut oil over medium heat. Add the onion and garlic and cook, stirring, until just soft, 3 to 4 minutes.
2. Add the zucchini, salt, black pepper, and red pepper flakes (if using) and cook, stirring, until the zucchini starts to become tender and turns golden brown, 5 to 7 minutes.
3. Stir in the cherry tomatoes and cook for 2 to 3 minutes. Add the basil and stir to combine.
4. Transfer to a serving platter and serve warm.

1 tablespoon coconut oil or ghee

1 small sweet onion, chopped

2 garlic cloves, minced

2 medium zucchini, cut into ½-inch chunks

½ teaspoon sea salt

¼ teaspoon freshly ground black pepper

⅛ teaspoon red pepper flakes (optional)

1¼ cups cherry tomatoes, halved

1 tablespoon chopped fresh basil

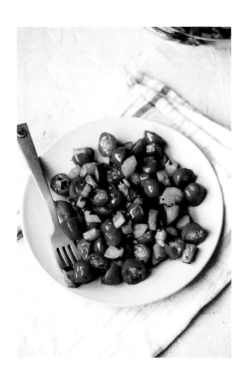

Jalapeño-Lime Cauliflower Rice

EGG-FREE, NUT-FREE, VEGETARIAN

Cauliflower rice has a light and fluffy texture that serves as the perfect companion to a variety of dishes. Lightly sautéing the cauliflower brings out a slightly nutty flavor, which pairs beautifully with jalapeño and lime.

Makes 4 servings

Prep time: **15 minutes**

Cooking time: **about 10 minutes**

1. Working in two or three batches, pulse the cauliflower in a large food processor until broken down into small pieces resembling grains of rice.

2. In a large skillet, melt the coconut oil over medium heat. Add the jalapeño and garlic and cook, stirring often, until tender, 3 to 4 minutes.

3. Add the riced cauliflower, salt, and pepper and cook until the cauliflower is just cooked through, 5 to 7 minutes. Remove the skillet from the heat and stir in the lime juice and cilantro. Serve warm.

1 large head cauliflower, cut into small florets
2 tablespoons coconut oil or ghee
1 jalapeño, seeded and finely chopped
1 garlic clove, minced
½ teaspoon sea salt
¼ teaspoon freshly ground black pepper
Juice of ½ lime
3 tablespoons minced fresh cilantro

Noelle's tip: For even chopping, fill the food processor only about half full of cauliflower for each batch.

Prep ahead: Rice the cauliflower ahead of time and store it in an airtight container in the refrigerator for up to 3 days, or in the freezer for up to a month.

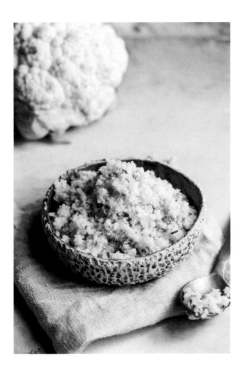

Easy Apple "Cookies"

EGG-FREE, NIGHTSHADE-FREE, VEGETARIAN

These apple "cookies" are a super-satisfying snack that both kids and kids at heart will love. They taste great with just about any nut butter and can be further customized depending on your favorite type of apple—whether you prefer Pink Lady (like Noelle) or Fuji (like Stef).

1. Place the apple slices on a tray or baking sheet. Spread the nut butter on one side of each apple slice and sprinkle with the cinnamon.
2. Top the slices with the coconut flakes, pecans, and chocolate (if using). Serve immediately.

Makes 4 servings (12 to 14 "cookies")

Prep time: 15 minutes

Cooking time: none

2 large sweet apples, such as Pink Lady or Fuji, cored with an apple corer and sliced crosswise into thin rings

½ cup almond butter

Dash of ground cinnamon

½ cup unsweetened coconut flakes

½ cup chopped raw pecans

½ ounce unsweetened baking chocolate, finely chopped (optional)

Special equipment: Apple corer

Noelle's tip: Coarsely chop the coconut flakes if you have some extra-long pieces.

Change it up: Use another nut butter, such as cashew or sunflower seed butter. Swap out the pecans for another nut, such as walnuts or cashews.

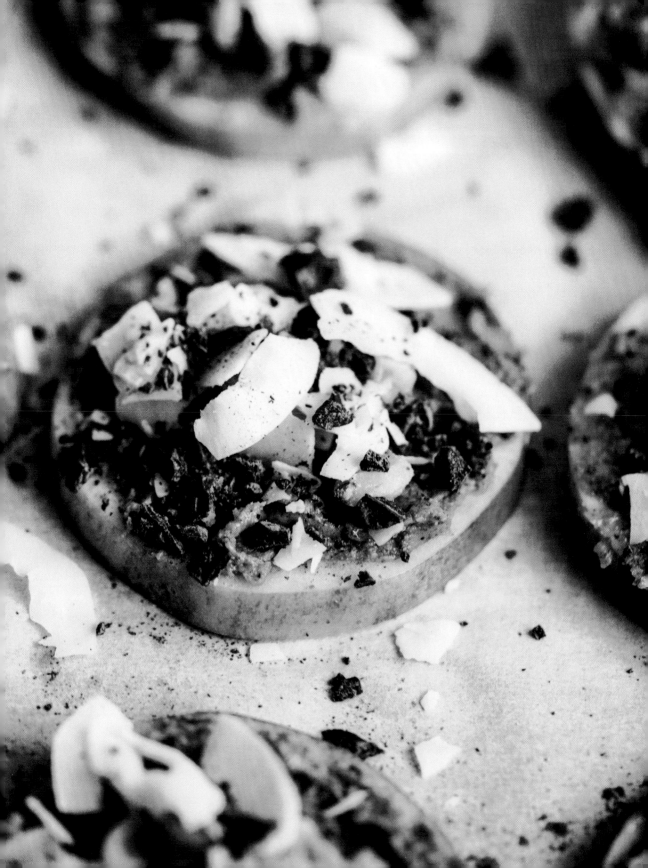

Baked Plantain Chips

EGG-FREE, NUT-FREE, VEGETARIAN

This snack has it all—it's crispy, crunchy, and slightly salty, with a hint of spice. To get uniform slices that crisp up with ease, I highly recommend using a mandoline or box grater slicing blade. It makes prepping super easy, which means there are bound to be plenty of plantain chips in your future.

Makes 3 or 4 servings
Prep time: **15 minutes**
Cooking time: **25 minutes**

2 large green plantains
2 tablespoons coconut oil or
  ghee, melted
¾ teaspoon sea salt
½ teaspoon chili powder
¼ teaspoon freshly ground
  black pepper
Juice of ½ lime

1. Preheat the oven to 350°F. Line two baking sheets with parchment paper or aluminum foil.

2. Cut the ends off each plantain. Make a shallow slit lengthwise along the skins and peel them off with your fingers.

3. Using a mandoline slicer, the slicing edge on a box grater, or a small paring knife, slice the plantains into discs as thin and uniform as possible. Place the plantain discs in a large bowl and gently stir so the discs are loose and not sticking together.

4. Add the coconut oil, ½ teaspoon of the salt, the chili powder, and the pepper and toss gently until the plantains are well coated.

5. Spread the plantains in a single layer on the prepared baking sheets. Bake for 22 to 25 minutes, until the plantains start to crisp and lightly brown. Watch closely to prevent burning—the thinner the slices, the more quickly they will crisp up.

6. Remove the plantains from the oven and immediately sprinkle them with the lime juice and remaining ¼ teaspoon salt. Let the chips cool before serving.

Noelle's tip: Plantain chips are best eaten the day they're made, as they'll lose their crispness over time.

Serve it with: Everyone's Favorite Guacamole (page 184) or Mango-Jalapeño Salsa (page 185)

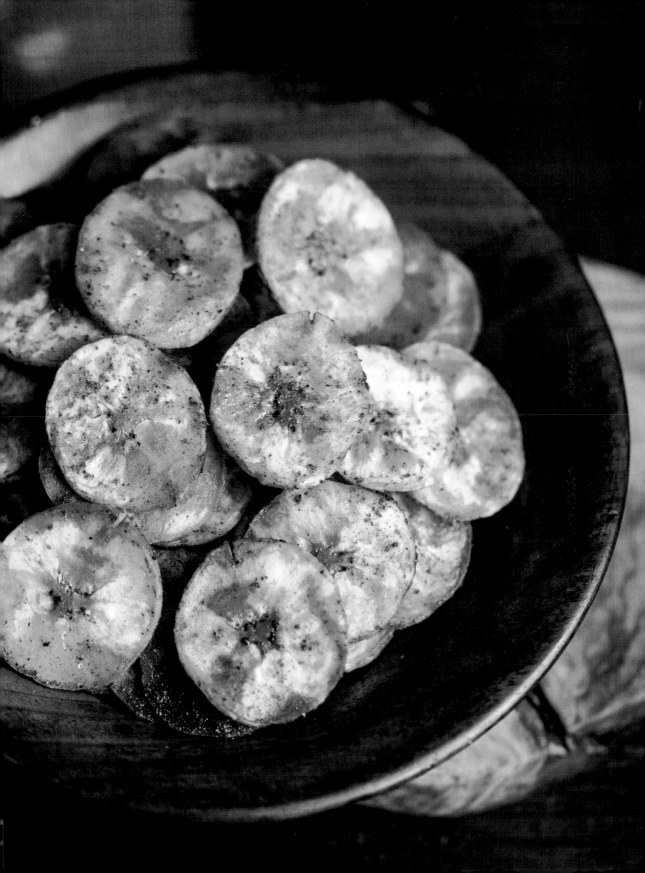

Chocolate-Cherry Energy Bites

EGG-FREE, NIGHTSHADE-FREE, VEGETARIAN

If you're a fan of prepackaged fruit and nut bars, you'll be pleasantly surprised at how easy they are to make at home. While rolling them into bite-size balls makes them easy to eat, you can also spread the dough in a standard loaf pan lined with parchment paper, chill, and cut them into bars.

Makes 12 servings (2 energy bites per serving)
Prep time: **15 minutes, plus 1 hour chilling time**
Cooking time: **none**

1. Line a baking sheet with parchment paper. Place the dates and dried cherries in a food processor and pulse until broken down into small pieces. Add the almonds, pecans, cacao powder, and salt and pulse until the mixture resembles bread crumbs.

2. Add the honey and vanilla and process until the mixture becomes sticky and binds together. Roll the mixture into about twenty-four 1½-inch balls and place them on the prepared baking sheet.

3. Freeze the bites until set, about 1 hour. Store in an airtight container in the refrigerator for up to 3 weeks or in the freezer for up to 6 months.

10 Medjool dates, pitted
1 cup unsweetened dried cherries
1 cup raw almonds
¼ cup raw pecans
2 tablespoons cacao powder or unsweetened cocoa powder
⅛ teaspoon sea salt
1 tablespoon raw honey
2 teaspoons pure vanilla extract

Noelle's tip: These bites will maintain a slightly soft texture right out of the freezer.

Cinnamon-Toasted Coconut "Chips"

EGG-FREE, NIGHTSHADE-FREE, NUT-FREE, VEGETARIAN

These crunchy and slightly sweet coconut "chips" are a staple snack in our home. My husband and I typically double the recipe and keep our stash stored in large mason jars. We eat them by the handful, add them to homemade nut mixes, or sprinkle them on top of treats.

Makes 12 servings
  (¼ cup per serving)
Prep time: **5 minutes**
Cooking time: **20 minutes**

3 cups unsweetened coconut
  flakes
2 tablespoons pure maple
  syrup
2 teaspoons ground cinnamon
¼ teaspoon sea salt

Noelle's tip: These chips crisp up as they cool, so resist the urge to grab a handful right out of the oven.

1. Preheat the oven to 300°F. Line a baking sheet with parchment paper.

2. Spread the coconut flakes in a single layer on the prepared baking sheet. Drizzle the flakes with the maple syrup and stir gently with a spatula until coated.

3. Sprinkle the coconut flakes with the cinnamon and salt and toss gently to coat.

4. Bake for 18 to 20 minutes, until lightly golden brown, stirring every 5 to 7 minutes.

5. Let the coconut chips cool completely before serving or storing. Store in an airtight container.

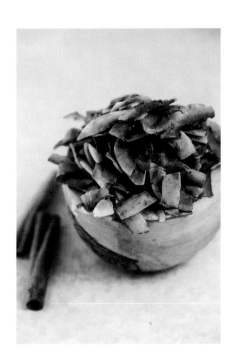

Spiced Rosemary Roasted Nuts

EGG-FREE, VEGETARIAN

My sister, who just so happens to be the queen of holiday parties, first introduced me to this recipe at a party we threw together. After realizing no one could stop hovering over the bowl—including myself—I immediately gave her a pen and paper and had her write down the recipe for me. Now I make these regularly to jazz up our snack options and serve them when hanging out with family or friends.

Makes about 22 servings (5½ cups; ¼ cup per serving)

Prep time: **5 minutes**

Cooking time: **12 minutes**

2 cups raw almonds
1½ cups raw walnut halves
1 cup raw cashews
1 cup raw pumpkin seeds
2 tablespoons coconut oil or ghee, melted
2 tablespoons finely chopped fresh rosemary
2 teaspoons raw honey
1 teaspoon sea salt
½ teaspoon cayenne pepper
¼ teaspoon ground cinnamon

1. Preheat the oven to 375°F.

2. Spread the almonds, walnuts, cashews, and pumpkin seeds in a single layer on a large baking sheet. Roast for 12 minutes. Remove from the oven and set aside.

3. In a small bowl, combine the coconut oil, rosemary, honey, salt, cayenne, and cinnamon. Pour the oil mixture over the nuts and stir with a spatula until coated.

4. Let the nuts cool completely before serving or storing. Store in an airtight container.

Change it up: Use other nuts or seeds, such as pecans or hazelnuts.

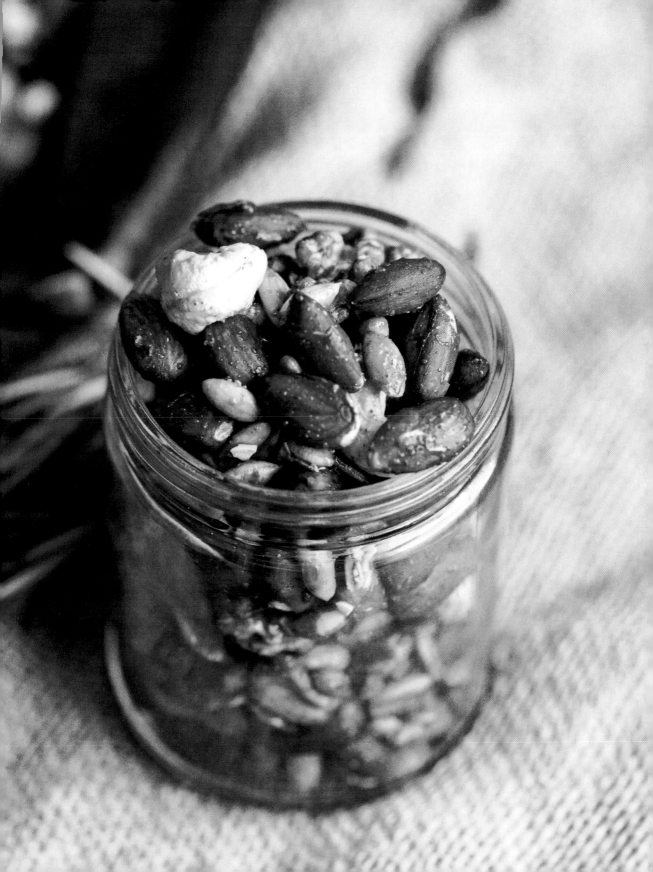

9

SALADS, DRESSINGS, AND DIPS

Apple, Avocado, and Chicken Salad

EGG-FREE, NIGHTSHADE-FREE, NUT-FREE

Having easy-to-grab protein sources on hand is an absolute must in our home for making it through the week. On Sunday afternoons, we bake chicken breasts in bulk, then use them in quick, simple recipes like this one for lunches or afternoon snacks throughout the week.

Makes 5 servings
(1 cup per serving)

Prep time: **15 minutes**
(not including chicken)

Cooking time: **none**

1. Place the avocado in a medium bowl and gently break it up with a fork until slightly mashed and chunky. Fold in the chicken, apple, celery, and onion.

2. Add the cilantro, lemon juice, olive oil, salt, garlic powder, and pepper and stir until combined. Taste and add more salt, if desired.

3. Serve alone, with lettuce leaves, or over mixed baby greens. Store in an airtight container in the refrigerator for up to 2 days.

1 large ripe avocado, diced
2 cups diced cooked chicken breast
1 sweet apple, such as Pink Lady or Fuji, cored and diced
1 celery stalk, finely chopped
¼ cup finely diced red onion
2 tablespoons finely chopped fresh cilantro
1 tablespoon fresh lemon juice
1 tablespoon extra-virgin olive oil
½ teaspoon sea salt, or more to taste
¼ teaspoon garlic powder
¼ teaspoon freshly ground black pepper
Lettuce leaves or mixed baby greens, for serving (optional)

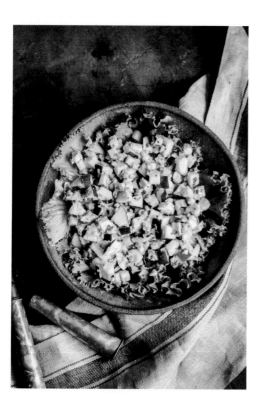

Chili-Lime Shrimp Salad

EGG-FREE, NUT-FREE

Jicama is a crispy and slightly sweet root vegetable. It pairs perfectly with chili-lime shrimp and gives this salad a nice crunch. If you're new to jicama, there's no better way to test it out.

1. To marinate the shrimp, place all the shrimp ingredients in a bowl and toss to coat evenly. Cover the bowl and marinate in the refrigerator for 30 minutes.

2. Meanwhile, preheat the oven to 425°F. Line a baking sheet with parchment paper or aluminum foil.

3. To make the salad, in a large bowl, combine the greens, avocado, jicama, cherry tomatoes, and onion. Toss gently to combine.

4. Remove the shrimp from the marinade and place them in a single layer on the prepared baking sheet. Roast for 10 to 12 minutes, until the shrimp are pink and opaque.

5. Arrange the salad on a large serving platter and top with the shrimp. Serve with the Honey-Lime Dressing.

Makes 4 servings

Prep time: 15 minutes (not including dressing), plus 30 minutes marinating

Cooking time: 12 minutes

Shrimp

1 pound large shrimp, peeled and deveined
½ cup extra-virgin olive oil
Juice of 2 limes
1 tablespoon chili powder
½ teaspoon sea salt
¼ teaspoon garlic powder
¼ teaspoon freshly ground black pepper

Salad

6 cups mixed baby greens
1 large avocado, diced
½ jicama, peeled and diced
10 cherry tomatoes, cut into slices
¼ cup diced onion
½ cup Honey-Lime Dressing (page 193)

Change it up: Swap out the jicama for ½ red bell pepper, sliced.

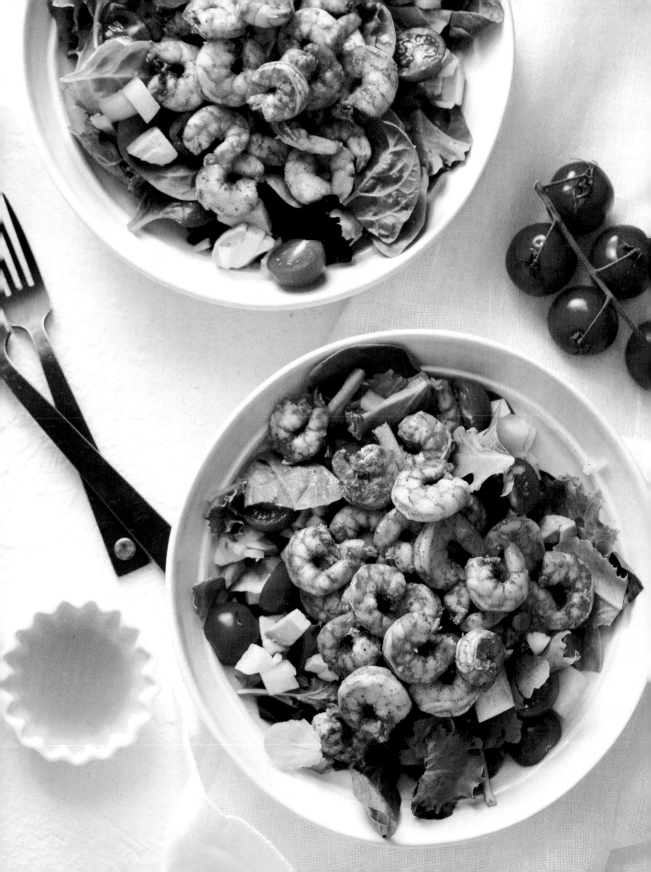

Roasted Beets and Berries Salad

EGG-FREE, NIGHTSHADE-FREE, VEGETARIAN

The beet is a nutrient-packed superhero vegetable that often doesn't get the attention it deserves. The easiest way to eat beets regularly is to roast them in bulk ahead of time and eat them throughout the week, tossed with a little olive oil and salt or incorporated into flavorful salads like this one.

Makes 4 servings

Prep time: **15 minutes (not including dressing)**

Cooking time: **1 hour**

2 medium beets
Extra-virgin olive oil
6 cups baby arugula
¾ cup fresh blueberries
¾ cup fresh raspberries
½ avocado, sliced
⅓ cup coarsely chopped raw walnuts
½ cup Raspberry Apple Cider Vinaigrette (page 191)

1. Preheat the oven to 400°F.
2. Trim off the beet ends and greens. Rub the beets with a little olive oil and wrap them individually in aluminum foil. Place them on a baking sheet and roast until fork-tender, about 1 hour. Let cool, then peel the beets (the skins should rub off easily) and cut them into 1-inch chunks.
3. Arrange the arugula on a platter and scatter with the beets, blueberries, and raspberries. Top with the avocado slices and walnuts and serve with the vinaigrette.

Prep ahead: Roast the beets up to 5 days ahead of time and store them in an airtight container in the refrigerator.

Change it up: Use chopped almonds or pecans instead of walnuts; use other berries, such as strawberries or blackberries.

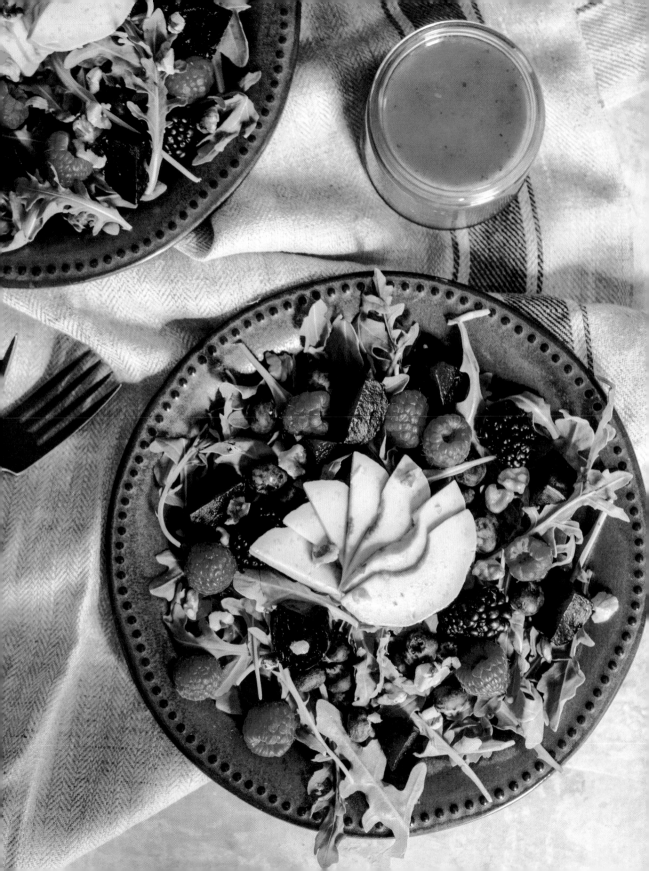

Strawberry Cobb Salad

This salad is my rendition of a traditional Cobb salad. Straw-berries and pecans are one of my favorite combinations, and the duo is elevated to a whole new level when balanced with the savoriness of bacon and tossed in my Dairy-Free Ranch Dressing. If you're looking to impress a crowd, this is your dish.

1. In a large skillet, melt the coconut oil over medium heat. Add the bacon and cook until crisp, 4 to 5 minutes on each side. Set the bacon aside on a paper towel to cool, then chop it into small pieces.

2. Arrange the lettuce on a large platter and spread the chopped bacon, eggs, avocado, cherry tomatoes, straw-berries, and pecans in rows over the lettuce.

3. Serve with the ranch dressing.

Makes 4 servings

Prep time: **15 minutes (not including dressing)**

Cooking time: **10 minutes**

1½ teaspoons coconut oil
8 bacon slices
1 large head romaine lettuce, coarsely chopped
3 large eggs, hard-boiled, peeled, and sliced
1 large avocado, diced
1 cup chopped cherry tomatoes
1 cup sliced strawberries
½ cup raw pecan halves
½ cup Dairy-Free Ranch Dressing (page 192)

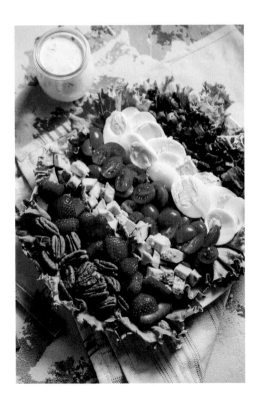

Buffalo Chicken Dip

NUT-FREE (IF DRESSING IS MADE WITH NUT-FREE OIL)

Hands-down, this is my favorite dish to take to tailgates and game-day celebrations. It's quick and easy to whip up and has the perfect balance of coolness and heat.

1. Preheat the oven to 350°F.
2. In a medium bowl, fold together the chicken, dressing, and hot sauce until combined.
3. Spread the mixture in an even layer in an 8 x 8-inch glass baking dish (or similar dish) and bake for 30 minutes, until the edges are lightly golden brown and bubbling.
4. Garnish with the scallions and serve with celery or carrot sticks.

Makes 4 to 6 servings

Prep time: **5 minutes (not including chicken or dressing)**

Cooking time: **30 minutes**

3 cups shredded cooked chicken (use leftovers from Slow Cooker Chicken, page 204)
1 cup Dairy-Free Ranch Dressing (page 192)
½ cup hot sauce (see tip)
1 scallion, finely chopped, for garnish
Celery or carrot sticks, for serving

Noelle's tip: I recommend using Tessemae's All-Natural Hot Buffalo Sauce or Frank's RedHot.

Prep ahead: Prepare Slow Cooker Chicken for dinner a few days prior and store the leftover shredded chicken in an airtight container in the refrigerator until ready to use. Make the dressing a few days prior and store it in a separate airtight container in the refrigerator.

Serve it with: Baked Plantain Chips (page 170)

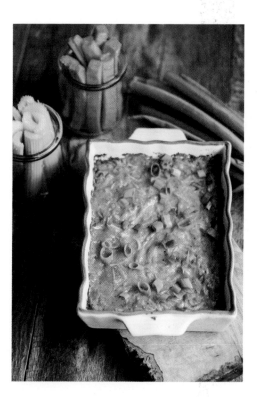

Everyone's Favorite Guacamole

EGG-FREE, NUT-FREE, VEGETARIAN

As the name suggests, this recipe is always a hit. It has the perfect balance of flavors, which keeps just about everyone coming back for more. If you're hoping for leftovers, you'll likely be disappointed.

Makes 10 to 12 servings
(about 4 cups)
Prep time: 10 minutes,
plus 1 hour chilling time
Cooking time: none

1. Put the avocado in a large bowl. Add the lime juice and mash the avocado with a potato masher or large fork, leaving it slightly chunky.

2. Add the onion, jalapeño, tomato, cilantro, salt, black pepper, cayenne, and cumin and fold until combined.

3. Cover the bowl and refrigerate for 1 hour to chill before serving.

4 ripe avocados, diced
Juice of 1 lime
½ medium onion, diced
½ jalapeño, seeded and
  minced
1 vine-ripe tomato, finely
  chopped
3 tablespoons coarsely
  chopped fresh cilantro
½ teaspoon sea salt
½ teaspoon freshly ground
  black pepper
¼ teaspoon cayenne pepper
¼ teaspoon ground cumin

Change it up: Use a whole jalapeño for a spicy kick.

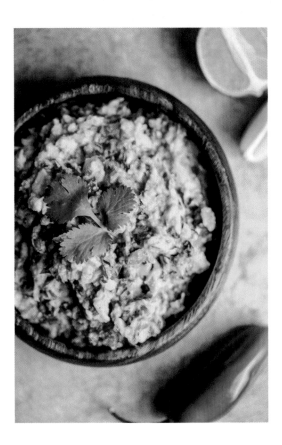

Mango-Jalapeño Salsa

EGG-FREE, NUT-FREE, VEGETARIAN

This sweet and spicy salsa is great for summer barbecues. Use it as a garnish on top of grilled meats or serve it as a dip with Baked Plantain Chips (page 170).

Makes 8 to 10 servings (about 3½ cups)

Prep time: 15 minutes, plus 10 minutes resting time

Cooking time: none

1. In a medium bowl, combine the mangoes, jalapeños, bell pepper, onion, and cilantro.
2. Drizzle with the lime juice and season with the salt. Toss to combine.
3. Let the salsa rest for 10 minutes before serving. Store in an airtight container in the refrigerator for up to 3 days.

2 large ripe mangoes, diced
1½ jalapeños, seeded and finely diced
1 red bell pepper, diced
½ small onion, diced
3 tablespoons chopped fresh cilantro
3 tablespoons fresh lime juice
⅛ teaspoon sea salt

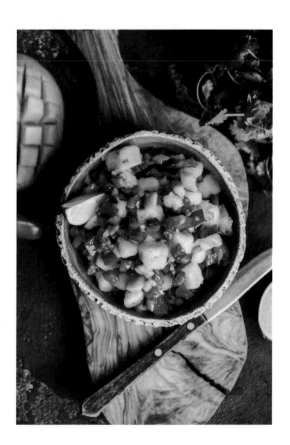

Avocado Butter

EGG-FREE, NIGHTSHADE-FREE, NUT-FREE, VEGETARIAN

This avocado butter has an endless number of uses and gives a delicious, flavorful kick to just about anything it adorns. Melt it on top of potatoes or cooked vegetables, or use it to finish grilled fish, steak, or chicken.

Makes 6 servings

Prep time: 5 minutes, plus 3 to 4 hours chilling time

Cooking time: none

1. Place all the ingredients in a food processor and blend until smooth.
2. Transfer the mixture to a sheet of parchment paper and form it into a log shape. Take an end of the parchment paper parallel to the log and pull it over so it covers the top of the log. Take the edge of the parchment paper and tuck it under the log, trimming the excess paper if necessary, and roll the log so it is encased in parchment paper. Twist the ends of the paper to make a large "Tootsie Roll." Tighten the twists to pack the mixture together in the center if necessary.
3. Refrigerate the log until it solidifies, 3 to 4 hours.
4. To serve, simply unwrap the parchment paper and cut the log into slices. Store leftovers in an airtight container in the refrigerator for up to 3 days.

1 medium avocado, halved, pitted, and peeled (about 5 ounces avocado flesh)

¼ cup unsalted ghee, at room temperature

1 tablespoon fresh lime juice

1 garlic clove, minced

1 tablespoon chopped fresh cilantro

1 teaspoon chopped fresh parsley

½ teaspoon ground cumin

¼ teaspoon sea salt

⅛ teaspoon freshly ground black pepper

Noelle's tip: You can also transfer the avocado butter to a round airtight container or jar for storage in the refrigerator. Simply use a spoon or knife to spread and serve.

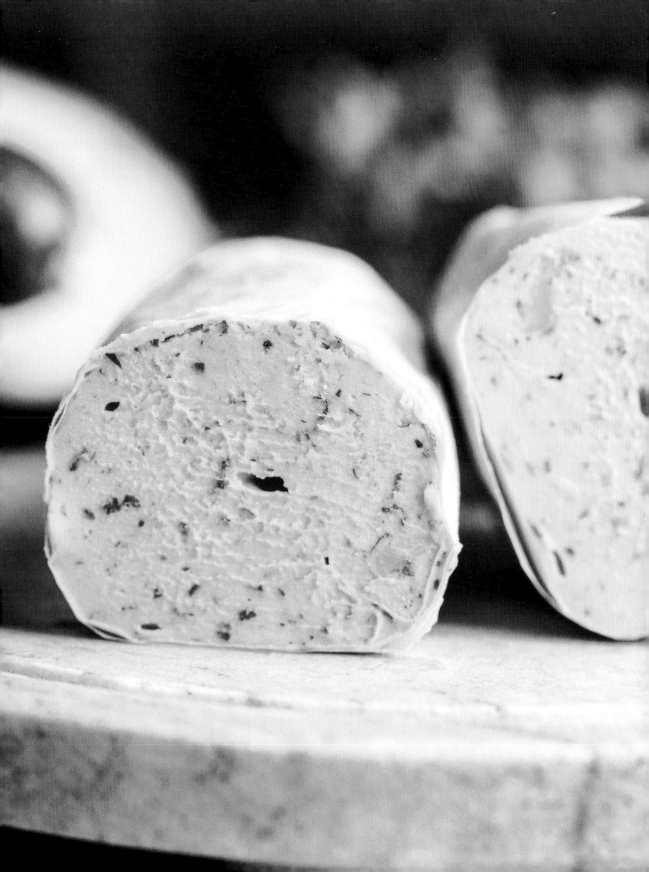

Simple Homemade Mayonnaise

NIGHTSHADE-FREE (IF USING NIGHTSHADE-FREE DIJON MUSTARD),
NUT-FREE (IF USING AVOCADO OIL), VEGETARIAN

For years I thought homemade mayonnaise had something against me. No matter how much I'd troubleshoot, I just couldn't seem to get it to emulsify. Thanks to this simple recipe, homemade mayo is now a regular staple in our household, which is great, because it goes with just about everything. When making mayonnaise, (1) be sure all your ingredients are at room temperature, and (2) be patient. Pouring the oil in slowly is key to the emulsion forming and holding, which means you'll be working your biceps and making mayo at the same time. How very efficient of you!

Makes 8 servings
(2 tablespoons per serving)
Prep time: **10 minutes,**
plus 1 hour chilling time
Cooking time: **none**

1 large egg
1 tablespoon Dijon mustard
1 tablespoon fresh lemon juice
¼ teaspoon sea salt
1 cup cold-pressed avocado
oil or macadamia nut oil

1. Make sure all the ingredients are at room temperature. Place the egg, mustard, lemon juice, and salt in a blender and blend on low speed until combined and frothy, about 20 seconds.

2. With the blender running on low, add the oil very slowly, pouring it in tiny, steady drops until you have added about ¼ cup. At this point, the mixture will start to thicken and emulsify.

3. Continue adding the oil in a very thin stream until combined and emulsified, 4 to 5 minutes. Resist the urge to rush when pouring, especially at the end.

4. Transfer the mixture to a glass container and refrigerate for 1 hour. The mayonnaise will thicken slightly when chilled.

5. Whip the mayonnaise with a spoon before serving. Store in the refrigerator for up to 5 days.

Noelle's tip: Extra-virgin avocado oil has an intense green hue, which will make the mayo a lightish green color. If you want a more traditional yellow mayo color, I recommend using a cold-pressed and lightly refined avocado oil, such as Primal Kitchen Avocado Oil, or macadamia nut oil.

Change it up: To make this painfully easy, you can also use an immersion blender. Simply combine all the ingredients in a tall, narrow jar and wait a few seconds for the egg to settle at the bottom. Place the immersion blender in the jar so the blade is situated at the bottom, power it on, and hold it in place until the emulsion begins to form and spread, about 20 seconds. Slowly move the blade up and down to fully incorporate and emulsify.

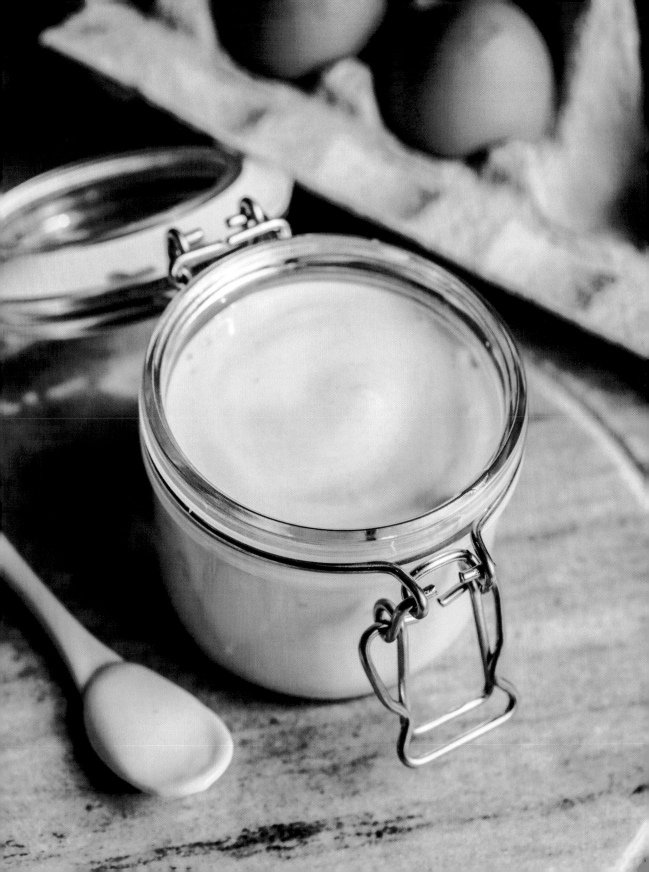

Cranberry-Apple Relish

EGG-FREE, NIGHTSHADE-FREE, VEGETARIAN

Cranberry-apple relish has been a part of our Thanksgiving tradition for years. It's a well-received alternative to the jellied sauces that typically come in a can, and can also serve as a sweet and tangy side dish to fall-inspired meals.

1. Place the apples and celery in a food processor and pulse until coarsely chopped. Add the remaining ingredients and pulse until finely chopped, stopping before the mixture becomes too mushy.

2. Transfer to a bowl, cover, and refrigerator for at least 1 hour before serving. Store in the refrigerator for up to 5 days.

Makes 8 servings
(¼ cup per serving)

Prep time: **10 minutes,**
plus 1 hour chilling time

Cooking time: **none**

2 large sweet apples, such
  as Pink Lady or Fuji,
  peeled, cored, and coarsely
  chopped
1 celery stalk, cut into 1-inch
  slices
1 cup fresh cranberries
  (see tip)
3 Medjool dates, pitted and
  coarsely chopped
¼ cup raw walnuts
2 tablespoons raw honey
¼ teaspoon ground cinnamon
⅛ teaspoon ground ginger

Noelle's tip: If you can't find fresh cranberries, use whole frozen cranberries. Simply thaw them, rinse, and drain before using.

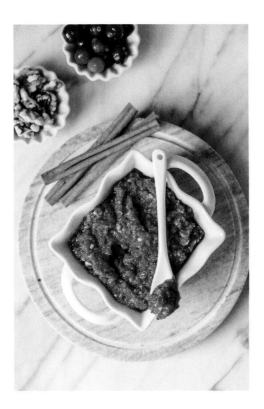

Raspberry Apple Cider Vinaigrette

EGG-FREE, NIGHTSHADE-FREE, NUT-FREE, VEGETARIAN

Slightly tart and sweet, this dressing pairs great with salads adorned with fresh berries, and can also be used as a marinade for a variety of meats.

Makes 10 servings
(2 tablespoons per serving)
Prep time: **5 minutes**
Cooking time: **none**

1. Place all the ingredients in a blender with 2 tablespoons water and blend on low speed until smooth, about 20 seconds.
2. Transfer to an airtight container and store in the refrigerator for up to 1 week.

¾ cup extra-virgin olive oil
¼ cup apple cider vinegar
⅓ cup fresh raspberries
1½ tablespoons raw honey
½ teaspoon sea salt
½ teaspoon dried basil

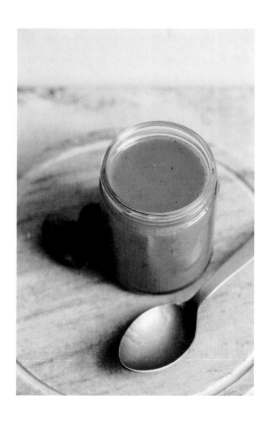

Dairy-Free Ranch Dressing

NIGHTSHADE-FREE (IF THE MAYO WAS MADE WITH NIGHTSHADE-FREE DIJON MUSTARD),
NUT-FREE (IF THE MAYO WAS MADE WITH AVOCADO OIL),
VEGETARIAN

As many times as I've served this dressing, no one has ever suspected it's completely dairy-free. It's super thick and creamy, which makes it great for serving as a dip or on top of salads.

Makes 10 servings (about 2 tablespoons per serving)

Prep time: 10 minutes (not including mayonnaise)

Cooking time: none

1. Place the coconut milk and lemon juice in a small glass measuring cup and stir. Let the mixture sit for 5 to 10 minutes.

2. In a large bowl, whisk together the coconut milk mixture and the remaining ingredients.

3. Serve or transfer to an airtight container and store in the refrigerator for up to 5 days.

¼ cup canned full-fat coconut milk

1½ teaspoons fresh lemon juice

1 cup Simple Homemade Mayonnaise (page 188; see tip)

1 teaspoon apple cider vinegar

2 tablespoons finely chopped fresh parsley

2 teaspoons finely chopped fresh chives

½ teaspoon dried dill

½ teaspoon garlic powder

¼ teaspoon onion powder

⅛ teaspoon sea salt

⅛ teaspoon freshly ground black pepper

Noelle's tip: To save time, you can use store-bought mayonnaise for this recipe, as mayonnaise made with healthier oils is now more widely available. I recommend using Primal Kitchen Avocado Oil Mayo.

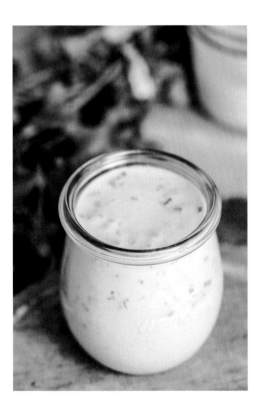

Honey-Lime Dressing

EGG-FREE, NIGHTSHADE-FREE, NUT-FREE, VEGETARIAN

This is my go-to "any salad" dressing that's always in the refrigerator because it's full of flavor and easy to throw together.

1. Place all the ingredients in a blender and blend on low speed until smooth, about 20 seconds.

2. Transfer to an airtight container and store in the refrigerator for up to 2 weeks.

Makes 6 servings
(2 tablespoons per serving)

Prep time: **5 minutes**

Cooking time: **none**

½ cup extra-virgin olive oil
¼ cup fresh lime juice
1½ tablespoons raw honey
½ teaspoon garlic powder
¼ teaspoon sea salt
⅛ teaspoon freshly ground
   black pepper

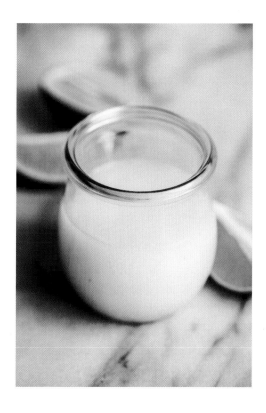

10

MAIN DISHES

Spiced Potato Soup

EGG-FREE, VEGETARIAN (IF USING VEGETABLE BROTH)

This hearty potato soup is a version of my mom's special recipe. After years of looking forward to having it when I visited home (and begging for the leftovers), I finally had her write it down for me. It's now our favorite soup to make in bulk because it stores great in the freezer, making busy nights a breeze.

Makes 8 to 10 servings

Prep time: 30 minutes (not including broth), plus more to soak the cashews

Cooking time: 30 minutes

1 cup raw cashews
Filtered water
8¼ cups Homemade Bone Broth (page 222)
1 tablespoon coconut oil or ghee
1 medium sweet onion, diced
4 garlic cloves, minced
¾ cup chopped white mushrooms
1 orange or red bell pepper, diced
2 carrots, finely diced
2 celery stalks, finely diced
Pinch of sea salt
Pinch of freshly ground black pepper
1 medium sweet potato, peeled and chopped
½ pound small white potatoes, chopped
1 (14.5-ounce) can diced tomatoes, with their juices

Spices

1 tablespoon paprika
1 teaspoon dried oregano
½ teaspoon dried basil
½ teaspoon onion powder
½ teaspoon sea salt
½ teaspoon freshly ground black pepper
¼ teaspoon cayenne pepper
⅛ teaspoon freshly ground white pepper

1. Place the cashews in a bowl and cover with filtered water. Soak for at least 2 hours and up to 12 hours. Drain the cashews and rinse well.

2. Place the cashews in a high-speed blender with 1¼ cups of the broth and blend until very smooth, 45 to 60 seconds (or longer, if you're not using a high-speed blender). Set the cashew cream aside.

3. In a large soup pot, melt the coconut oil over medium heat. Add the onion and garlic and cook until just soft, 3 to 4 minutes.

4. Add the mushrooms, bell pepper, carrots, celery, salt, and black pepper and cook until the vegetables start to soften, 4 to 5 minutes. Add the sweet potato, white potatoes, tomatoes with their juices, remaining 7 cups broth, cashew cream, and spices. Bring the soup to a boil, then reduce the heat to maintain a simmer and cook uncovered until the vegetables are soft, about 20 minutes.

5. Ladle the soup into bowls and serve warm. Store leftovers in airtight containers in the refrigerator for up to 4 days or in the freezer for up to 3 months.

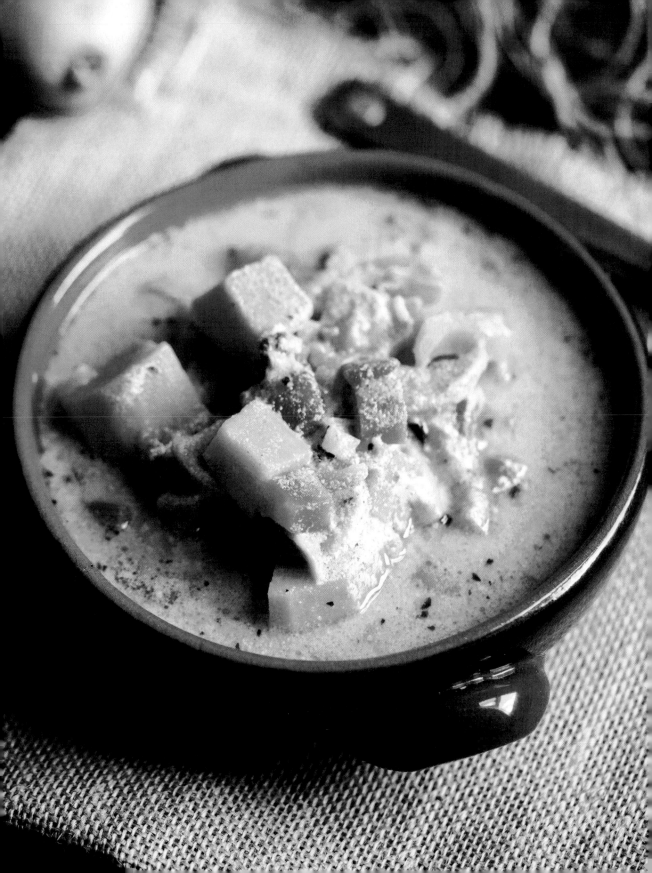

Baked Ratatouille

EGG-FREE, NUT-FREE, VEGETARIAN

When I made ratatouille for the first time, I was pleasantly surprised at how easy it was to prepare. It's a great dish to serve during the summer when vegetables are plentiful and flavorful, and according to my husband, it tastes just like pizza without the dough. I think that means it's a winner.

1. Preheat the oven to 375°F.

2. Spread 1 cup of the marinara sauce over the bottom of a 6 x 9-inch baking dish (or similar-size dish). Sprinkle the onion over the marinara sauce.

3. Using a mandoline slicer or sharp knife, slice the eggplant, zucchini, squash, and tomatoes crosswise about ¾ inch thick, making the slices as uniform as possible. Arrange the vegetables sideways in rows in an alternating pattern (1 slice eggplant, zucchini, squash, tomato, and repeat) on top of the onion. Fit in as many slices as possible. Pour the remaining ½ cup marinara sauce over the vegetables.

4. In a small bowl, whisk together the olive oil, garlic, basil, oregano, and red pepper flakes. Spoon the mixture evenly over the vegetables.

5. Sprinkle the vegetables with the salt and black pepper and cover the dish with foil. Bake for 30 minutes, remove the foil, and bake for 15 minutes more, until the sauce is bubbling and the vegetables are cooked through. Serve warm.

Makes 3 servings
Prep time: **20 minutes**
Cooking time: **45 minutes**

1½ cups marinara sauce
½ medium onion, sliced
1 small eggplant, such as Japanese or Italian
1 medium zucchini (see tip)
1 medium yellow squash (see tip)
3 Roma (plum) tomatoes
3 tablespoons extra-virgin olive oil
1 garlic clove, minced
1 tablespoon chopped fresh basil
½ teaspoon dried oregano
⅛ teaspoon red pepper flakes
Pinch of sea salt
Pinch of freshly ground black pepper

Noelle's tip: Because vegetable sizes can vary, especially when purchased from the farmers' market, I recommend having another zucchini or squash on hand in case you have extra space in your baking dish.

Change it up: Use an oval baking dish or deep pie dish about 10 inches in diameter. Depending on the dish you use, you can get creative with how you stack the vegetables.

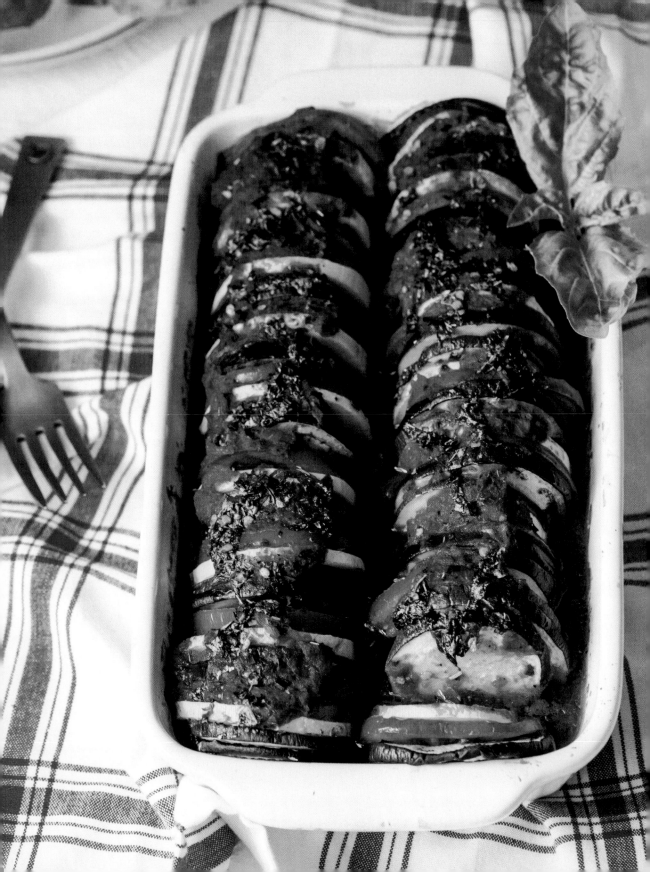

Apple-Chicken Skillet

EGG-FREE, NIGHTSHADE-FREE, NUT-FREE

After I made this dish for the first time, it instantly became one of our regular meals. The combination of apples, onion, and spices makes the chicken super flavorful, and cooking it all up in one skillet makes cleanup incredibly easy.

Makes 4 servings

Prep time: **10 minutes (not including broth)**

Cooking time: **less than 30 minutes**

1. In a large skillet, melt 1 tablespoon of the coconut oil over medium-high heat. Season the chicken breasts with the salt and pepper and sear until golden brown on both sides, about 3 minutes per side. Remove the chicken from the skillet and set aside.

2. Melt the remaining 1 tablespoon coconut oil in the skillet. Add the apples, onion, thyme, garlic powder, and allspice and cook until the apples and onion are just soft, 5 to 6 minutes.

3. Return the chicken breasts to the skillet and nestle them into the apples and onion. Add the broth and vinegar and stir gently to incorporate. Bring the mixture to a boil, then reduce the heat to maintain a simmer and cover the skillet. Cook until the chicken is cooked through, 10 to 15 minutes, depending on thickness.

4. To serve, place each chicken breast on a plate and spoon the apples and onion on top.

2 tablespoons coconut oil or ghee

4 boneless, skinless chicken breasts

½ teaspoon sea salt

½ teaspoon freshly ground black pepper

2 large sweet apples, such as Pink Lady or Fuji, cored and sliced

1 sweet onion, chopped

1 teaspoon dried thyme

½ teaspoon garlic powder

¼ teaspoon ground allspice

1 cup Homemade Bone Broth (page 222)

1 tablespoon apple cider vinegar

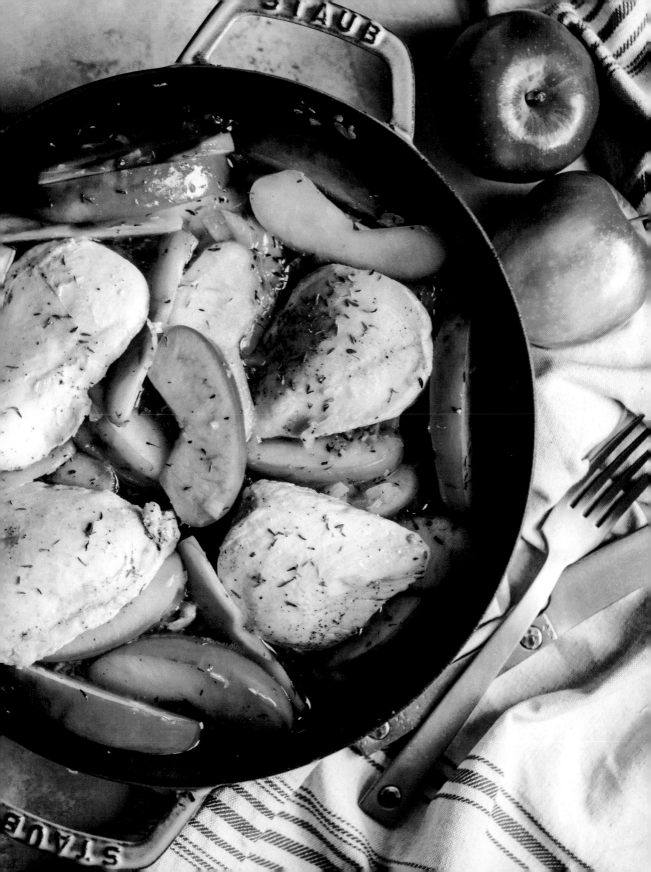

Baked Sriracha Chicken Wings

EGG-FREE, NUT-FREE

These oven-baked chicken wings are the perfect combination of spicy and sweet. By boiling the chicken wings prior to roasting them, they end up tender on the inside and nice and crispy on the outside.

Makes 3 or 4 servings
Prep time: **10 minutes**
Cooking time: **50 minutes**

1. Preheat the oven to 450°F. Line a baking sheet with parchment paper or aluminum foil.

2. Bring a large pot of water to a boil and add the salt. Add the chicken wings and boil for 10 minutes. Drain the wings and pat them dry. The drier they are, the better they will crisp up.

3. Arrange the wings in a single layer on the prepared baking sheet. Roast for 35 to 40 minutes, flipping once halfway through to crisp them evenly.

4. While the wings are roasting, combine all the sauce ingredients in a small saucepan over medium heat. Warm the sauce through, stirring to combine, then set the pan aside off the heat.

5. Transfer the wings to a large bowl. Pour the sauce over the wings and toss until coated evenly. Serve warm.

½ teaspoon sea salt
2 pounds chicken wing
   sections (see tip)

Sauce

¼ cup coconut oil or ghee
3 tablespoons sriracha sauce
2 tablespoons raw honey
1 tablespoon coconut aminos
Juice of ½ lime
½ teaspoon garlic powder

Noelle's tip: If starting with whole wing sections that have to be cut, save the wing tips and throw them in the freezer to use the next time you make Homemade Bone Broth (page 222).

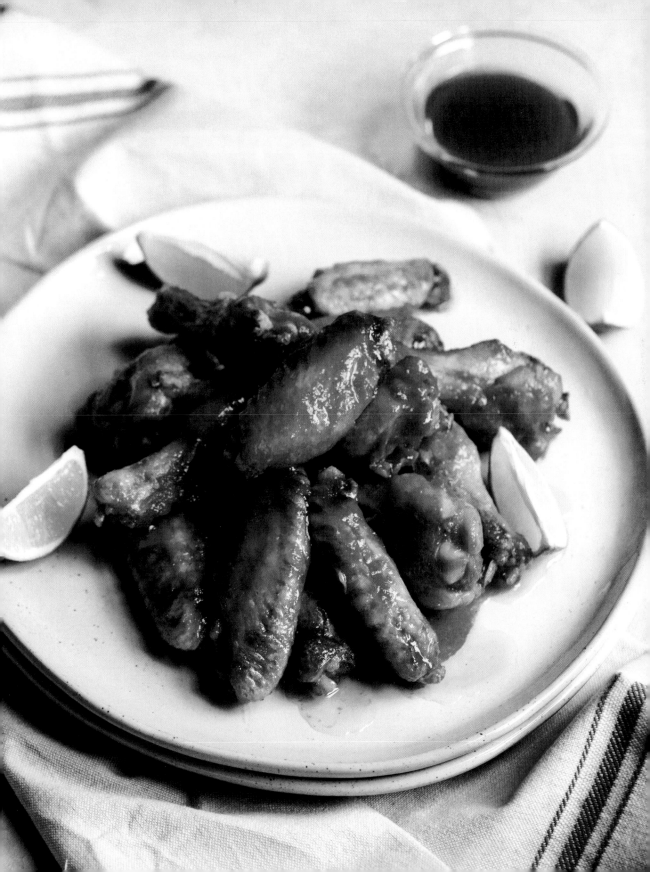

Slow Cooker Chicken

EGG-FREE, NUT-FREE

Out of all the appliances in my kitchen, my slow cooker sees the most action because of recipes like this one. I throw everything together in the morning while making coffee, and have a nice warm meal (with leftovers!) waiting for me at dinnertime.

1. Scatter the onion, carrots, and potatoes in a 6-quart (or larger) slow cooker.

2. In a small bowl, combine all the spices for the spice rub. Rub the mixture all over the chicken, including inside the cavity.

3. Place the chicken on top of the vegetables in the slow cooker, breast side down. Cover and cook on Low for 7 to 8 hours, or until the chicken is cooked through and tender.

4. To make the skin slightly crispy, preheat the broiler about 10 minutes before the chicken is ready to come out of the slow cooker. Transfer the whole chicken to a glass baking dish and finish it under the broiler, about 5 minutes.

5. Place the chicken on a cutting board and let it rest for 10 minutes. To serve, cut it up into serving pieces or debone the chicken and shred the meat. Serve with the vegetables.

Makes 6 servings
Prep time: 15 minutes
Cooking time: 7 to 8 hours

1 medium onion, sliced into thick wedges
3 carrots, sliced lengthwise and cut into 2-inch pieces
4 or 5 medium red potatoes, quartered
1 large (4-pound) whole chicken, giblets removed

Spice rub

1 teaspoon smoked paprika
1 teaspoon paprika
1 teaspoon dried oregano
1 teaspoon sea salt
1 teaspoon dried thyme
½ teaspoon ground sage
½ teaspoon garlic powder
½ teaspoon freshly ground black pepper
¼ teaspoon ground turmeric

Noelle's tip: To make this even easier, you can eliminate the chopped veggies and simply place the spice-rubbed chicken in the slow cooker for the same amount of time. Nothing else needed!

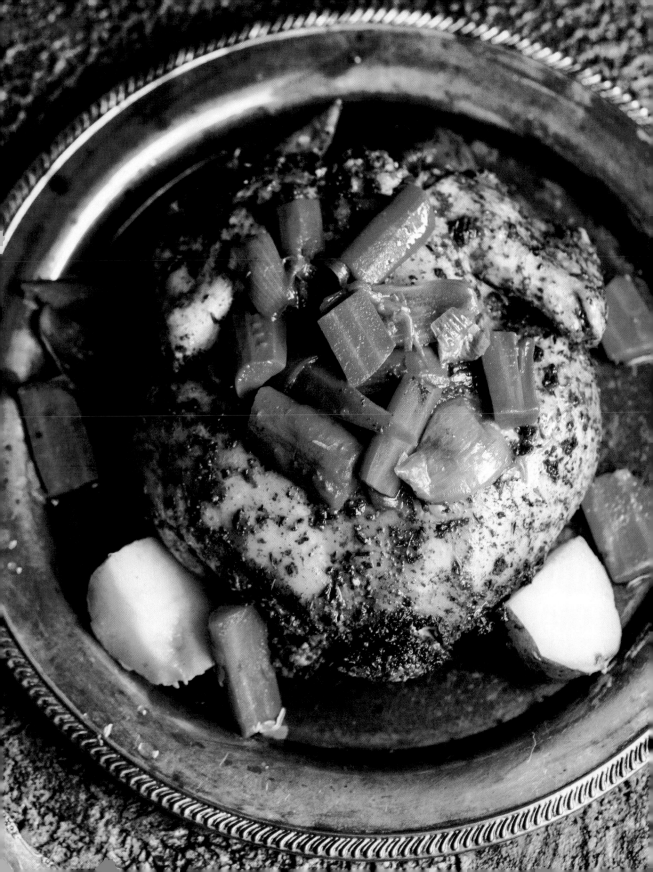

Chicken-Sage Meatballs

NIGHTSHADE-FREE

This dish is one of my favorite weeknight meals to make. The meatballs are not only super flavorful, they're also easy to cook in bulk and store well in the freezer, giving you more bang for your dinner-making buck.

Makes about 6 servings (around thirty-two 1½-inch meatballs)

Prep time: **15 minutes**

Cooking time: **20 minutes**

1. Preheat the oven to 400°F. Line a baking sheet with parchment paper or aluminum foil.
2. In a large skillet, melt the coconut oil over medium heat. Add the onion and cook until soft, 4 to 5 minutes. Remove the onion from the skillet and let it cool.
3. In a large bowl, combine the onion, chicken, egg, almond flour, sage, parsley, garlic powder, salt, and pepper. Form the mixture into about thirty-two 1½-inch balls (1.2 ounces each) and place them on the prepared baking sheet.
4. Bake for 18 to 20 minutes, or until fully cooked inside.

1½ teaspoons coconut oil or ghee
½ medium sweet onion, diced
2 pounds ground chicken
1 large egg, lightly beaten
¼ cup almond flour
1½ teaspoons ground sage
1 teaspoon dried parsley
1 teaspoon garlic powder
½ teaspoon sea salt
½ teaspoon freshly ground black pepper

Serve it with: Creamy Mashed Cauliflower (page 157)

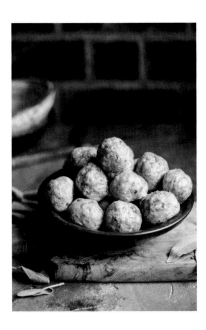

Bacon-Guacamole Chicken Rolls

EGG-FREE, NUT-FREE

This dish was one of the first meals I ever experimented with on my own in the kitchen. My then boyfriend (now husband) was on a seven-month deployment, and I wanted to have some recipes under my belt that would blow him away when he came home. In short, this recipe totally nailed it.

Makes 4 servings
(2 rolls per serving)
Prep time: 15 minutes
(not including guacamole)
Cooking time: 35 minutes

1. Preheat the oven to 400°F. Line a baking sheet with parchment paper or aluminum foil.

2. Slice each chicken breast horizontally through the center, to create two thin breasts.

3. Season the meat with the salt and pepper. Lay each breast flat and spread about 1 tablespoon of the guacamole on top. Roll up each breast with the guacamole inside, secure each roll with a toothpick, and place the rolls on the prepared baking sheet.

4. Wrap 1 piece of bacon around each roll, using the toothpick as an anchor for the ends.

5. Bake for 30 to 35 minutes, depending on the thickness of the rolls, until the chicken is cooked through. Remove the toothpicks before serving.

4 boneless, skinless chicken breasts
¼ teaspoon sea salt
¼ teaspoon freshly ground black pepper
½ cup Everyone's Favorite Guacamole (page 184; see tip)
8 bacon slices

Noelle's tip: Use your favorite store-bought fresh guacamole to make this dish quick and easy.

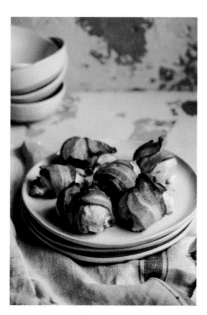

Cilantro-Lime Turkey Burgers

EGG-FREE (WITHOUT MAYO), NUT-FREE

Yes, it is possible for turkey burgers to be full of flavor and downright delicious. The combination of cilantro, lime, and spices makes these burgers irresistible, especially when topped with guacamole. (Because, obviously.)

1. In a large bowl, combine the turkey, onion, cilantro, lime juice, cumin, chili powder, garlic powder, and pepper. Form the mixture into 4 equal-size patties.

2. In a large skillet, melt the coconut oil over medium heat. Season both sides of the patties with salt and cook them until the center is no longer pink and the juices run clear, 5 to 6 minutes per side.

3. Serve the burgers warm, wrapped in crispy lettuce leaves and topped with your favorite toppings.

Makes 4 servings

Prep time: **10 minutes (not including guacamole or mayo)**

Cooking time: **12 minutes**

1 pound ground turkey
¼ cup diced onion
¼ cup fresh cilantro, finely chopped
Juice of ½ lime
1 teaspoon ground cumin
½ teaspoon chili powder
¼ teaspoon garlic powder
¼ teaspoon freshly ground black pepper
1 tablespoon coconut oil or ghee
Sea salt
Lettuce leaves, for serving

Toppings

Sliced tomato
Sliced red onion
Everyone's Favorite Guacamole (page 184) or Simple Homemade Mayonnaise (page 188; optional)

Change it up: Use ground chicken instead of turkey.

Serve it with: Parsnip and Carrot Fries (page 160)

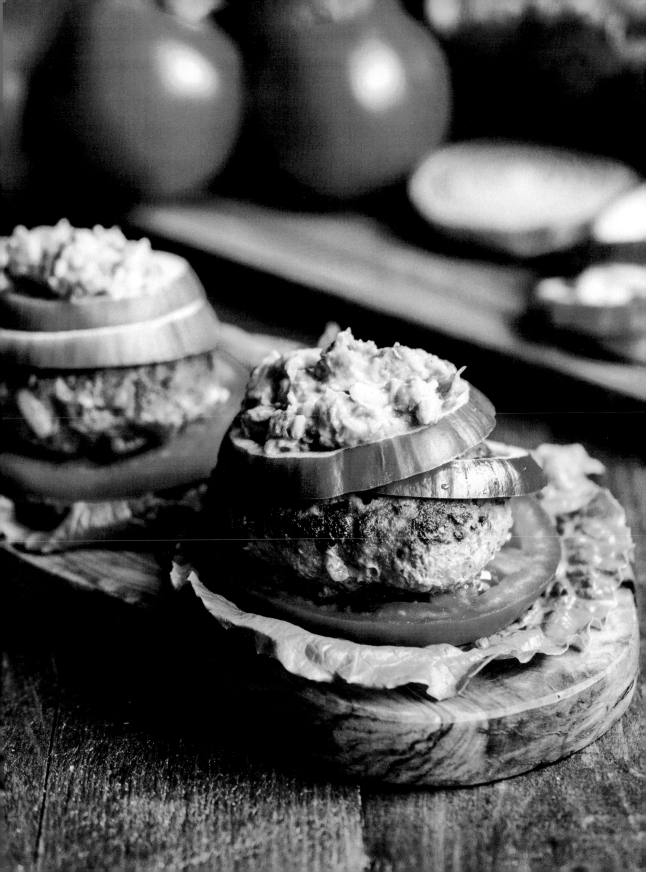

Classic Italian Turkey Meatballs

Whenever I make this recipe, my husband somehow instantly develops an Italian accent. It must be the delicious combination of olive oil, tomatoes, and fresh basil, which makes us all temporarily a little Italian.

Makes 3 or 4 servings (about eighteen 1½-inch meatballs)

Prep time: **10 minutes**

Cooking time: **less than 25 minutes**

1. Preheat the oven to 400°F. Line a baking sheet with parchment paper or aluminum foil.

2. In a large bowl, combine all the ingredients for the meatballs. Form the mixture into about eighteen 1½-inch balls (1.2 ounces each) and place them on the prepared baking sheet. Bake for 15 minutes, or until fully cooked inside.

3. Meanwhile, to make the tomato sauce, heat the olive oil in a large, deep skillet over medium heat. Add the onion, garlic, salt, and pepper and cook until the vegetables are just soft, 3 to 4 minutes.

4. Add the tomatoes and oregano and stir. Bring the sauce to a boil, then reduce the heat to maintain a simmer and cook until the sauce thickens slightly, 12 to 15 minutes. Stir in the basil.

5. Nestle the meatballs into the sauce and simmer until heated through, 2 to 3 minutes. Serve warm.

Meatballs

1 pound ground turkey
1 large egg, lightly beaten
2 tablespoons almond flour
¼ cup chopped onion
1 tablespoon tomato paste
2 tablespoons chopped fresh parsley
1 tablespoon chopped fresh basil
1 garlic clove, minced
½ teaspoon sea salt
¼ teaspoon freshly ground black pepper

Tomato sauce

2 tablespoons extra-virgin olive oil
½ medium onion, finely chopped
2 garlic cloves, minced
½ teaspoon sea salt
¼ teaspoon freshly ground black pepper
1 (28-ounce) can crushed tomatoes
1 teaspoon dried oregano
¼ cup chopped fresh basil

Change it up: If you're short on time, use a store-bought tomato-basil sauce instead of making it yourself.

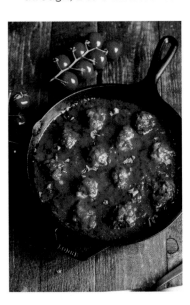

Bacon-Liver Meatballs

EGG-FREE, NUT-FREE

If liver isn't at the top of your favorite foods list, these meatballs just might make you a fan. They have a hint of liver's richness, making them a great (and sneaky) way to incorporate organ meats into your diet.

Makes 3 or 4 servings (eighteen 1½-inch meatballs)

Prep time: 10 minutes

Cooking time: 25 minutes

1. Preheat the oven to 400°F. Line a baking sheet with parchment paper or aluminum foil.

2. In a medium skillet, melt the coconut oil over medium heat. Add the bacon and cook until just crisp, 4 to 5 minutes. Set the bacon aside on a paper towel to cool.

3. In a large bowl, use a silicone spatula or large spoon to fold together the bacon, ground beef, liver, onion, thyme, paprika, oregano, garlic, salt, and pepper. When the mixture starts to come together, continue to mix it with your hands until well combined.

4. Form the mixture into about eighteen 1½-inch balls (1.2 ounces each) and place them on the prepared baking sheet.

5. Bake for 15 to 20 minutes, or until fully cooked inside. Serve warm.

1½ teaspoons coconut oil or ghee
4 bacon slices, finely diced
1 pound ground beef
4 ounces beef liver, finely chopped
½ small onion, diced
1 teaspoon dried thyme
1 teaspoon paprika
½ teaspoon dried oregano
2 garlic cloves, minced
½ teaspoon sea salt
¼ teaspoon freshly ground black pepper

Noelle's tip: To make these easier to prepare, break down the beef liver in a food processor until mushy, then combine it with the rest of the ingredients.

Serve it with: Creamy Mashed Cauliflower (page 157)

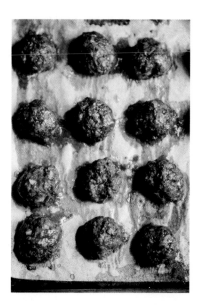

Asian Beef Stir-Fry

EGG-FREE, NUT-FREE

With this quick and simple stir-fry, the secret's in the sauce. It creates a savory glaze that coats the meat and vegetables and melds all the flavors together in the pan.

1. To make the stir-fry, freeze the steak for 20 to 30 minutes. Trim the excess fat away and cut the steak across the grain into very thin slices, ¼ to ½ inch thick.

2. In a large skillet, melt 2 tablespoons of the coconut oil over medium-high heat. When the oil is hot, add the steak slices and cook until browned, 1 to 2 minutes on each side. Cook the beef in two batches, if needed, to avoid crowding the pan. Remove the steak and set aside.

3. Reduce the heat to medium and add the remaining 1 tablespoon coconut oil to the skillet. Add the mushrooms, zucchini, bell pepper, onion, parsley, and salt and cook, stirring, until the vegetables are just tender, 5 to 6 minutes.

4. Meanwhile, to make the sauce, in a medium bowl, whisk together all the sauce ingredients.

5. Return the beef to the skillet and pour the sauce over the meat and vegetables. Stir and cook until the meat is heated through, 2 to 3 minutes.

6. Transfer to a serving platter and garnish with the scallions and sesame seeds. Serve warm.

Makes 3 or 4 servings

Prep time: 20 minutes, plus 30 minutes chilling time

Cooking time: less than 15 minutes

Stir-fry

1½ pounds sirloin steak (see tip)
3 tablespoons coconut oil or ghee
10 ounces white mushrooms, sliced
1 small zucchini, halved crosswise and sliced into ¼-inch-thick strips
1 red bell pepper, sliced into ¼-inch-thick strips
½ medium onion, sliced
½ teaspoon dried parsley
Pinch of sea salt

Sauce

½ cup coconut aminos
3 garlic cloves, minced
1 tablespoon raw honey
1 tablespoon pure toasted sesame oil
1 teaspoon sriracha sauce
¼ teaspoon ground ginger

2 scallions, chopped, for garnish
2 teaspoons sesame seeds, for garnish

Noelle's tip: When cutting the steak, don't stress over making the slices perfectly uniform and even. Smaller slices and steak "pieces" can all be included in the stir-fry.

Change it up: Use top sirloin or flank steak instead of sirloin steak, or swap out the beef for chicken.

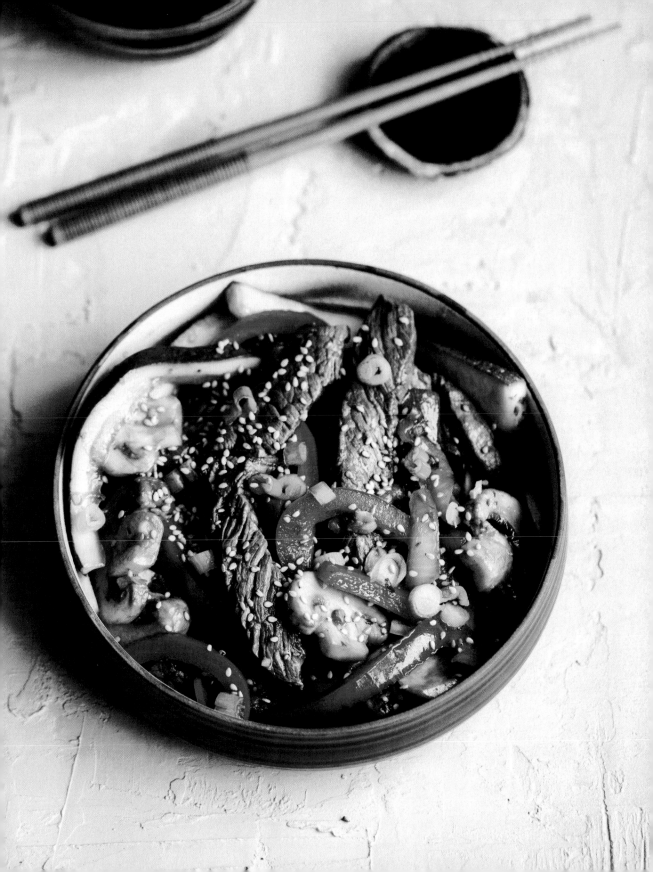

Zucchini-Beef Taco Skillet

EGG-FREE, NUT-FREE

Long live Taco Tuesday! This dish combines all the fresh-ness and flavors of tacos with the special addition of zuc-chini. Not only is it incredibly delicious, it's also super easy to cook up and can be served straight out of the skillet.

1. To make the taco seasoning, in a small airtight container, combine all the seasoning ingredients. Set aside 1 table-spoon for the taco skillet and store the rest in a cool, dark place for another use.

2. In a large skillet, melt the coconut oil over medium heat. Add the onion and cook until just soft, 3 to 4 minutes. Add the ground beef and taco seasoning, stirring to break up and crumble the meat as it cooks. Cook until the beef is lightly browned.

3. Add the bell pepper and zucchini and cook until the veg-etables are cooked but still firm, 5 to 6 minutes. Add the to-mato and stir. Cover the skillet and cook for 2 to 3 minutes more.

4. Remove the skillet from the heat and garnish with the ci-lantro and avocado. Serve straight from the skillet, in crispy lettuce leaves.

Makes 3 or 4 servings
Prep time: 15 minutes
Cooking time: 25 minutes

Taco seasoning

2 tablespoons chili powder
1 tablespoon ground cumin
2 teaspoons paprika
1½ teaspoons sea salt
1 teaspoon dried oregano
1 teaspoon garlic powder
1 teaspoon onion powder
½ teaspoon freshly ground black pepper

Taco skillet

1 tablespoon coconut oil or ghee
1 small sweet onion, diced
1 pound ground beef
1 bell pepper, diced
1 small zucchini, diced
1 medium tomato, diced
2 teaspoons chopped fresh cilantro, for garnish
¼ avocado, diced, for garnish
Lettuce leaves, for serving

Noelle's tip: Many companies are now making grain-free coconut and cassava flour tortillas, which are another great way to serve up this dish. Check the fridge section at your local specialty grocery store to see if they're available.

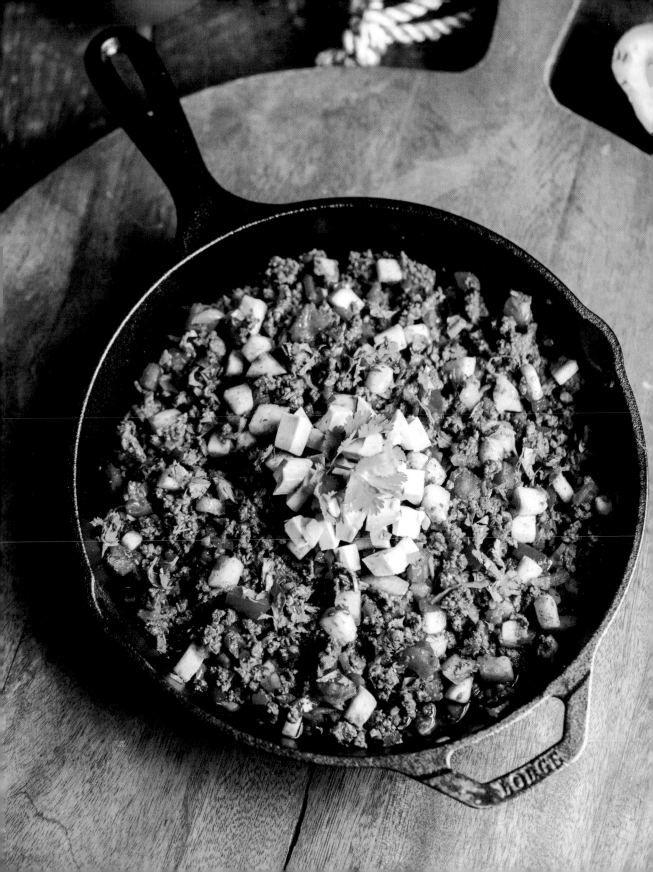

Slow Cooker Garlic-Thyme Pot Roast

EGG-FREE, NUT-FREE

Want to come home to a pot full of fork-tender meat that melts in your mouth? With the slow cooker, it's as easy as hitting the "on" button.

Makes 6 to 8 servings

Prep time: 15 minutes (not including broth)

Cooking time: 8 hours

1. In a large skillet, melt the coconut oil over medium-high heat. Season the roast with the salt and pepper, using more salt as needed if the roast is large, and brown it on all sides in the skillet, 6 to 8 minutes.

2. Place the roast in a 6-quart (or larger) slow cooker. Season the roast evenly on all sides with the garlic, thyme, paprika, and oregano. Arrange the potatoes and carrots around the roast and add the broth.

3. Cover the slow cooker and cook on Low for 8 hours.

4. Transfer the roast to a cutting board and let it rest for 5 to 10 minutes. Slice the roast across the grain and arrange it on a platter with the vegetables. Garnish with a few tablespoons of the juices from the slow cooker and serve.

1½ tablespoons coconut oil or ghee
1 (3- to 4-pound) chuck roast
1 teaspoon sea salt, or more as needed
½ teaspoon freshly ground black pepper
4 garlic cloves, minced
2 teaspoons dried thyme
1 teaspoon paprika
½ teaspoon dried oregano
4 or 5 medium red potatoes, quartered
2 or 3 carrots, unpeeled, sliced lengthwise and cut into 2-inch pieces
1 cup Homemade Bone Broth (page 222)

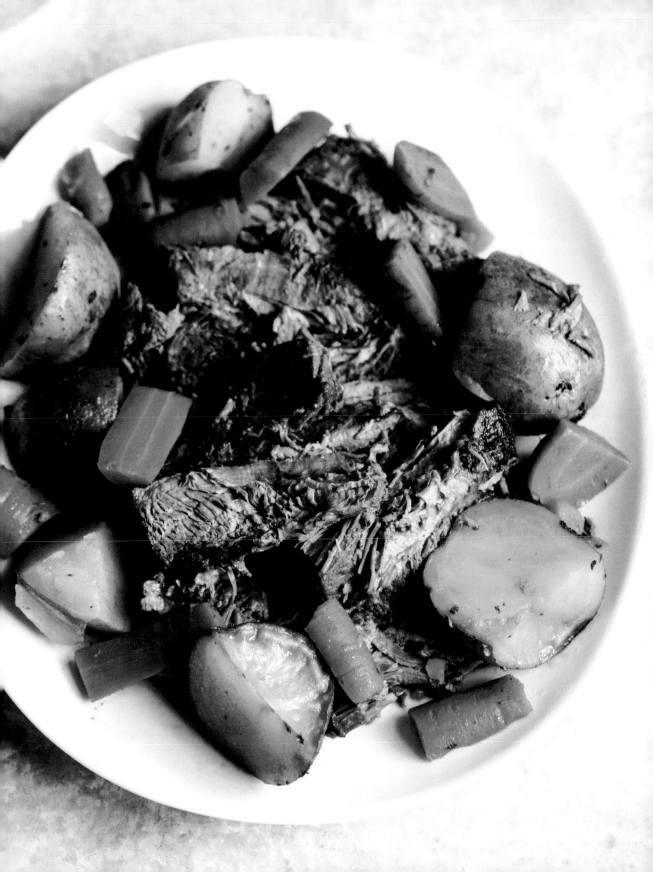

Shepherd's Pie

EGG-FREE, NUT-FREE

Japanese sweet potatoes have purple/reddish skin and creamy white flesh. They're more starchy and denser than traditional sweet potatoes, which makes this pie hearty and irresistible.

1. Place the potatoes in a medium saucepan and cover with cool water. Bring the water to a boil over medium-high heat, reduce the heat to maintain a simmer, and cook the potatoes until fork-tender, 10 to 12 minutes. Drain the potatoes and transfer to a large bowl or the bowl of a stand mixer fitted with the paddle attachment.

2. Whip the potatoes with a handheld mixer or with the stand mixer on medium-low speed until smooth, 1 to 2 minutes. With the mixer running, add the coconut milk, coconut oil, salt, and pepper and whip until combined. Set aside.

3. Preheat the oven to 375°F.

4. In a 10-inch cast-iron skillet, melt the coconut oil over medium heat. Add the bacon and cook until just crisp, 4 to 5 minutes. Set the bacon aside on a paper towel to cool.

5. Place the celery, carrots, onion, and mushrooms in the skillet and cook until the vegetables are soft, 5 to 7 minutes. Add the ground beef, paprika, salt, thyme, garlic powder, and pepper, stirring to break up and crumble the meat as it cooks. Cook until the beef is lightly browned, 7 to 8 minutes.

6. Stir in the broth and tomato paste and press the mixture down with a spatula to spread it evenly over the skillet. Cook until the liquid has reduced slightly, about 5 minutes. Remove the skillet from the heat.

7. Fold two-thirds of the bacon into the whipped potatoes. Top the meat with spoonfuls of the potatoes and gently spread the potatoes to cover the meat.

8. Sprinkle the pie with the remaining bacon and place the skillet on a baking sheet to catch any drips. Bake for 20 to 25 minutes, until the potatoes are lightly golden brown.

9. Spoon the pie directly out of the skillet to serve.

Makes 6 servings

Prep time: **25 minutes (not including broth)**

Cooking time: **50 minutes**

Potatoes

2 large Japanese sweet potatoes, peeled and cut into large chunks
2 tablespoons canned full-fat coconut milk
1 tablespoon coconut oil
¼ teaspoon sea salt
⅛ teaspoon freshly ground black pepper

Meat filling

1½ teaspoons coconut oil or ghee
4 bacon slices, finely diced
2 celery stalks, chopped
2 carrots, chopped
½ medium onion, diced
½ cup chopped white mushrooms
1½ pounds ground beef or lamb
1 teaspoon paprika
1 teaspoon sea salt
½ teaspoon dried thyme
¼ teaspoon garlic powder
¼ teaspoon freshly ground black pepper
¾ cup Homemade Bone Broth (page 222)
2 tablespoons tomato paste

Prep ahead: Double the recipe for the potatoes and make them a day or two ahead of time as a side dish for another meal. Store the extra in an airtight container in the refrigerator until ready to use.

Change it up: To reduce the cooking time, eliminate the bacon and simply cook the vegetables in coconut oil or ghee.

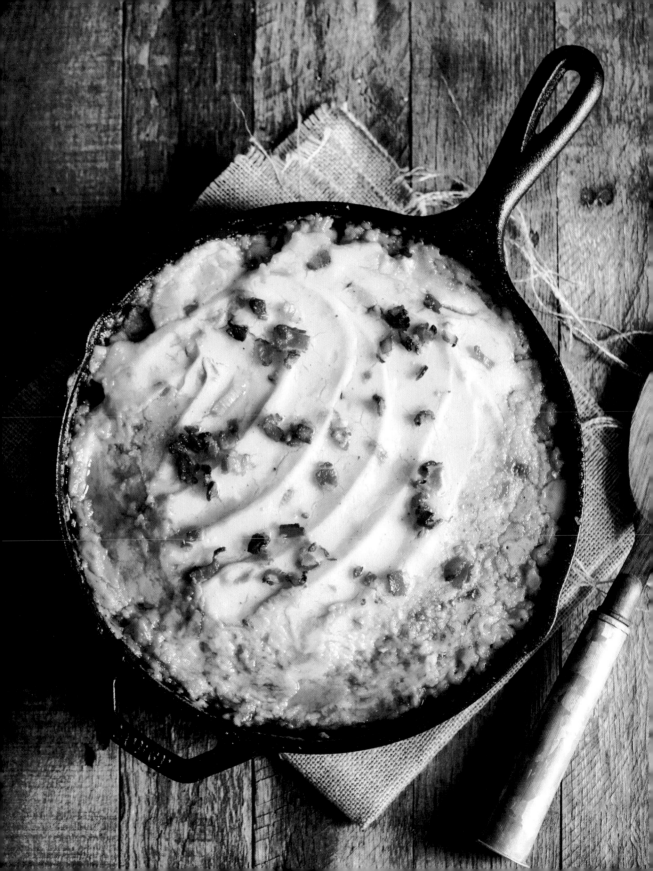

Grilled Balsamic Flank Steak

EGG-FREE, NIGHTSHADE-FREE, NUT-FREE

This recipe's quick and simple balsamic marinade ensures you'll get tender, juicy flank steak every time. For mouth-watering texture, make sure your grill is nice and hot, which will quickly sear the steak on the outside without overcooking the inside.

Makes 4 to 6 servings
Prep time: **5 minutes, plus 4 to 6 hours marinating time**
Cooking time: **10 minutes**

⅓ cup balsamic vinegar
¼ cup extra-virgin olive oil
2 garlic cloves, minced
1 tablespoon chopped fresh basil
1 teaspoon dried thyme
1 (1½- to 2-pound) flank steak
Sea salt and freshly ground black pepper

Serve it with: Lemon-Garlic Roasted Broccoli (page 163)

Change it up: Swap out the basil for fresh parsley or oregano.

1. In a medium bowl, whisk together the vinegar, olive oil, garlic, basil, and thyme. Place the steak in a glass or ceramic baking dish and pour the marinade over the top, making sure to coat both sides. Cover and marinate the steak in the refrigerator for 4 to 6 hours.

2. Preheat a grill to medium-high heat.

3. Remove the steak from the marinade and gently shake off the excess. Season both sides of the steak with salt and pepper and place it on the grill. Grill to your desired doneness, 4 to 5 minutes on each side for medium-rare, depending on thickness.

4. Transfer the steak to a cutting board, cover it with aluminum foil, and let it rest for 5 to 10 minutes. Slice thinly across the grain and serve.

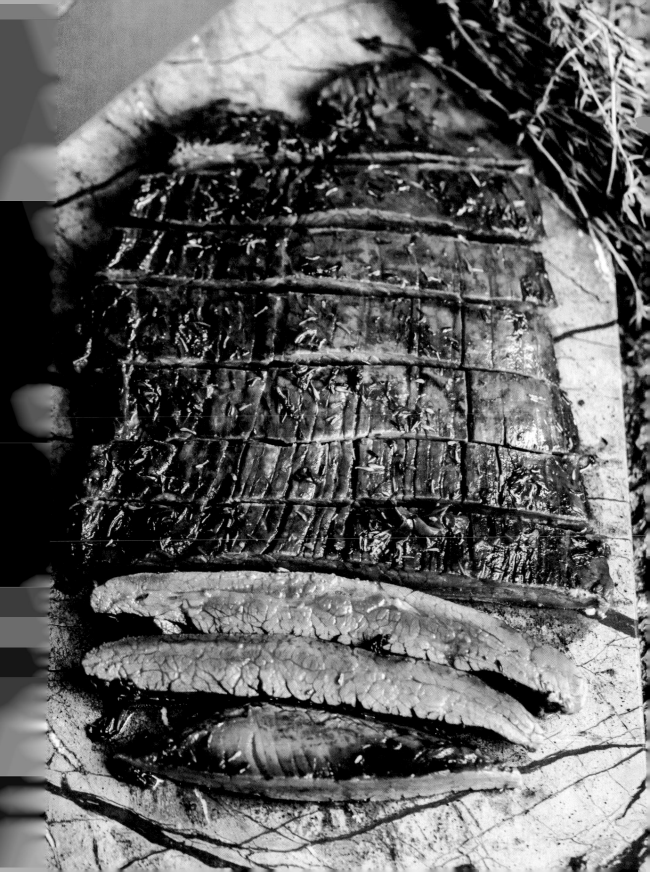

Homemade Bone Broth

EGG-FREE, NIGHTSHADE-FREE, NUT-FREE

Homemade bone broth, also known as liquid gold, is great to cook in bulk and stash in the freezer. You can sip it on its own or use it in soups or stews. While roasting the bones may seem like an unnecessary step, don't skip it. Doing so gives the broth a much heartier flavor, which will enhance any recipe it's used in.

Makes about 10 cups
Prep time: 10 minutes
Cooking time: 24 hours

3 to 4 pounds mixed beef
 bones (see tip)
1 onion, quartered
5 garlic cloves, minced
1 teaspoon whole black
 peppercorns
1 teaspoon sea salt
2 bay leaves (optional)
Filtered water
2 tablespoons apple cider
 vinegar

1. Preheat the oven to 425°F.

2. Place the bones in a single layer on a baking sheet or roasting pan. Roast for 40 minutes, flipping the bones once halfway through to brown them evenly.

3. Place the bones, onion, garlic, peppercorns, salt, and bay leaves (if using) in a 6-quart (or larger) slow cooker. Add 10 to 12 cups filtered water, enough to cover the bones but no higher than 1 inch from the top of the slow cooker insert. Add the vinegar.

4. Cover the slow cooker and cook on Low for at least 12 hours and up to 24 hours.

5. When the broth has cooled slightly, strain it through a fine-mesh strainer into a large heat-safe bowl and let cool. Discard the solids.

6. When the broth is cool enough, pour it into smaller jars for storing. Store in the refrigerator for up to 5 days or in the freezer for up to a year.

Noelle's tip: To get the most out of your broth, use a combination of meaty bones, like soup or marrow bones, and bones with more cartilage, such as oxtails or knuckle bones. The best place to get grass-fed bones is from local farms, which will have a variety of bones for relatively cheap.

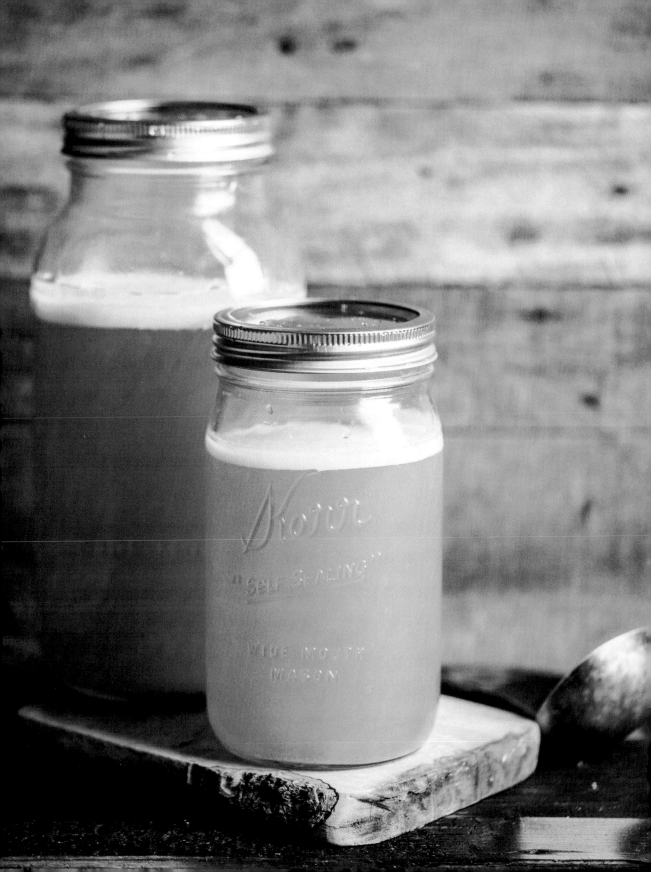

Sweet Potato Chipotle Bison Sliders

EGG-FREE, NUT-FREE

You could have a burger, or you could have perfectly sized chipotle bison burgers sandwiched between two thick-cut roasted sweet potato rounds and topped with avocado slices. To make this your own, add your favorite ingredients to the stack, such as onions, crispy bacon, or a fried egg.

1. To prepare the sweet potatoes, preheat the oven to 400°F. Line a baking sheet with parchment paper or aluminum foil.

2. Slice the potatoes crosswise into ½-inch-thick rounds (you will need 12 fairly even-size rounds). In a large bowl, toss the sweet potatoes with the coconut oil until well coated. Arrange the potatoes in a single layer on the prepared baking sheet and season both sides with the salt and pepper. Roast for 25 to 30 minutes, or until lightly golden brown and tender, flipping the rounds once halfway through to ensure even cooking. Set aside.

3. Meanwhile, to make the burgers, in a medium bowl, combine the bison, chipotle, cumin, garlic powder, and pepper. Form the mixture into 6 patties.

4. In a large skillet, melt the coconut oil over medium heat. Season both sides of the patties with salt and cook until browned and to your desired doneness, 4 to 5 minutes on each side for medium. Remove the patties from the skillet.

5. Assemble the burger stacks by topping a sweet potato slice with arugula, 1 tomato slice, 1 bison burger, avocado, and another sweet potato slice. Secure with a wooden skewer and serve.

Makes 3 servings (2 sliders each)

Prep time: **15 minutes**

Cooking time: **30 minutes**

Sweet potato rounds

2 large sweet potatoes
1½ tablespoons coconut oil, melted
½ teaspoon sea salt
¼ teaspoon freshly ground black pepper

Burgers

1 pound ground bison
½ teaspoon ground chipotle chile
¼ teaspoon ground cumin
¼ teaspoon garlic powder
¼ teaspoon freshly ground black pepper
1 tablespoon coconut oil
Sea salt

Toppings

Handful of baby arugula
1 medium tomato, cut into 6 slices
1 avocado, thinly sliced

Special equipment: 4-inch wooden skewers

Change it up: Use ground beef instead of bison.

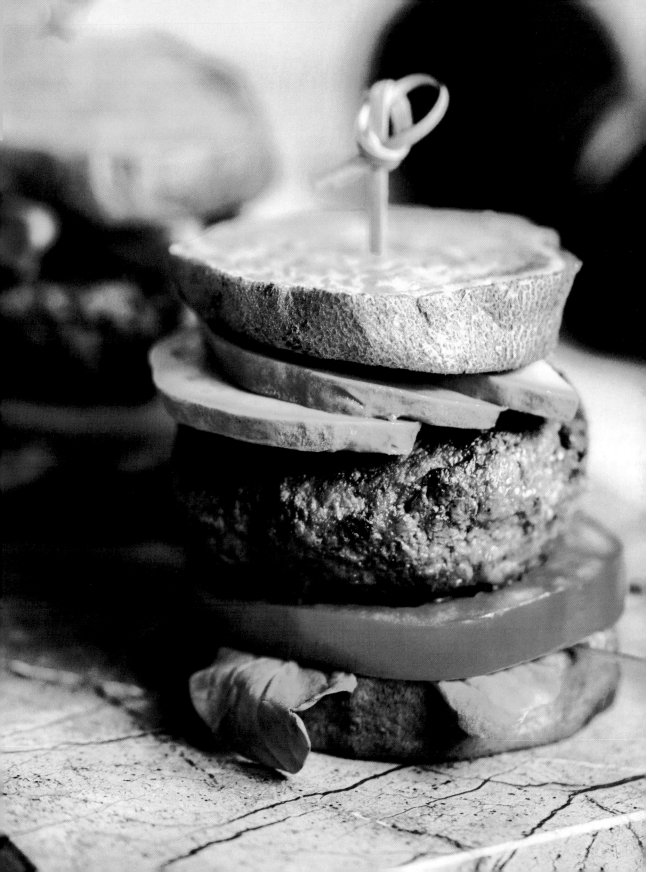

Slow Cooker Bison Chili

EGG-FREE, NUT-FREE

This chili is the ultimate "set it and forget it" recipe. Simply throw all the ingredients into the slow cooker in the morning, and by dinnertime you'll have a warm and hearty chili cooked to perfection. I make this recipe often using bison or ground beef, depending on what's in the freezer—and both are always a hit.

1. In a large skillet, melt the coconut oil over medium heat. Add the onion and garlic and cook until just soft, 3 to 4 minutes. Add the bison and stir to break up and crumble the meat as it cooks. Cook until the meat is no longer pink, 7 to 8 minutes.

2. Transfer the bison mixture from the skillet to the slow cooker. Add the sweet potato, bell pepper, jalapeño, tomatoes, broth, chili powder, cumin, salt, black pepper, cinnamon, and cayenne (if using) and stir.

3. Cover the slow cooker and cook on Low for 6 to 8 hours.

4. Serve garnished with the cilantro.

Makes 4 servings

Prep time: **20 minutes (not including broth)**

Cooking time: **6 to 8 hours**

2 tablespoons coconut oil or ghee
1 medium onion, diced
2 garlic cloves, minced
1 pound ground bison
1 large sweet potato, peeled and cut into ½-inch cubes
1 bell pepper, diced
1 jalapeño, seeded and diced
1 (28-ounce) can crushed tomatoes
1 cup Homemade Bone Broth (page 222)
2 tablespoons chili powder
2 teaspoons ground cumin
1 teaspoon sea salt
½ teaspoon freshly ground black pepper
¼ teaspoon ground cinnamon
¼ teaspoon cayenne pepper (optional)
¼ cup fresh cilantro leaves, for garnish

Change it up: Use ground beef instead of bison. Swap out the sweet potato for ½ pound butternut squash.

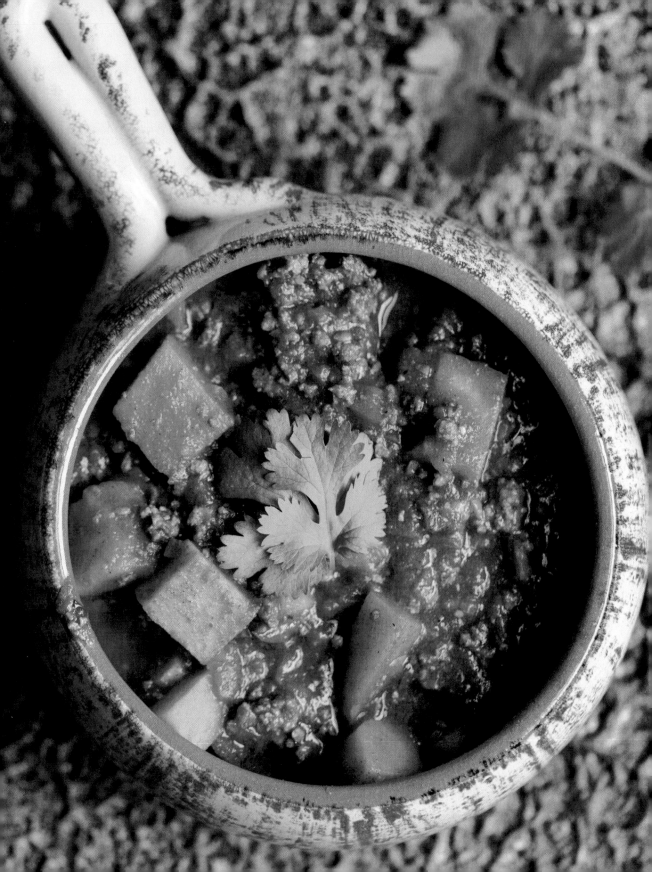

Pan-Seared Lamb Chops with Sage-Apple-Mint Puree

EGG-FREE. NIGHTSHADE-FREE, NUT-FREE

I'm always blown away by how easy it is to make delicious, perfectly seared lamb chops at home. While the lamb chop is a very tender cut of meat you don't have to do much to, the sage-apple-mint puree adds a savory finish that makes the chops melt in your mouth. This is a great dinner for two—especially when celebrating a special occasion.

1. In a small bowl, combine the olive oil, rosemary, garlic, salt, and pepper. Place the lamb chops in a shallow baking dish and spoon the olive oil mixture over the chops, making sure to coat both sides. Cover and marinate the lamb in the refrigerator for 1 hour.

2. Meanwhile, to make the puree, place all the ingredients for the puree in a food processor and process until combined. Set aside.

3. In a large skillet with a lid, melt the coconut oil over medium-high heat. When the oil is hot, add the chops and sear until golden brown on both sides, 2 to 3 minutes per side. Remove the skillet from the heat, cover the skillet, and let it sit for 2 to 3 minutes.

4. Remove the chops from the skillet and let them rest for 5 to 10 minutes. Serve topped with the sage-apple-mint puree.

Makes 2 or 3 servings

Prep time: 15 minutes, plus 1 hour marinating time

Cooking time: less than 10 minutes

3 tablespoons extra-virgin olive oil
1 tablespoon finely chopped fresh rosemary
3 garlic cloves, minced
½ teaspoon sea salt
⅛ teaspoon freshly ground black pepper
8 lamb chops, each about ¾ inch thick
2 tablespoons coconut oil or ghee

Sage-apple-mint puree

1 Granny Smith apple, cored and sliced
⅓ cup extra-virgin olive oil
¼ cup packed fresh mint leaves
1 tablespoon chopped fresh sage
2 teaspoons apple cider vinegar
Pinch of sea salt

Change it up: For rarer lamb chops, remove the chops from the skillet and let them rest immediately after searing.

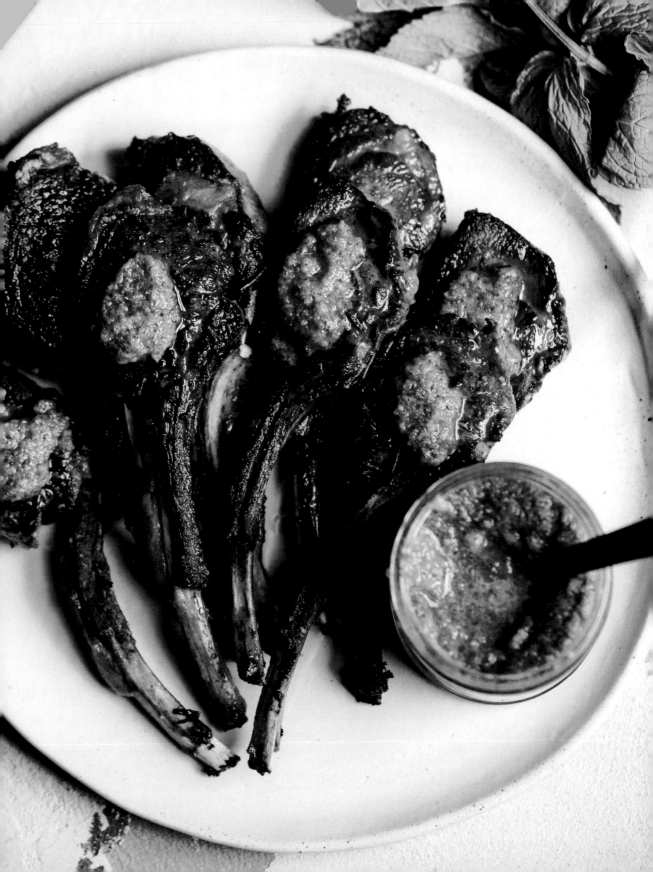

Moroccan Lamb Meatballs

EGG-FREE, NUT-FREE

I love it when I can take a simple recipe, such as classic meatballs in a red sauce, and create an entirely new dish using a different set of spices. For this recipe, the Moroccan-inspired blend of spices takes center stage and gives the dish a sweet and savory flavor.

Makes about 3 servings (around twenty 1¼-inch meatballs)

Prep time: 10 minutes

Cooking time: less than 20 minutes

1. To make the meatballs, in a large bowl, combine the lamb, parsley, paprika, coriander, cinnamon, cumin, salt, and pepper. Form the mixture into about twenty 1¼-inch meatballs (about 1 ounce each) and set aside on a platter.

2. In a large skillet, melt the coconut oil over medium heat. Add the meatballs and cook until lightly browned on all sides, 3 to 4 minutes. Remove the meatballs from the skillet and set aside. Drain all but 1 tablespoon of the fat from the skillet and place the skillet back on the heat.

3. To make the sauce, add the olive oil to the fat in the skillet. When the oil is hot, add the onion and garlic and cook until just soft, 3 to 4 minutes. Add the diced tomatoes with their juices, tomato paste, cinnamon, coriander, salt, and pepper and stir.

4. Bring the sauce to a boil, then reduce the heat to maintain a simmer and return the meatballs to the skillet, turning them several times to coat them in the sauce. Cover the skillet and cook until the meatballs are cooked through, 5 to 7 minutes.

5. Garnish with the parsley and serve warm.

Meatballs

1 pound ground lamb
1 tablespoon chopped fresh parsley
½ teaspoon paprika
½ teaspoon ground coriander
½ teaspoon ground cinnamon
½ teaspoon ground cumin
½ teaspoon sea salt
¼ teaspoon freshly ground black pepper
1 tablespoon coconut oil or ghee

Sauce

1 tablespoon extra-virgin olive oil
½ medium onion, diced
2 garlic cloves, minced
1 (14.5-ounce) can diced tomatoes, with their juices
1 tablespoon tomato paste
½ teaspoon ground cinnamon
¼ teaspoon ground coriander
¼ teaspoon sea salt
¼ teaspoon freshly ground black pepper

1 tablespoon chopped fresh parsley, for garnish

Change it up: Use ground beef instead of lamb. Swap out the parsley for fresh cilantro.

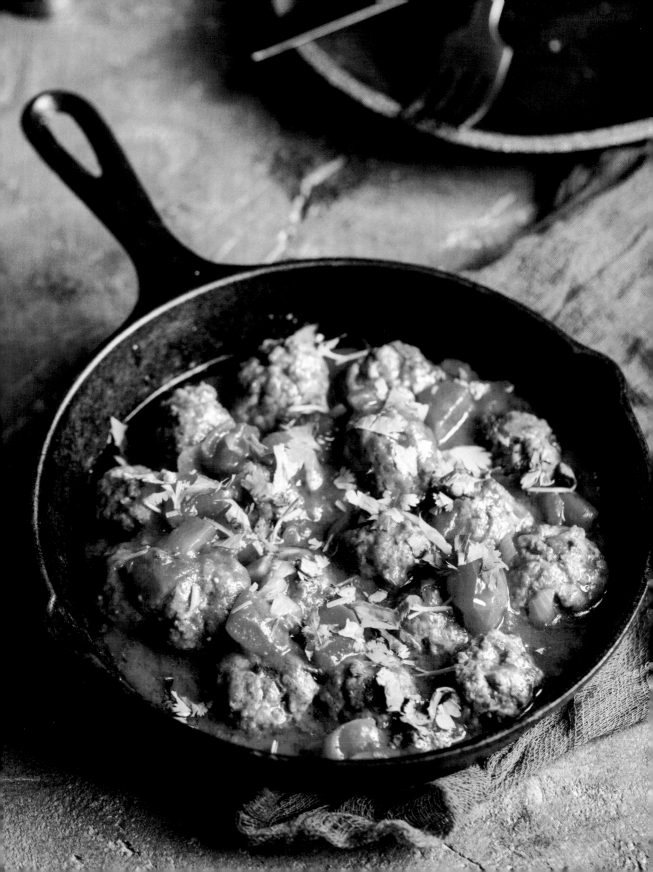

Oven-Roasted Spareribs

EGG-FREE, NUT-FREE

Don't be intimidated by the long cooking time. These ribs are not only super easy to prepare, they're also fall-off-the-bone delicious. By finishing them under the broiler, you create the perfect amount of crispiness on the outside.

Makes 3 or 4 servings

Prep time: 10 minutes, plus 20 minutes resting time

Cooking time: about 2 hours

3 to 4 pounds pork spareribs

Rub

1 tablespoon paprika
1 tablespoon chili powder
1 teaspoon sea salt
1 teaspoon onion powder
1 teaspoon garlic powder
½ teaspoon cayenne pepper
½ teaspoon freshly ground black pepper

Serve it with: Rosemary Roasted Potatoes (page 164)

1. Preheat the oven to 275°F.

2. Rinse the ribs and pat them dry. Place each rack of spareribs on a sheet of heavy-duty aluminum foil that's large enough to enclose it.

3. In a small bowl, combine the spices for the rub. Season the ribs evenly with the rub.

4. Seal each rack of spareribs in the foil by bringing the two long edges of the foil together and rolling the seal down toward the meat. Roll the two opposite ends toward the meat, making sure each rib is completely enclosed in foil.

5. Place the ribs on a large baking sheet and let them sit undisturbed for at least 20 minutes.

6. Roast the ribs for 2 hours. Remove the baking sheet from the oven and let the ribs cool in the foil; switch the oven to broil. When the foil is cool to the touch, remove it and transfer the ribs to a broiler pan.

7. Broil the ribs for 2 to 3 minutes on each side, until slightly crisp. Watch closely to prevent burning.

8. Cut the ribs into sections and serve.

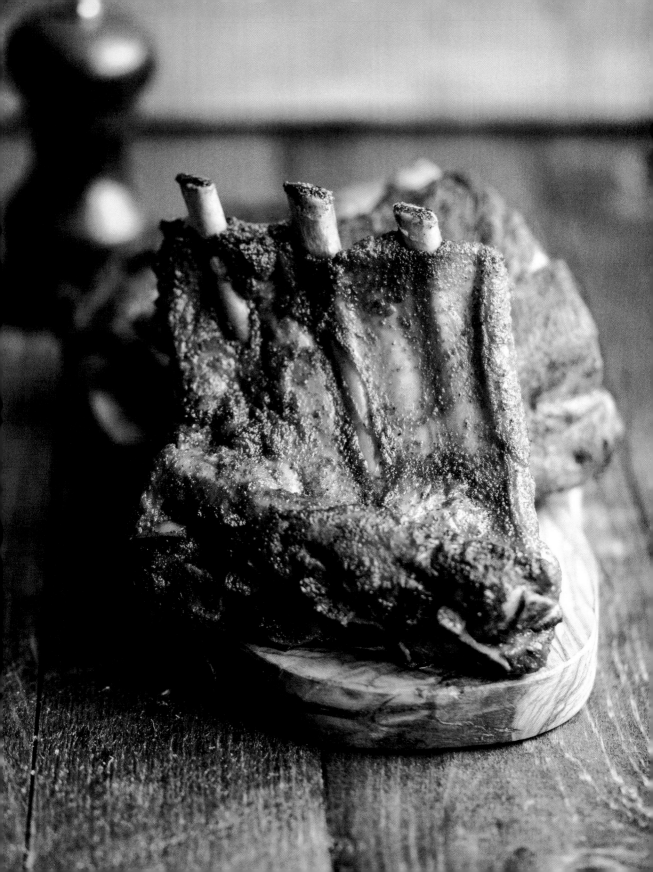

Balsamic Wine Pork Chops

EGG-FREE, NIGHTSHADE-FREE, NUT-FREE

Gone are the days of tough, dry pork chops. By simmering the chops in broth and wine, they come out flavorful, savory, and juicy. And—bonus—the entire dish is cooked in a single pan.

Makes 4 servings

Prep time: 10 minutes (not including broth)

Cooking time: less than 25 minutes

1. In a large skillet, melt 1 tablespoon of the coconut oil over medium-high heat. Season the pork chops with the salt and pepper and sear until golden brown on both sides, about 2 minutes per side. Remove the pork chops from the skillet and set aside.

2. Reduce the heat to medium and add the remaining 1 tablespoon coconut oil to the skillet. Add the mushrooms, onion, and garlic and cook until the vegetables are soft, 5 to 6 minutes.

3. Pour the wine into the skillet and cook for 1 minute. Add the broth and thyme and stir. Return the pork chops to the skillet and nestle them into the sauce. Spoon the mushrooms and onion over the pork, cover the skillet, and cook for 10 minutes over medium heat.

4. Uncover the skillet and drizzle the pork chops with the vinegar. Cook, uncovered, for 2 minutes more.

5. To serve, place each pork chop on a plate and spoon some of the mushrooms, onion, and sauce on top. Garnish with the parsley.

2 tablespoons coconut oil or ghee
4 boneless pork chops
½ teaspoon sea salt
½ teaspoon freshly ground black pepper
8 ounces white mushrooms, sliced
1 medium sweet onion, sliced
3 garlic cloves, minced
½ cup red wine or 100 percent red grape juice
½ cup Homemade Bone Broth (page 222)
1 teaspoon dried thyme
2 tablespoons balsamic vinegar
1 tablespoon chopped fresh parsley, for garnish

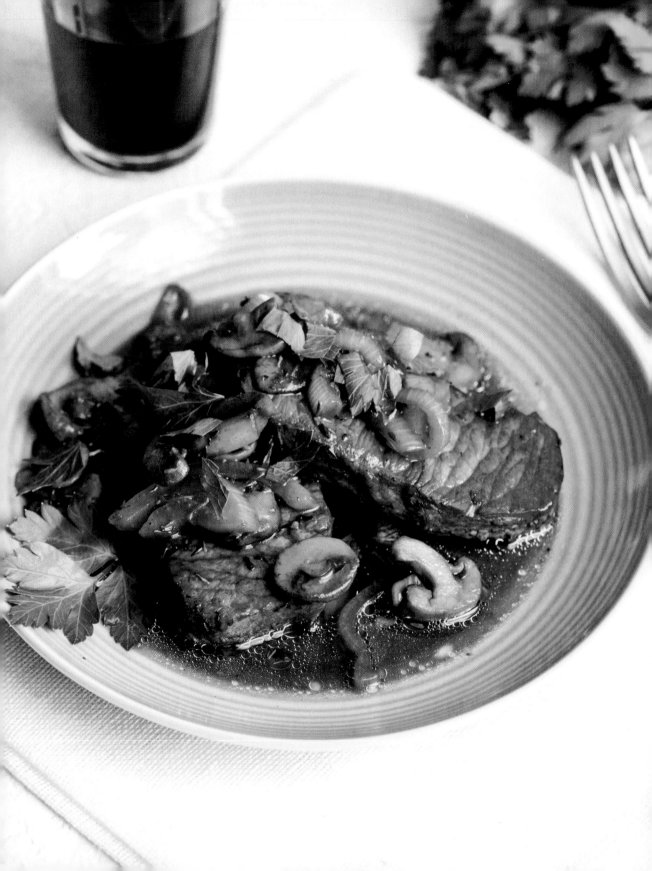

Firecracker Salmon

EGG-FREE, NUT-FREE

Appropriately named for its delicious glaze, this recipe is one of the dishes I make when I have zero time to prep a meal at night. I marinate the salmon in the morning and shift it over to the oven to cook at dinnertime. The result is flaky and moist salmon that's fiery and sweet.

1. In a medium bowl, whisk together all the marinade ingredients. Place the salmon in shallow bowl and pour the marinade on top, making sure to coat both sides. Cover and marinate the salmon in the refrigerator for 4 to 6 hours.

2. Preheat the oven to 400°F.

3. Remove the salmon from the marinade and place it skin-side down in a baking dish. Pour the marinade from the bowl over the salmon.

4. Bake for 18 to 20 minutes, or until the thickest part of salmon is no longer translucent.

5. Transfer the salmon to a large serving platter and garnish with the scallions.

Makes 4 servings

Prep time: **5 minutes, plus 4 to 6 hours marinating time**

Cooking time: **20 minutes**

Marinade

¼ cup extra-virgin olive oil
¼ cup coconut aminos
1 tablespoon balsamic vinegar
1 tablespoon raw honey
3 garlic cloves, minced
1 teaspoon sriracha sauce
½ teaspoon ground ginger
½ teaspoon red pepper flakes
½ teaspoon freshly ground black pepper
½ teaspoon onion powder

Salmon

1½ pounds wild-caught salmon fillet (coho or sockeye work best; see tip)
2 scallions, finely sliced, green ends only, for garnish

Noelle's tip: You can use one large salmon fillet for this recipe, or four smaller fillets that add up to 1½ pounds.

Serve it with: Lemon-Garlic Roasted Broccoli (page 163)

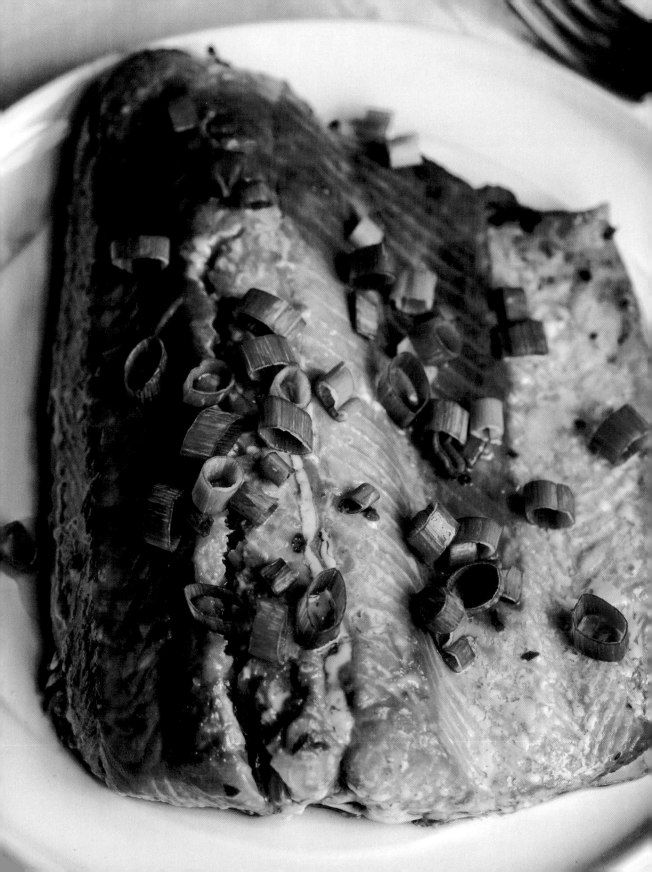

Coconut Macadamia Nut–Crusted Mahimahi

EGG-FREE, NIGHTSHADE-FREE

There's nothing quite like the combination of coconut and lime, except for when it's combined with macadamia nuts and turned into a golden brown crust. As a result, you may find that even the pickiest of eaters will gobble up this dish and request seconds.

1. Place the mahimahi in a shallow baking dish and pour the coconut milk over the fillets, making sure to coat both sides. Cover and marinate the fish in the refrigerator for 1 hour.

2. Preheat the oven to 425°F. Line a baking sheet with parchment paper or aluminum foil.

3. In a medium bowl, combine the macadamia nuts, almond flour, shredded coconut, and coconut oil. Set aside.

4. Remove the fish from the coconut milk and place the fillets on the prepared baking sheet. Season both sides with salt and pepper and bake for 5 minutes.

5. Remove the baking sheet from the oven and let the fish cool slightly. Spread the nut mixture evenly over the top and sides of each fillet, patting and pressing down to make it stick.

6. Sprinkle the fillets with the lime juice and bake for 8 to 10 minutes, until the crust is golden brown. Serve warm.

Makes 4 servings

Prep time: **15 minutes, plus 1 hour marinating time**

Cooking time: **15 minutes**

4 (6-ounce) mahimahi fillets
1 (13.5-ounce) can full-fat coconut milk
1¼ cups coarsely ground roasted macadamia nuts (see tip)
¼ cup almond flour
¼ cup unsweetened shredded coconut
¼ cup coconut oil or ghee, melted
Sea salt and freshly ground black pepper
Juice of ½ lime

Noelle's tip: The best way to coarsely grind the macadamia nuts is in a food processor. If you don't have one on hand, you can place the nuts in a zip-top bag, seal the bag, and pound them gently with a rolling pin.

Change it up: Use another white-fleshed fish like sole or halibut. Swap out the lime juice for lemon juice.

Serve it with: Mango-Jalapeño Salsa (page 185)

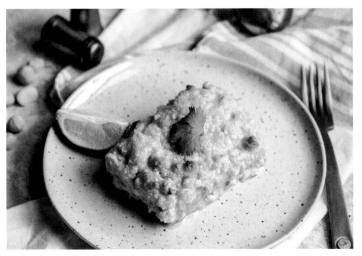

Shrimp and Cabbage Stir-Fry

EGG-FREE, NUT-FREE

While shrimp is great because it cooks so quickly, you have to watch it closely to make sure it doesn't become over-cooked and rubbery. The shrimp is done when the exterior is pink and the center is opaque with just a little white color. Using a large pan is crucial for this dish, as it helps the shrimp cook evenly and allows all the flavors to meld together at the end.

1. In a large skillet, melt 1 tablespoon of the coconut oil over medium heat. Add the onion, garlic, and ginger and cook, stirring, for 2 to 3 minutes.

2. Add the shrimp, salt, black pepper, and sriracha and cook, stirring, until the shrimp are pink and opaque, 3 to 4 minutes. Remove the mixture from the skillet and set aside.

3. Melt the remaining 1 tablespoon coconut oil in the skillet. Add the cabbage and bell pepper and stir. Stir in the coconut aminos and cook, stirring, until the cabbage softens and wilts, 5 to 6 minutes.

4. Return the shrimp mixture to the skillet and stir until combined and warm, 1 to 2 minutes. Remove the skillet from the heat and stir in the cilantro. Serve warm.

Makes 4 servings

Prep time: 15 minutes

Cooking time: less than 15 minutes

2 tablespoons coconut oil or ghee
1 medium onion, diced
3 garlic cloves, minced
½ teaspoon ground ginger
1 pound large shrimp, peeled and deveined
Sea salt and freshly ground black pepper
1 teaspoon sriracha sauce
½ head cabbage, cut into 1-inch pieces
1 red bell pepper, diced
2 tablespoons coconut aminos
1 tablespoon chopped fresh cilantro

Change it up: Swap out the shrimp for diced chicken.

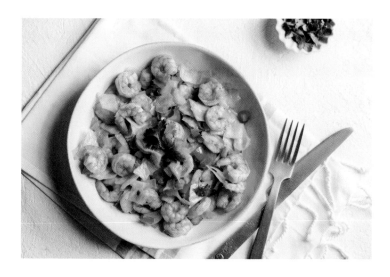

Thai Coconut Curry Shrimp

EGG-FREE, NUT-FREE

If food could give you a hug, this Thai coconut curry would wrap you in its arms and encase you in warmth. The savory spices of red curry combined with the sweetness of smooth coconut milk create a perfectly balanced bowl of nourishment that tastes just as beautiful as it looks.

Makes 4 or 5 servings

Prep time: 15 minutes
(not including broth or cauliflower rice)

Cooking time: less than 25 minutes

1. In a large skillet, melt 1 tablespoon of the coconut oil over medium heat. Add the shrimp, salt, and black pepper and cook until the shrimp are pink and opaque, 3 to 4 minutes. Remove the shrimp from the skillet and set aside.

2. Melt the remaining 1 tablespoon coconut oil in the skillet. Add the onion, bell pepper, and garlic and cook until the vegetables are just soft, 4 to 5 minutes. Add the curry paste and stir until fragrant, about 30 seconds.

3. Add the coconut milk, broth, fish sauce, and sriracha and stir until combined. Bring the mixture to a boil, then reduce the heat to maintain a simmer and cook until the sauce thickens slightly, 5 to 7 minutes. Return the shrimp to the skillet and stir until coated in the sauce and warm, 1 to 2 minutes.

4. Remove the skillet from the heat and stir in the cilantro and lime juice. Serve warm in a shallow bowl over cauliflower rice, if desired.

2 tablespoons coconut oil or ghee
1½ pounds large shrimp, peeled and deveined
Sea salt and freshly ground black pepper
1 small onion, thinly sliced
1 red bell pepper, sliced into thin strips
2 garlic cloves, minced
2 tablespoons Thai red curry paste
1 (13.5-ounce) can full-fat coconut milk
1 cup Homemade Bone Broth (page 222)
2 tablespoons Red Boat Fish Sauce
1 teaspoon sriracha sauce
3 tablespoons finely chopped fresh cilantro
Juice of ½ lime
1 recipe Jalapeño-Lime Cauliflower Rice (page 167), for serving (optional)

Change it up: Use diced chicken instead of shrimp. Swap out the cilantro for fresh basil.

Prep ahead: Double the recipe for the Jalapeño-Lime Cauliflower Rice. Make it 2 or 3 days ahead of time as a side dish for another meal. Store the extra in an airtight container in the refrigerator until ready to use.

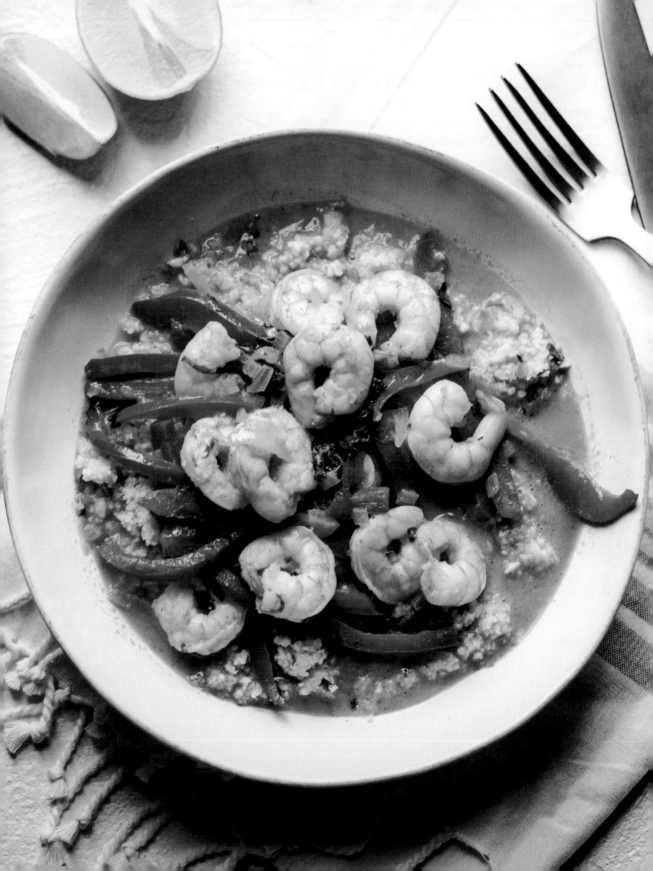

Caribbean Grilled Tuna Steaks

EGG-FREE, NUT-FREE

Tuna is a fantastic fish for grilling because it's dense and holds together well when placed directly on the grill grate. This Caribbean-inspired marinade gives the steaks a punch of spice and tang while also adding moisture.

Makes 4 servings

Prep time: 10 minutes (not including salsa)

Cooking time: less than 10 minutes

1. In a small bowl, whisk together the olive oil, lime juice, garlic, onion powder, smoked paprika, salt, cumin, ginger, pepper, and cinnamon. Place the tuna steaks in a shallow baking dish and spread the seasoning mixture all over the steaks, turning them to coat both sides. Cover and marinate the tuna in the refrigerator for 30 minutes.

2. Preheat a grill to medium-high heat.

3. When the grill is hot, place the steaks on the grill and cook for 4 to 5 minutes on each side for medium, or to your desired doneness.

4. Garnish the steaks with the salsa and serve.

2 tablespoons extra-virgin olive oil
1 tablespoon fresh lime juice
1 garlic clove, minced
2 teaspoons onion powder
1 teaspoon smoked paprika
½ teaspoon sea salt
½ teaspoon ground cumin
¼ teaspoon ground ginger
¼ teaspoon freshly ground black pepper
⅛ teaspoon ground cinnamon
4 (6- to 8-ounce) tuna steaks
½ cup Mango-Jalapeño Salsa (page 185), for serving

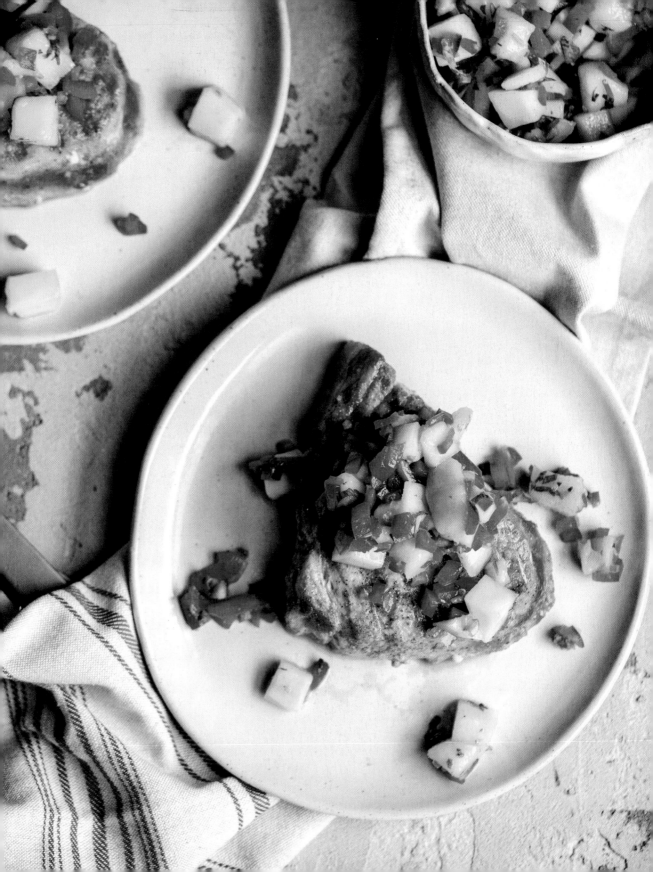

11

TREATS

Chocolate Coconut Bombs

EGG-FREE, NIGHTSHADE-FREE, NUT-FREE, VEGETARIAN

When you're craving chocolate, these nutrient-dense bombs are the perfect poppable solution. To make them more fun to eat, use silicone candy molds in different shapes and sizes.

Makes 20 servings
(1 bomb per serving)

Prep time: **5 minutes, plus 1 hour chilling time**

Cooking time: **none**

1. In a small saucepan, heat the coconut butter and coconut oil over medium-low heat, stirring continuously, until just melted.

2. Remove the pan from the heat and stir in the honey and vanilla. Fold in the cacao powder and stir until no lumps remain.

3. Place a silicone mini-muffin pan on a baking sheet (or use a mini-muffin pan lined with silicone baking cups). Pour the mixture evenly into 20 wells of the muffin pan, filling each one about half full with the chocolate mixture. Refrigerate until the chocolate is set, about 1 hour.

4. Pop the bombs out of the molds and store in an airtight container in the refrigerator for up to 2 weeks or in the freezer for up to 2 months.

½ **cup coconut butter**
½ **cup coconut oil**
2 **tablespoons raw honey**
½ **teaspoon pure vanilla extract**
¼ **cup cacao powder or unsweetened cocoa powder**

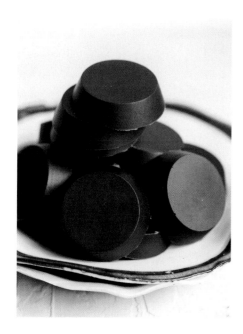

Salted Dark Chocolate Almond Butter Cups

EGG-FREE, NIGHTSHADE-FREE, VEGETARIAN

I keep a stash of these mini almond butter cups in the freezer at all times. They're super rich and satisfying, with a creamy, melt-in-your-mouth texture.

Makes 12 servings
(2 mini cups per serving)

Prep time: 20 minutes, plus
1 hour chilling time

Cooking time: none

Chocolate cups

¾ cup coconut oil

3 tablespoons pure maple
syrup or raw honey

¾ teaspoon pure vanilla
extract

¾ cup cacao powder or
unsweetened cocoa powder

Coarse sea salt

Filling

⅓ cup unsalted creamy
almond butter

1 teaspoon coconut flour

1 teaspoon pure maple syrup

½ teaspoon pure vanilla
extract

*Change it up: Use another nut
butter, such as cashew butter, for
the filling.*

1. Line a 24-cup mini-muffin pan with silicone or parchment paper baking cups.

2. To make the chocolate cups, in a small saucepan, melt the coconut oil, maple syrup, and vanilla over medium-low heat. As soon as the coconut oil is melted, immediately remove the pan from the heat and gently fold in the cacao powder, stirring until no lumps remain. Let cool slightly.

3. Spoon about 1 teaspoon of the chocolate mixture into each muffin liner so the bottom is coated. Set the saucepan with the remaining chocolate aside and refrigerate the muffin pan until the chocolate sets, about 10 minutes.

4. Meanwhile, to make the filling, combine all the filling ingredients in a food processor and process until smooth, scraping down the sides of the bowl as necessary.

5. Remove the muffin pan from the refrigerator and scoop about ½ teaspoon of the filling into each cup. Gently press the filling down with the back of the measuring spoon to smooth it into an even layer.

6. If the remaining chocolate in the saucepan is too thick, reheat it for a few seconds and stir. Pour the chocolate into each cup to cover the filling, using 1½ to 2 teaspoons per cup. Sprinkle the cups with salt and place the pan back in the refrigerator until the chocolate is solid, about 1 hour. Store in an airtight container in the refrigerator for up to a month or in the freezer for up to 2 months.

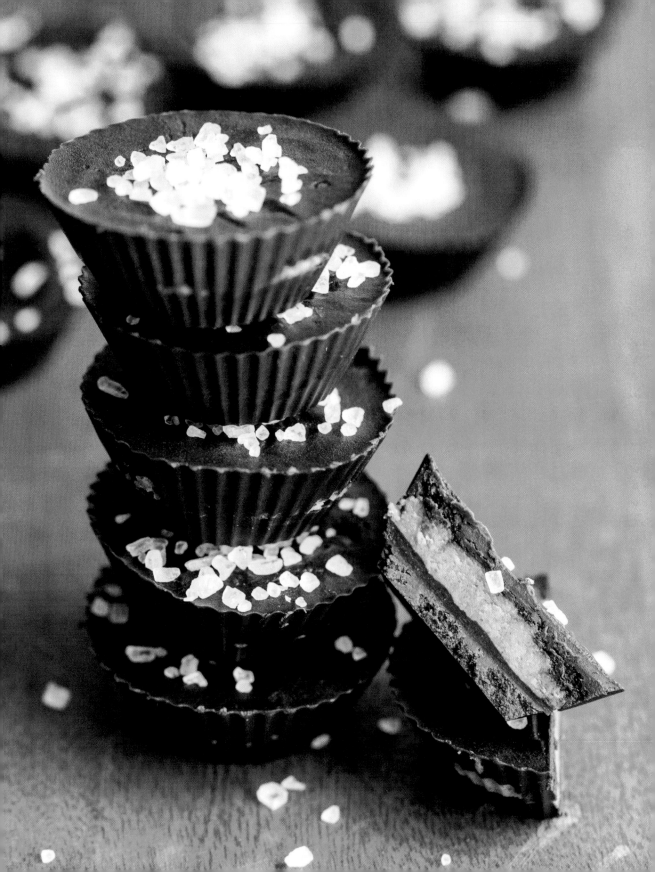

Whipped Coconut Cream

EGG-FREE, NIGHTSHADE-FREE, NUT-FREE, VEGETARIAN

Whipped coconut cream can be enjoyed on top of fruit, smoothies, and desserts—or straight out of a bowl with a spoon. When making this whipped coconut cream, do not use "lite" coconut milk or other canned coconut products such as coconut cream. You'll be left with a not-so-whipped liquidy coconut mess.

1. Open the can of coconut milk and scoop out the solid cream into a large bowl or the bowl of a stand mixer fitted with the whisk attachment. Pour the coconut water that remains in the can into a separate bowl and set aside (see tip).

2. Using a handheld mixer or the stand mixer, beat the coconut cream on low speed for 3 to 5 minutes. Add the honey and vanilla, increase the speed to medium, and continue to whip. If you'd like to make the cream slightly softer, add 1 or 2 teaspoons of the coconut water while whipping.

3. Once the cream starts to have a uniform texture, increase the speed to high and whip until it holds soft peaks.

4. Serve with fruit or on top of treats. Store any leftovers in an airtight container in the refrigerator for up to 4 days.

Makes 6 servings
(about ¾ cup)

Prep time: **10 minutes**

Cooking time: **none**

1 (13.5-ounce) can full-fat coconut milk, refrigerated overnight
1½ teaspoons raw honey
½ teaspoon pure vanilla extract

Noelle's tip: Store the leftover coconut water in the fridge and use it to make smoothies or for cooking.

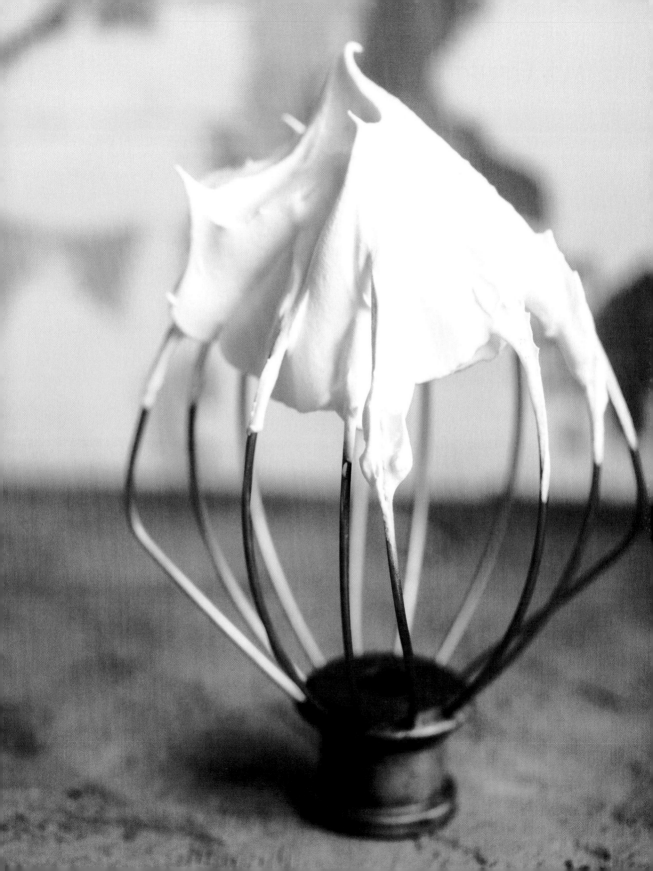

Dark Chocolate Mug Cake

NIGHTSHADE-FREE, NUT-FREE, VEGETARIAN

This dark chocolate mug cake is my go-to on-the-fly dessert. It's moist and full of decadence, and brings a whole new twist to making a cake from scratch.

1. In a microwave-safe mug, combine the coconut flour, cacao powder, and baking powder. Stir in the coconut milk, honey, coconut oil, and vanilla, making sure no lumps remain.

2. Add the egg and gently whisk it into the mixture until a gooey, chocolaty batter forms.

3. Microwave on high for 2 to 2½ minutes. Remove the mug from the microwave and let it sit for 1 or 2 minutes.

4. Serve with your toppings of choice.

Makes 1 or 2 servings (1 mug cake)

Prep time: **5 minutes**

Cooking time: **2½ minutes**

Mug cake

2 tablespoons coconut flour
2 tablespoons cacao powder or unsweetened cocoa powder
¼ teaspoon baking powder
¼ cup canned full-fat coconut milk
1½ tablespoons raw honey
2 teaspoons coconut oil, melted
¼ teaspoon pure vanilla extract
1 large egg, lightly beaten

Toppings (optional)

Whipped Coconut Cream (page 248)
Homemade Chocolate Shell Topping (page 252)
Fresh strawberries or raspberries

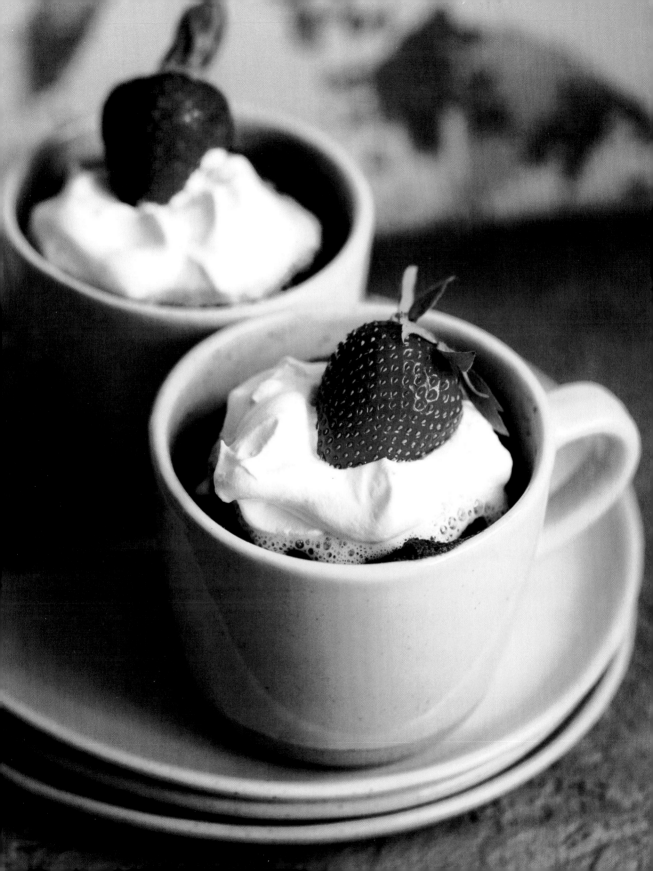

Homemade Chocolate Shell Topping

EGG-FREE, NIGHTSHADE-FREE, NUT-FREE, VEGETARIAN

I first published this recipe on the Coconuts and Kettlebells website years ago after attempting to create a chocolate dip for fruit. I had some extra strawberry slices in the freezer, and thanks to my impatient personality, I ended up pouring the mixture over the slices while they were still slightly frozen. Much to my surprise, the chocolate hardened instantly, which reminded me of the Magic Shell I used to have on my ice cream at my grandma's house as a kid. Now it's one of the most popular recipes on my blog and makes it into a variety of recipes (for obvious reasons).

Makes 3 or 4 servings

Prep time: **5 minutes**

Cooking time: **None**

¼ cup coconut oil, melted

1 tablespoon pure maple syrup or raw honey

¼ teaspoon pure vanilla extract

¼ cup cacao powder or unsweetened cocoa powder

1. In a small bowl, combine the coconut oil, maple syrup, and vanilla. Stir well.

2. Gently fold in the cacao powder and stir until no lumps remain.

3. Let the mixture cool slightly, then pour it on top of frozen fruit or cold desserts and watch as it hardens—like magic!

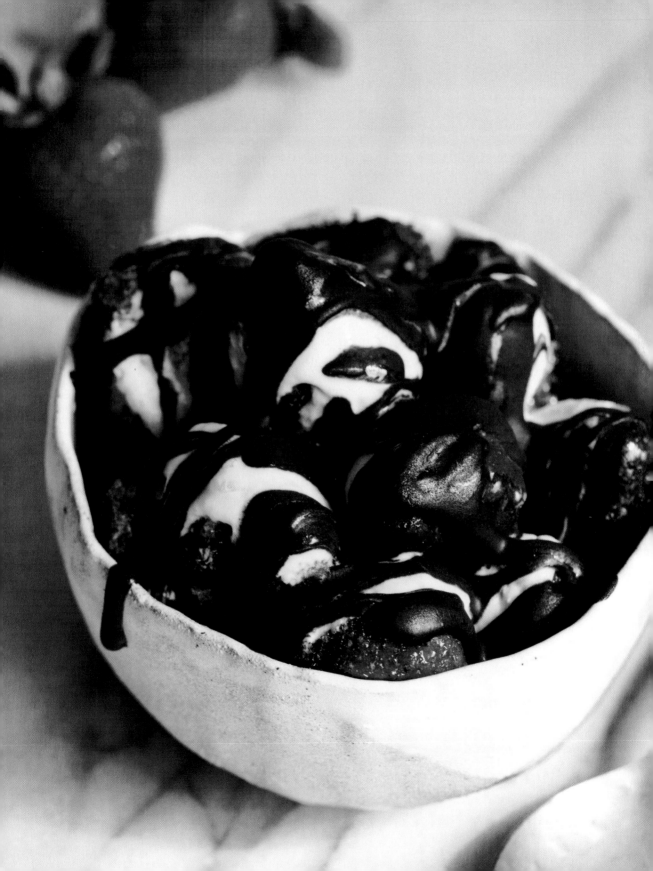

Banana Split Pops

EGG-FREE, NIGHTSHADE-FREE, NUT-FREE (WITHOUT THE CHOPPED WALNUTS), VEGETARIAN

These little banana splits on a stick are the perfect summer party treat. If you're making a bunch ahead of time for a large group, simply wrap them individually in parchment paper and store in an airtight container in the freezer.

1. Line a baking sheet with parchment paper. Slide the fruit onto each ice pop stick in this order: 1 banana slice, 1 pineapple chunk, 1 strawberry slice, 1 cherry.

2. Transfer the fruit pops to the prepared baking sheet and freeze until the fruit is chilled, 15 to 20 minutes.

3. Pour the chocolate shell into a shallow baking dish for dipping. Place the chopped walnuts, if using, on a small plate.

4. Remove the baking sheet from the freezer. Dip one side of each fruit pop in the chocolate, holding it there for 2 to 3 seconds until the chocolate starts to harden. Sprinkle immediately with the chopped walnuts and return to the baking sheet.

5. Freeze the pops until the chocolate sets completely, about 15 minutes. Serve immediately.

Makes 6 servings
(2 pops per serving)

Prep time: 25 minutes, plus 15 minutes chilling time

Cooking time: none

2 small bananas, cut crosswise into six 1-inch slices (12 slices total)
12 (1-inch) pineapple chunks (about ¼ pound)
6 strawberries, halved
12 fresh cherries, pitted (see tip)
Homemade Chocolate Shell Topping (page 252)
¼ cup finely chopped raw walnuts (optional)

Special equipment: Ice pop sticks

Noelle's tip: If you can't find fresh cherries, use frozen pitted cherries. Simply lay them out to thaw for 5 to 10 minutes before assembling and slide the stick right into the small opening where the cherry was pitted.

Change it up: Use mango chunks instead of pineapple. Use unsweetened shredded coconut instead of walnuts to make them nut-free.

Serve it with: Whipped Coconut Cream (page 248) for dipping

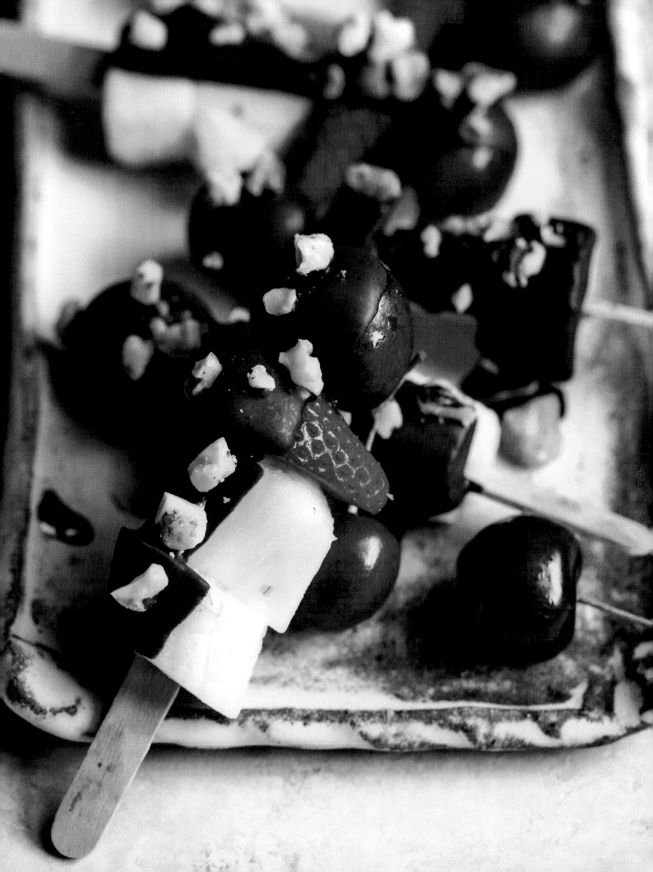

Chocolate-Covered Strawberry Ice Pops

EGG-FREE, NIGHTSHADE-FREE, NUT-FREE (WITHOUT THE NUT TOPPING), VEGETARIAN

As a superfan of frozen fruit, I've always loved making (and eating) homemade ice pops. These pops are a rendition of one of my favorite fruit treats—chocolate-covered strawberries. If you're short on time or just want a fruity treat, simply skip the chocolate shell topping and enjoy.

Makes 6 servings (1 ice pop per serving)

Prep time: 10 minutes, plus 15 minutes chilling time

Cooking time: none

1. Place all the ingredients for the ice pops in a blender or food processor and blend until smooth.

2. Pour the mixture evenly into ice pop molds and insert ice pop sticks (see tip). Place the ice pops in the freezer until frozen solid, about 6 hours.

3. Pour the chocolate shell into a shallow baking dish for dipping.

4. Line a baking sheet with parchment paper. Remove the ice pops from the molds by running the molds under warm water for a few seconds. Dip each ice pop in the chocolate shell topping, holding it there for 2 to 3 seconds until the chocolate starts to harden. Sprinkle immediately with your toppings of choice and place on the prepared baking sheet.

5. Freeze the ice pops until the chocolate sets completely, about 15 minutes. Serve immediately.

Ice pops

1¼ cups sliced strawberries

1 large banana, peeled, frozen, and sliced

½ cup canned full-fat coconut milk

Homemade Chocolate Shell Topping (page 252)

Toppings (optional)

Unsweetened shredded coconut

Finely chopped raw nuts, such as pistachios, pecans, or almonds

Freeze-dried fruit pieces

Special equipment: Ice pop molds

Noelle's tip: If your ice pop molds don't come with sticks that are secured in place, simply insert an ice pop stick into the center of each pop after they've been in the freezer for about 45 minutes.

Change it up: Swap out the strawberries for fresh mango chunks.

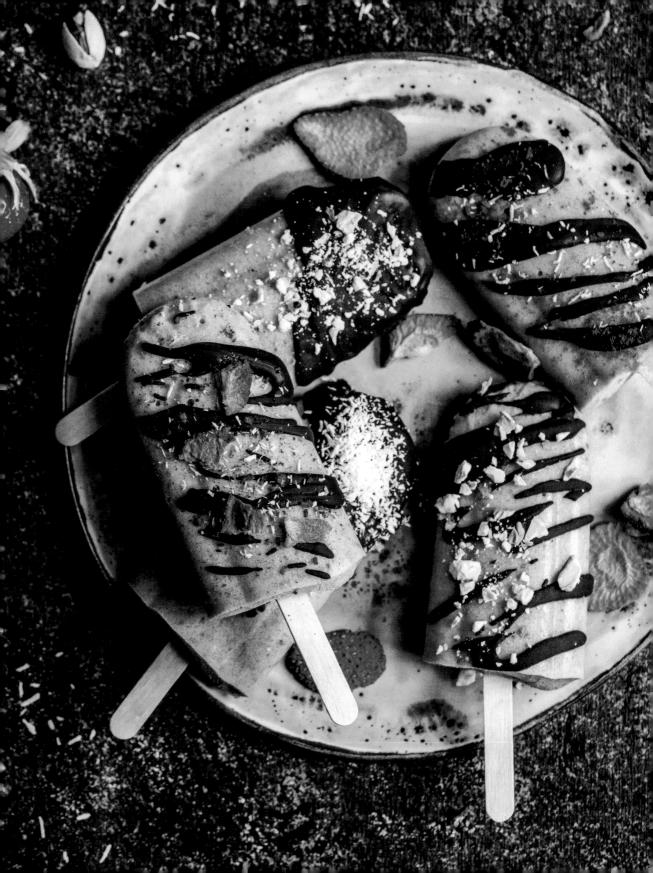

Almond Shortbread Cookies

EGG-FREE, NIGHTSHADE-FREE, VEGETARIAN

With just a few simple ingredients, these shortbread cookies are hard to beat. They're slightly crisp on the outside and buttery soft in the center, and have the perfect amount of sweetness. If they stick around longer than a day or two, it's likely because you were smart enough to hide them from the others. Well done.

1. Preheat the oven to 350°F. Line a baking sheet with parchment paper.

2. In a large bowl, fold all the ingredients together until combined. Roll the dough into about twelve 1¼-inch balls and place them on the prepared baking sheet (see tip).

3. Gently flatten each cookie using a fork. Turn the fork perpendicular to the first indentation and lightly press down to create a crosshatch design.

4. Bake for 9 to 10 minutes, until the edges turn lightly golden brown. Remove the cookies from the baking sheet and let them cool completely on a wire rack before serving. Store in an airtight container at room temperature for up to 1 week.

Makes 6 servings (2 cookies per serving)
Prep time: 15 minutes
Cooking time: 10 minutes

1 cup almond flour
3 tablespoons ghee, at room temperature (not melted)
2 tablespoons pure maple syrup
½ teaspoon pure vanilla extract
⅛ teaspoon ground cinnamon
Pinch of sea salt

Noelle's tip: To make the dough easy to flatten, place it in the refrigerator for 30 minutes before rolling it into balls.

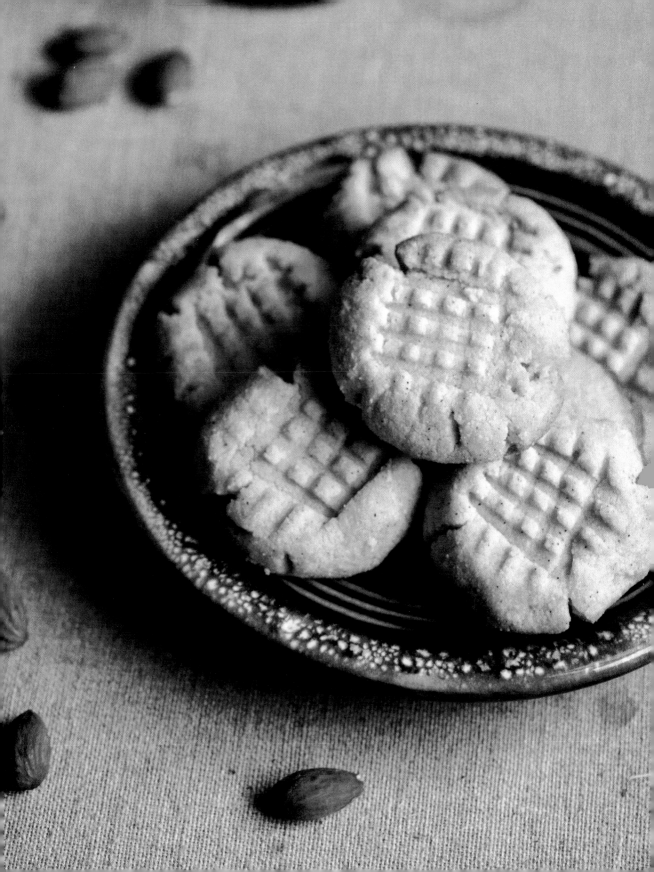

No-Bake Almond-Coconut Cookie Bars

EGG-FREE, NIGHTSHADE-FREE, VEGETARIAN

It doesn't get much better than coconut candy adorned with almonds and smothered in chocolate—except when it's reinvented as a no-bake, triple-layer cookie bar using nourishing ingredients.

Makes 18 servings
(1 bar per serving)
Prep time: **30 minutes,**
  plus 1 hour chilling time
Cooking time: **none**

Crust
4 Medjool dates, pitted
1 cup almond flour
2 tablespoons coconut oil

Coconut layer
3 tablespoons coconut butter
2 tablespoons coconut oil
1½ tablespoons pure maple syrup
½ teaspoon pure vanilla extract
1 cup unsweetened shredded coconut

Chocolate layer
¼ cup coconut oil, melted
1 tablespoon pure maple syrup or raw honey
¼ teaspoon pure vanilla extract
¼ cup cacao powder or unsweetened cocoa powder

1. Line an 8½ x 4½-inch loaf pan with parchment paper so that it presses evenly into the corners and comes up the sides.

2. To prepare the crust, place the dates in a food processor and pulse until broken down into small pieces. Add the almond flour and pulse until combined. Add the coconut oil and process until a loose dough forms. The mixture should stick together when you squeeze it between your fingers.

3. Spread the dough evenly over the bottom of the prepared loaf pan, pressing it down firmly to flatten it.

4. To make the coconut layer, in a small saucepan, warm the coconut butter and coconut oil over medium-low heat until just melted. Remove the pan from the heat and stir in the maple syrup and vanilla. Fold in the shredded coconut until combined.

5. Spread the coconut layer over the crust, gently pressing it down to flatten and spread it evenly. Place the pan in the freezer to chill, about 15 minutes.

6. Meanwhile, to make the chocolate layer, in a glass measuring cup, combine the coconut oil, maple syrup, and vanilla. Gently fold in the cacao powder and stir until no lumps remain.

7. Remove the pan from the freezer and slowly pour the chocolate mixture over the coconut layer. Spread it evenly with a silicone spatula and return the pan to the freezer to set, about 1 hour.

8. Remove the pan from the freezer and pull up on the parchment paper to lift the solid bar out of the pan and onto a cutting board. Let the bar thaw slightly, then use a sharp knife to cut it into 18 small squares.

9. Store the bars in an airtight container in the refrigerator for slightly softer texture for up to 2 weeks, or in the freezer for up to 2 months.

Change it up: Skip the almond crust and prepare the coconut and chocolate layers to make dark chocolate coconut bars.

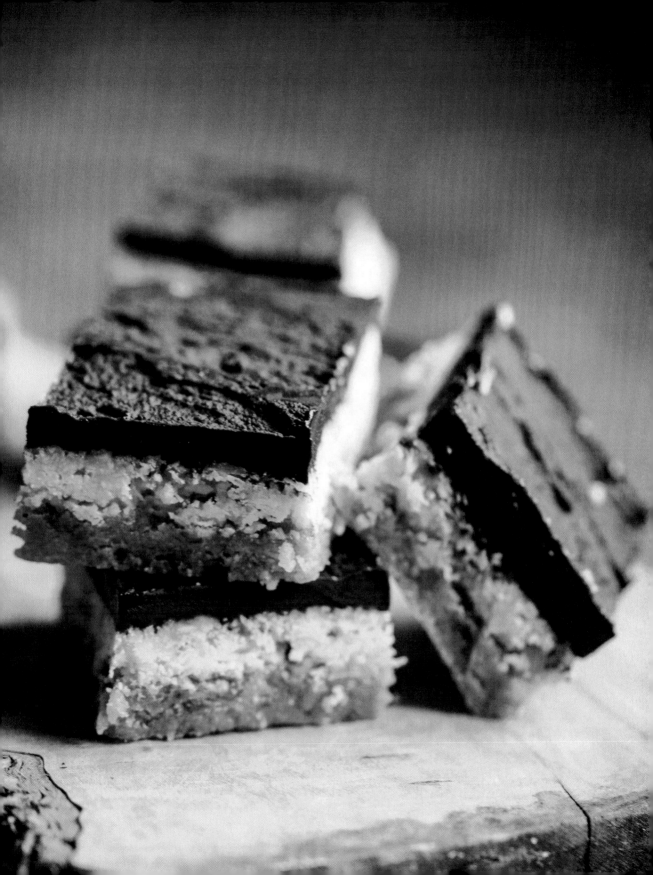

Lemon-Raspberry Mini Cheesecakes

EGG-FREE, NIGHTSHADE-FREE, VEGETARIAN

For years, my mom would order a professionally made raw cheesecake for me for my birthday. Everyone in our family loved it so much that it quickly became the cake we got for all special occasions. One year, being the amazing wife that I am, I forgot to order a cake for my husband's birthday and was left to take the task to the kitchen. I'm happy to say that thanks to this recipe, his birthday was not ruined, and the mini cheesecakes have now taken over as the preferred option in the family.

1. Bring 1½ cups water to a boil in a small saucepan. Place the cashews in a glass bowl and pour the boiling water over them. Soak the cashews for 1 hour, then drain and rinse.

2. Meanwhile, to make the crust, place the dates in a food processor and pulse until broken down into small pieces. Add the pecans and salt and process until a loose dough forms. The mixture should stick together when you squeeze it between your fingers.

3. Place a standard 12-cup silicone muffin pan on a baking sheet, or use a standard 12-cup muffin tin lined with silicone or parchment paper baking cups.

4. Spoon 1 heaping tablespoon of the crust mixture into each well of the pan, pressing firmly to flatten it evenly. Use the back of the measuring spoon to pack the crust down. Set aside.

5. To make the filling, place the cashews, honey, lemon juice, coconut milk, coconut oil, lemon zest, and vanilla in a blender and blend on high speed until very smooth, scraping down the sides of the blender as necessary.

6. Pour the filling evenly over the crusts. Lightly tap the baking sheet or muffin tin against a hard surface to smooth the filling and remove any bubbles. Place 1 raspberry on top of each cheesecake.

7. Freeze the cheesecakes until they solidify, 4 to 6 hours.

8. Pop the cheesecakes out of the molds and serve chilled. Store in an airtight container in the freezer.

Makes 12 servings (1 mini cheesecake per serving)

Prep time: 15 minutes, plus 1 hour soaking time and 4 to 6 hours chilling time

Cooking time: none

Filling

1½ cups raw cashews
⅓ cup raw honey
½ cup fresh lemon juice
½ cup canned full-fat coconut milk
¼ cup coconut oil, melted
1 teaspoon lemon zest
1 teaspoon pure vanilla extract
12 fresh raspberries

Crust

1 cup pitted dates
1 cup raw pecans
Pinch of sea salt

Noelle's tip: You can serve these right out of the freezer, or let them thaw for 10 minutes before serving so they have a softer texture.

Change it up: Use fresh blueberries instead of raspberries.

Serve it with: Whipped Coconut Cream (page 248) for topping

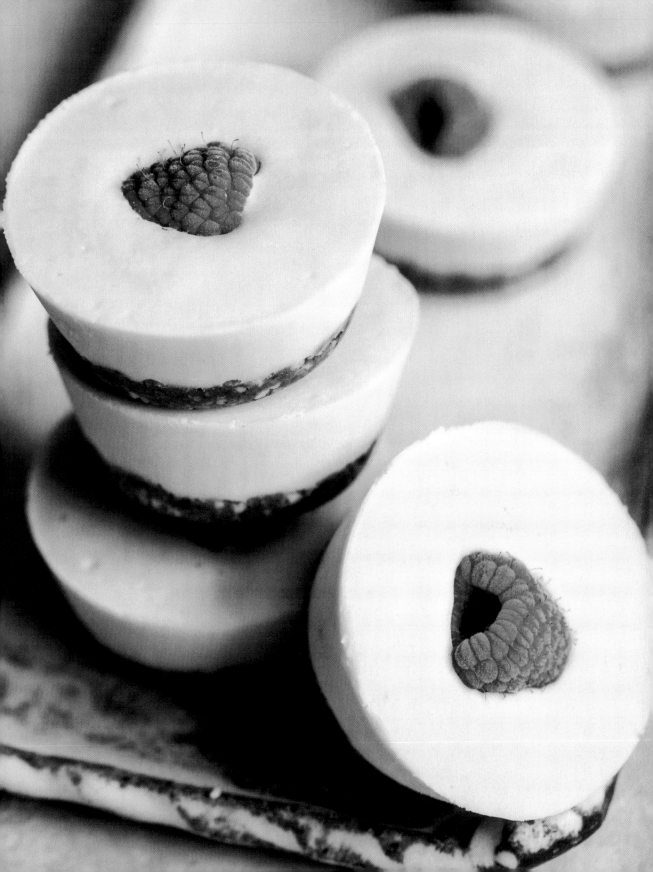

Avocado Chocolate Mousse

EGG-FREE, NIGHTSHADE-FREE, VEGETARIAN

This decadent dessert uses the creaminess of avocado to create a silky-smooth chocolaty mousse. While it's delicious on its own, you can also serve it as a dip for fruit or layer it in small glass jars with whipped coconut cream, fruit, and crushed nuts to make mini trifles.

Makes four ½-cup servings

Prep time: 5 minutes, plus 1 hour chilling time

Cooking time: none

1. Place all the ingredients for the mousse in a food processor and blend until smooth, scraping down the sides of the bowl as necessary. Refrigerate the mousse for 1 hour.

2. Spoon into bowls and serve chilled with the toppings of your choice. Store leftover mousse in an airtight container in the refrigerator for up to 2 days.

1 large avocado, refrigerated until cold, halved, pitted, and peeled

3 tablespoons cacao powder or unsweetened cocoa powder

½ cup canned full-fat coconut milk

2½ tablespoons raw honey

1 tablespoon almond butter

1 teaspoon pure vanilla extract

¼ teaspoon ground cinnamon

Pinch of sea salt

Toppings (optional)

Whipped Coconut Cream (page 248)

Fresh raspberries

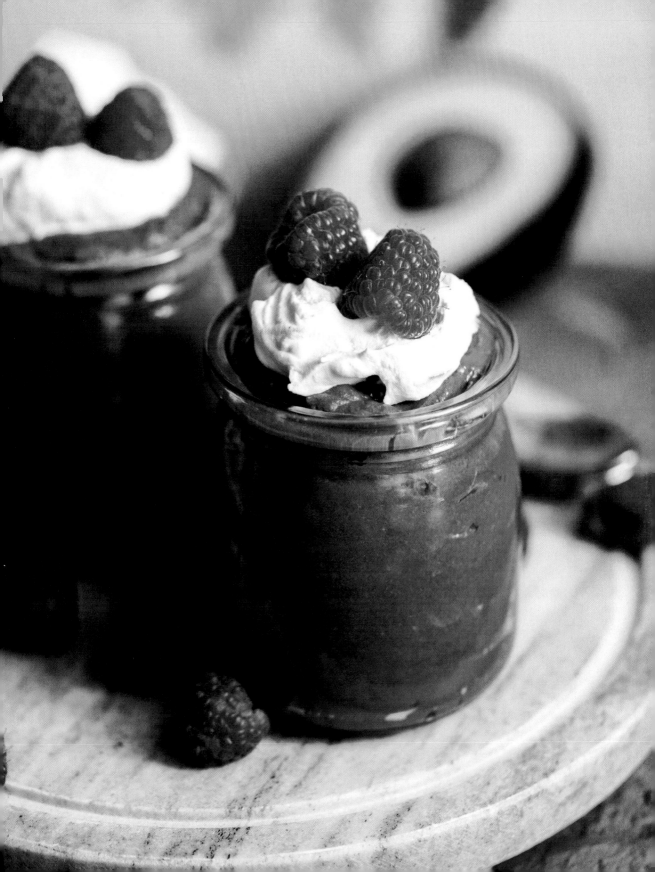

Watermelon-Lime Gummies

EGG-FREE, NIGHTSHADE-FREE, NUT-FREE

Gummies are a nutrient-dense snack that serve as a fun (and tasty) way to get more of the gut-healing benefits of gelatin into your diet. You can use a variety of silicone candy molds to make these gummies look like stars, hearts, gummy bears, or even Legos—so let your inner child come out and get creative!

Makes 8 servings (24 or more gummies, depending on mold size)

Prep time: **20 minutes, plus 2 hours chilling time**

Cooking time: **none**

1. If you're using watermelon chunks, place them in a blender and blend until liquefied. Strain the juice through a fine-mesh strainer and discard the pulp. Skim any white foam off the top of the strained juice and discard.

2. In a medium saucepan, combine the watermelon juice, lime juice, and honey and whisk over medium-low heat until combined. The mixture should be hot but not boiling.

3. While whisking, slowly add the gelatin to the saucepan, sprinkling it in 1 tablespoon at a time. Continue until the gelatin has completely dissolved, 5 to 7 minutes. Avoid adding the gelatin too quickly, which will result in larger clumps that are difficult to incorporate.

4. Remove the pan from the heat and pour the mixture into silicone candy molds set on a baking sheet (see tip). Refrigerate until firm, about 2 hours.

5. Pop the gummies out of the molds and store in an airtight container in the refrigerator for up to 1 week.

4 cups fresh watermelon chunks, or 2 cups 100 percent watermelon juice
½ cup fresh lime juice
¼ cup raw honey
6 tablespoons grass-fed gelatin

Special equipment: Silicone candy mold(s)

Noelle's tip: You can also pour the mixture into an 8 x 8-inch glass baking dish, refrigerate it until firm, 2 or 3 hours, then cut it into small squares.

Change it up: Swap out the lime juice for fresh lemon juice.

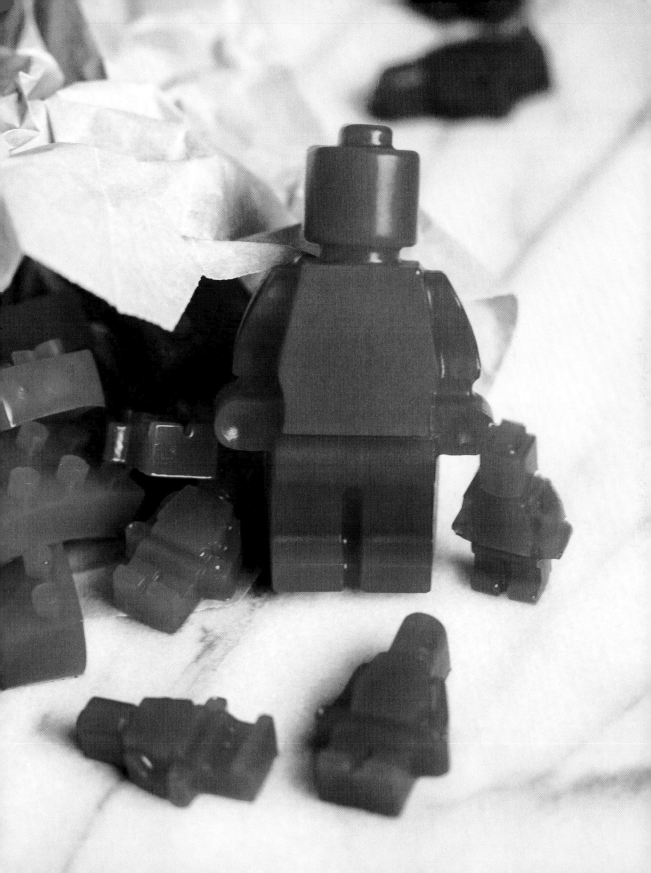

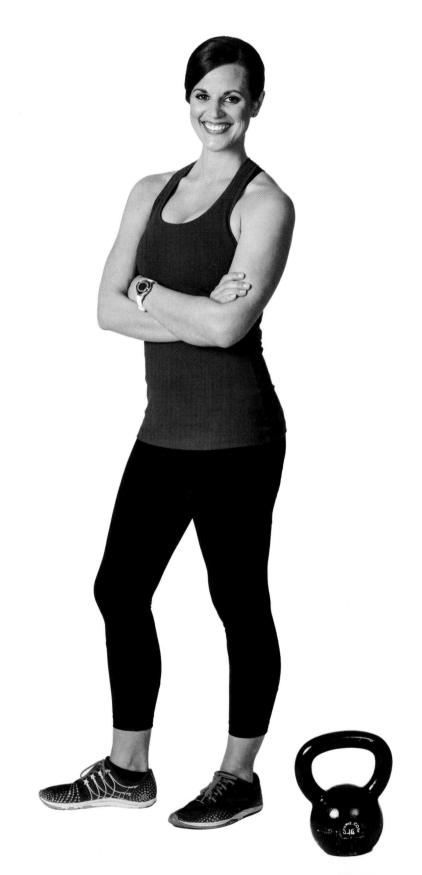

12

THE COCONUTS AND KETTLEBELLS
FITNESS PLAN

While this may come as a surprise, workouts don't have to be hard, time-consuming, or unenjoyable to be effective. In fact, you can build strength and improve your body's functional capacity just about anywhere with workouts that easily fit into your schedule. Sound too good to be true? The good news is—it's not. By ditching the idea that there is only *one* way to get fit, and instead pursuing what you enjoy and what works best for you, you'll be able to create a sustainable fitness plan that flows with your changing desires and needs.

You may notice this approach is incredibly similar to the recommendations made in Part I about how to figure out what macronutrient ratios and specific foods work best for your body. This is because bioindividuality—or the idea that you respond uniquely to different inputs depending on your genetics, background, and lifestyle—plays into *everything*, including your fitness. If a fitness program doesn't serve you physically, mentally, or emotionally, there's nothing wrong with you. It's simply a sign that whatever you're doing isn't the best fit. With this change in thinking, "shoulds" and shame take a back seat to "What is going to serve my body today?" What *will* serve your body on a given day will depend on a variety of factors, including your experience level, time constraints, injuries, current health conditions, sleep quality, and overall stress. All of these things can fluctuate both in the short and long term, which makes flexibility a necessary part of the pursuit of fitness.

With the Coconuts and Kettlebells Fitness Plan, you'll create a template that is structured and easy to follow while also learning how to incorporate the appropriate amount of flexibility when needed. By engaging with fitness in this way, it becomes a part of you. Depending on the day, movement can be restorative, a way to play and have fun, or an opportunity to push yourself and explore new boundaries. Your fitness template will serve as the perfect complement to the nutrition plan you chose to follow and the mind-set shifts you make as you pursue health. Instead of seeing health and fitness as a destination to be achieved, you'll be able to focus on the journey—and enjoy the process.

WHY MOVEMENT MATTERS

Before diving into the details of the plan, it's important to understand the benefits of movement. In recent years, the fitness industry has become inundated with special products, programs, and challenges that promise quick results and lasting happiness. By helping you get the "perfect" butt and achieve "a tight and toned midsection in 14 days!," you are guaranteed to *finally* love your body. While it's not always easy to see, these claims are designed to make you feel shame and judgment for not looking a specific way. If you believe you are inferior or not good enough, there's a good chance you'll buy whatever is being marketed and sold—no matter how unrealistic it seems. Unfortunately, these "solutions" have nothing to do with health and leave people feeling less happy with themselves than when they started.

Pursuing fitness because it makes your body healthy, strong, and resilient facilitates a much more empowering mind-set. Looking at the bigger picture, it's clear that movement positively impacts nearly every bodily system. Yes, regular exercise increases lean body mass and strengthens muscles and bones. But it also changes the way your genes function, including the ones that play a role in energy metabolism, insulin response, and inflammation. In addition to being able to carry all the groceries into the house in one trip, you'll also be better equipped to combat diseases such as cancer and depression. Here are some of the biggest reasons to make exercise a part of your weekly routine.

1. EXERCISE PREVENTS DISEASE

Regular exercise reduces your risk of developing a number of health conditions, including heart disease, cancer, Alzheimer's, and dementia. By decreasing chronic inflammation, it also helps the immune system fight off colds and other infections.

2. EXERCISE SUPPORTS MENTAL HEALTH

When you exercise, your brain releases neurotransmitters such as dopamine, norepinephrine, and serotonin. These chemical messengers improve cognitive function and boost overall mood. By changing your brain chemistry in both the short and long term, exercise can help combat anxiety and depression.

3. EXERCISE IMPROVES SLEEP

Exercise helps you fall asleep faster, improves sleep quality, and increases sleep duration. Given what we know about the importance of sleep, this can affect everything from alertness and productivity to tissue growth and repair.

4. EXERCISE MITIGATES STRESS

In appropriate doses, exercise releases endorphins, relaxes muscles, and relieves tension. It also provides an outlet for dealing with anxiety and worry, which improves your ability to cope with mental and emotional stress.

5. EXERCISE BUILDS CONFIDENCE

One of the most powerful benefits of exercise is improved self-esteem. It helps you feel empowered by what your body *does*, which is much more impactful than simply focusing on the way it looks. Engaging with activities that allow you explore what you can do makes you more confident in other areas of your life.

HOW TO USE THE COCONUTS AND KETTLEBELLS FITNESS PLAN

To help you engage with fitness in the way that works best for you, the plan has two components. First, you'll learn how to create your own fitness plan using easy-to-follow guidelines. The plan you create will serve as a template you can use long-term, as you'll be able to make adjustments to it when your goals change or you progress in your fitness. The second component is three done-for-you fitness plans you can start following immediately. Each four-week plan is designed to improve overall fitness according to your experience level and is great to do alongside the 4x4. You can use either of these options when pursuing fitness, or a combination of both. For example, you may chose to follow one of the four-week plans initially, and create your own template to follow after that. Do what works best for you and helps you move toward your goals.

CREATING YOUR OWN PLAN

Creating a fitness plan that is balanced, effective, and exciting begins with the star of the show—*you!* This means that how much, how often, and what you do as part of your workout routine may look different from what someone else is doing, and that's perfectly okay. Constantly comparing yourself to others or your "former" self does nothing more than cloud your ability to listen to your body. To achieve success, the best thing you can do is what fits your current needs and abilities. If that means simply doing one or two workouts per week, then that's a great place to start. Progress occurs in small, incremental shifts and doesn't need to be forced.

To create a plan that incorporates the right amount of stress for your body so that progress can occur, there are four key elements to consider: frequency, dose, type, and rest.

I. FREQUENCY

The first thing to determine when creating your own template is how many days you'll work out per week. While many things will affect how often you work out, a good place to start is your experience level. Here are some basic guidelines to follow when assessing how often you should be exposing your body to exercise:

- *2 or 3 workouts per week:* You're relatively new to working out or have taken an extended period of time off (more than 6 months) from any exercise.

- *3 or 4 workouts per week:* You've been working out for at least 6 months and have experience with low- to medium-intensity training.

- *4 or 5 workouts per week:* You've been working out for at least 12 months and have experience with high-intensity workouts and strength training.

A workout can be one from this book or another activity you enjoy doing that focuses on strength or conditioning, such as cycling or a group fitness class. (For more information about workout type, see page 275.) Your workout frequency may be slightly different from these guidelines if you have goals outside of improved health and fitness or certain limitations, such as injuries or chronic health conditions. Also, the number of times you work out each week may fluctuate, and that's perfectly okay. If you were able to get in only one or two workouts a few weeks in a row because of time constraints or additional stress, your efforts have *not* been in vain. To maintain fitness, your body needs consistent exposure to activity only in small doses. Focus on doing what you can, and increase the number of times you work out per week back to baseline when you are able to.

2. DOSE

Dose is simply the duration of your workouts. While fitness memes may convey otherwise, you do *not* need to "push through pain" or keep going until you "puke, faint, or die" in order to build fitness and strength. Furthermore, you don't need to work out for hours a day to see results. Studies show that doing shorter bouts of intense training greatly improves both aerobic and anaerobic capacity and increases lean body mass. We're talking *four-minutes-total* kind of short. This doesn't mean you should do only high-intensity workouts, or that longer, less-intense training isn't beneficial. It simply means that shorter workouts can be powerful and effective, especially when your time is limited. In short, there is no such thing as *"It's not worth it unless I can spend at least thirty minutes working out."* When pursuing fitness, assess the time you have and focus on making the most of that time.

AEROBIC CAPACITY: The maximum amount of oxygen the body can use while exercising. The more you exercise, the more efficient your cardiorespiratory system becomes and the more oxygen your body can utilize during workouts. This translates into being able to work out harder and longer.

ANAEROBIC CAPACITY: The maximum amount of energy the body can use *without* oxygen. You use your anaerobic system during short, intense exercise bouts. The more high-intensity activity you do, the quicker your muscles will be able to recover after hard lifting or sprint efforts and the more you'll be able to maintain speed and intensity.

A concept called the minimum effective dose can provide insight when assessing what dose is right for your body. The minimum effective dose is simply the smallest dose that will produce a desired outcome. An example of this concept can be found in boiling water. Water boils at 212°F at sea level. Applying more heat to water doesn't make it "boil more," and heat applied beyond what is needed to boil the water is redundant. When pursuing fitness, the minimum effective dose recognizes that workouts are a form of stress and that exposing your body to more of it comes at a price. This is especially true if you're already under a lot of stress in other areas of life. The body perceives all stress the same—whether it's from work, family issues, or workouts. By being intentional and purposeful with workout time, you'll eliminate unnecessary stress, which will allow you to recover and make adaptations more efficiently. In short, more is not inherently better, nor does it always lead to "more" results.

How to Find Your Ideal Dose

1. After figuring out which days are best for you to work out, determine how much time you have to dedicate to each workout.

2. Choose either a workout from this book or another workout you enjoy that is specific to your goals and can be completed within your allotted time. Remember to also give yourself sufficient time to warm up and cool down.

3. If you have more time after the workout is completed, add a few mobility exercises that target your problem areas (see page 303).

3. TYPE

The type of workouts you choose to do will vary based on what you enjoy and your goals. In this book, workouts are categorized as strength workouts or conditioning workouts. Of course, many workouts facilitate adaptations in both areas; however, each category provides guidance as to which type is dominant. As a general baseline, if your goal is to improve overall health and fitness, you'll want to include a combination of strength and conditioning workouts each week. This will keep your workouts varied by challenging your body in different ways. Here are some basic guidelines to follow regarding what type of workouts to do each week depending on your workout frequency:

- 2 workouts per week ⟶ 1 strength workout, 1 conditioning workout
- 3 workouts per week ⟶ 2 strength workouts, 1 conditioning workout
- 4 workouts per week ⟶ 2 strength workouts, 2 conditioning workouts
- 5 workouts per week ⟶ 3 strength workouts, 2 conditioning workouts

If you have more specific goals or needs, you can shift the workouts you do to include more of one type of workout. For example, if you'd like to focus on building upper body strength, you can include more strength workouts in your routine. Or if you'd like to focus on being able to run three miles without stopping, you can include more conditioning workouts in your routine. Over time, the type of workouts you do will fluctuate as you pursue new goals and achieve them. This is a great way to pursue fitness long term and make improvements in a progressive, balanced way.

STRENGTH WORKOUTS: use resistance to make muscles, bones, joints, tendons, and ligaments stronger. For strength workouts, you'll use more challenging weights and perform repetitions with control.

CONDITIONING WORKOUTS: use structured patterns of work and rest periods to build aerobic and anaerobic capacity. In this book, conditioning workouts are typically higher in intensity and incorporate functional movements. As a result, you'll be using moderate loads in order to perform repetitions faster.

ADDING OTHER WORKOUTS

The workouts in this book are efficient and easy to do at home. While they are incredibly effective, they are by no means your only option for building fitness. For a fitness plan to be exciting and sustainable and serve you long term, it's important to include other types of movement you enjoy doing. This could include everything from martial arts to a pole-dancing class. If you're new to fitness, finding activities you enjoy may take some time and experimentation. A great place to start is to ask friends, family, or neighbors what they enjoy and would recommend. When trying a new activity, give yourself at least a week or two to get acclimated before deciding if it's right for you or not. Often, once you become more familiar with something, you start to gain confidence and have fun doing it.

When adding another workout, simply plug it into your template according to what category it best fits under. If the workout demands intensity or includes periods of working hard and resting, it can be categorized as a *conditioning workout*. Some examples of conditioning workouts include CrossFit, indoor cycling, kickboxing, dancing, or playing soccer. If the workout exposes your body to challenging loads, it can be categorized as a *strength workout*. This could include weight training at the gym, a gymnastics class, Olympic lifting, TRX training, or Pilates.

RESTORATIVE MOVEMENT

An additional type of activity that will greatly benefit your body is restorative movement. Restorative movement helps to reduce pain, improve recovery, and mitigate stress. Examples include walking, gentle yoga, and mobility exercises (see page 303). You can do this type of movement the same day as your workouts, on rest days, or in place of a workout if your body needs more time to recover. During more stressful times, you can also shift to doing only restorative movement for as long as you need to until your body is ready to take on more vigorous activity. As a general recommendation, it's best to do some type of restorative movement one to three times a week. Think of it as an opportunity to add nourishment to your joints, muscles, and bones, and to improve your body's functional capacity. Restorative movement, like walking, has been shown to increase range of motion and circulation, improve mental health, boost immune function, and clear out accumulated waste product. For this reason, you will benefit from doing it whenever you want for as long as you like.

4. REST

Rest is one of the most important aspects of a fitness plan because it allows your body to adapt to the training it has been exposed to. In other words, training doesn't make you stronger—your *rest* does. Yes, there must be exposure to adequate intensity and frequency of training to initiate adaptation. But without appropriate rest, the body is unable to rebuild and repair the damage that has occurred. In short, to facilitate adaptation, work and rest have to be in balance. If you rest too much in between workouts, progress won't occur and you'll likely experience regular soreness. If you rest too little in between workouts, you'll eventually experience some of the signs and symptoms of overtraining, including decreased performance, sleep disturbances, decreased lean body mass, adrenal insufficiency, loss of motivation, mood disturbances such as depression and anxiety, or increased muscle soreness. Because overtraining has a high degree of variability and occurs gradually, it's easy to overlook. What your body needs will be unique to you and will fluctuate with your changing circumstances.

For many people, going "off plan" and taking an unscheduled rest day is hard to do. Most of us find comfort in having a routine, especially when improvements are happening and goals are being reached. Additionally, the conventional fitness industry has made "skipping" a workout seem like something you should feel shame or guilt for. Because of this, many people perceive that their self-worth as a human being is intertwined with their ability to maintain a workout plan. And if that's you, I have incredibly great news for you. Your self-worth as a human being is *not* related to your ability to follow a workout plan perfectly as prescribed. Furthermore, you are not a "good" or "bad" person based on the workouts you do or don't do. Some weeks, you'll need more rest than others—and that's perfectly okay. Stress is cumulative, and if your body is under stress from other areas of life, it may not respond positively to workouts.

While following the frequency guidelines on page 272 will help you establish a baseline for balancing workouts with rest, here are five questions that will help you determine if an extra rest day or two is a good idea:

1. ARE YOU EXCESSIVELY SORE?

Experiencing muscle soreness or tightness that inhibits proper mobility is a sign your muscles aren't ready to experience additional stress.

2. DO YOU HAVE A NAGGING PAIN?

The appearance of pain or a "twinge" that won't resolve, especially in the low back, knee, ankle, or foot, may indicate excessive inflammation and the need for more time to repair.

3. DO YOU FEEL WEAK OR "OFF"?

Decreased performance is one of the most common signs of overtraining. When your warm-up weight starts to feel like your max, or a 200-meter run feels like a mile, it's a good sign it's time to shift to a rest day (or week).

4. ARE YOU FEELING NOT THAT INTO IT?

Loss of interest, enthusiasm, and motivation for performing workouts you genuinely enjoy doing typically means it's time to take a step back. Generally, a few days off will help ignite excitement again.

5. ARE YOU OVERLY FATIGUED OR DRAINED?

The cumulative effective of a couple of bad nights of sleep, a big project at work, and family drama can expose the body to a high amount of stress in a short period of time. Adding a workout will likely push the body to experience a demand it's not capable of managing. Taking an extra day or two and prioritizing recovery and sleep is great during these times.

If you're relatively new to fitness, err on the side of rest if you answer yes to any of these questions. As you become more experienced with understanding how your body responds to fitness demands, you'll have a better idea of when you should push it and when you shouldn't.

READY, SET, GOAL!

Goals are incredibly helpful at providing vision and direction when making decisions about what you want to accomplish long term. They can boost short-term motivation and help you organize your resources and time. In order for goals to be effective, they do *not* need to be overly complicated or limiting. In fact, the best way to establish your goals is to first take a step back and figure out *why* you want to achieve the things you do. The why behind your desire to complete a goal is a powerful motivator. When you take your focus off of the *what* and connect it with your why, your goal takes on a life of its own. You're connected to the purpose rather than to the action itself.

To figure out your why, simply write down two or three general things you hope to accomplish with the Coconuts and Kettlebells Fitness Plan. Now ask yourself why it is you want to achieve those things. If it helps, write this down as well. Then take your answer and ask yourself why again. Continue to ask yourself why with each answer you give until you've done it a total of five times. Once you do, you will have gotten to the heart of your desire. For example, if you'd like to become stronger and build stamina, you may discover your final why is to spend more quality time playing outside with your kids.

When going through this process, be honest with yourself. It's easy to give the answer you think you should because you perceive it's the "right" one. By allowing yourself to dig deeper and evaluate the reasons behind your desires, you may find what you want changes. Once you've successfully developed your why, write it down on a sticky note and place it somewhere prominent. Connect with your why once a week and use it to evaluate whether a specific action or decision is aligned with your end goal.

Once you've figured out your why, it's time to create a few goals for yourself. First, create one long-term goal you'd like to achieve in the next six to twelve months. This should be related to your why, but more specific and measurable. Second, create one short-term goal you'd like to achieve in the next one to three months. Your short-term goal should be a stepping stone to achieving your long-term goal. For example, your short-term goal may be to perform your first modified push-up in six weeks, while your long-term goal is to do five regular push-ups in six to eight months. Your why behind your goals might be to feel stronger and more confident in your ability to defend yourself.

Just because you've created goals for yourself doesn't mean your success is now defined by whether you achieve them or not. Your goals are simply meant to focus your efforts and give you markers for measuring progress. You have the freedom to change your goals at any time based on the feedback your body is giving you. If you end up dealing with an unexpected injury or find that your body needs more time to adapt, you can shift your goals accordingly. Being flexible in this way allows you to see fitness as a *journey* rather than a destination. It gives you the freedom to celebrate small wins, and reevaluate your goals along the way instead of getting hung up on something that may not be right for you. In this environment, progress occurs gradually and with ease.

HOW TO TRACK YOUR PROGRESS

When you follow a fitness plan, tracking your progress gives you feedback about your efforts. Because progress occurs in small, incremental shifts, if you don't intentionally track your progress, you're likely to miss the improvements you are making. This can lead to loss of motivation, discouragement, and jumping from one plan to the next, which can inhibit progress altogether. To give you a clear picture of whether your plan is helping you achieve your goals, here are four measurable components of fitness you can track and evaluate regularly.

1. VOLUME

The number of workouts you're able to maintain each week. For example, if you perform three workouts per week and eventually work up to maintaining four workouts per week, that's measurable progress. If you're limited to a set number of workouts each week, you could also assess the total time spent working out. Going from doing three 20-minute workouts per week to three 30-minute workouts per week is also an increase in volume.

2. STRENGTH

How much force (weight in pounds or kilograms) your muscles can exert. In essence, this is the weight you're able to use in workouts. If you use a 12kg kettlebell for a workout and two months later use a 16kg kettlebell for the same workout, your strength has improved.

3. ENDURANCE

The number of repetitions you're able to do. This could include the number of push-ups or squats you're able to do within a given time period, how far you can run without stopping, or the number of sprints you can do in a specific workout.

4. SPEED

The rate at which you're able to perform a specific task. For example, you may perform a workout two minutes faster than you once did or cover more ground during a thirty-second sprint.

A Word on the Scale

$\mathcal{M}$any people make the mistake of using only the scale to track progress. The truth is, the scale doesn't show the status of your health or fitness or changes in lean body mass. Unfortunately, when the scale is the only marker of success, small fluctuations in weight can result in unnecessary stress, anxiety, and feelings of defeat, and the manipulation of a number becomes more important than improving the health of the body. This is why it's so important to track a variety of metrics that can be compiled to present a clearer picture. While numbers can be helpful for establishing a starting point, regular assessment of physical weight can be incredibly misleading. Your self-worth and success are not defined by a number, and health and happiness don't all of a sudden appear at a certain weight. Focusing on all the ways in which your quality of life is improving will allow you to focus on the journey rather than treating health as a destination.

In addition to tracking the metrics from your workouts, it's also important to assess how you feel overall. Do you have more energy? Are you less fatigued? Are you sleeping better? Recording how you feel before and after your workouts and making note of how your daily tasks are being impacted will help you assess these changes. While sometimes overlooked, small improvements in managing day-to-day activities is the result of your body becoming more capable.

To help you track your progress, you can download my free Coconuts and Kettlebells Progress Tracker at coconutsandkettlebells.com/bookdownloads.

EQUIPMENT GUIDE

All the workouts in the Coconuts and Kettlebells Fitness Plan use two specific tools: your body and kettlebells. As a result, the workouts are easy to implement and cost-effective. If you're new to kettlebells and plan to do these workouts at home, here's a quick rundown of what you'll need.

I. KETTLEBELLS

A kettlebell is a weighted ball with a flat bottom and a handle on top. They come in a variety of sizes and are used to build strength, power, and endurance. Kettlebells are incredibly versatile due to their shape and how you can manipulate them. They can be pressed, held, swung, thrown, and moved in hundreds of ways. When used properly, they teach the body how to move better by improving mobility, range of motion, and stability. Kettlebells are traditionally made from iron or steel and sold in 4kg weight increments.

WHICH WEIGHTS SHOULD YOU BUY?

If you're totally new to kettlebells or have limited experience with strength training, I recommend first purchasing a kettlebell that is around 8kg (or 17 pounds). Your first kettlebell will be what you use to learn different movements, including both upper- and lower-body movements. A good way to gauge how this will feel is to hold a 15-pound dumbbell in your hand at the gym or a sporting goods store. See how the weight feels and make sure you're comfortable pressing it overhead and stepping back into a lunge with it in your hand.

If you have experience with kettlebells and/or strength training, I recommend purchasing a 12kg (26-pound) kettlebell as your first kettlebell. This weight will be great for most upper- and total-body movements. As you become more proficient in kettlebell movements, you can purchase a 16kg (35-pound) or 20kg (44-pound) kettlebell as your second kettlebell for total- and lower-body movements. Purchasing a third kettlebell that weighs at least 24kg (52 pounds) for lower-body movements is great if you plan to get more serious about kettlebell training and want to work out exclusively at home.

Because kettlebells are growing in popularity, they are now available at some larger sporting goods stores. They are also available online from vendors like CFF Fit (cfffit.com) and Dragon Door (dragondoor.com), which offer high-quality kettlebells that have a money-back guarantee or lifetime warranty. I recommend getting classic cast-iron kettlebells over vinyl or plastic varieties, which tend to be less durable and have inconsistent sizing.

2. MAT

Although the purpose of an exercise mat is self-explanatory, it's a must-have when doing workouts at home. A high-quality, comfortable mat will allow you to perform stretches, mobility exercises, and other workout activities on a variety of surfaces, including tile and wood flooring, asphalt, or concrete. For high-intensity training and kettlebell workouts, I recommend getting an interlockng exercise mat, which can be found at sporting goods stores or online through retailers like Amazon. These mats provide a larger space to work out on (six tiles typically cover 24 square feet), and they stay put during workouts.

3. GYM CHALK

When using kettlebells, a little gym chalk goes a long way. While you'll likely be fine without this in the beginning, as you move on to doing more challenging workouts, gym chalk will help you maintain your grip on the kettlebell. This is especially important when it's hot or you're sweating a lot. A block of gym chalk can be found at most sporting goods stores or online through retailers like CFF Fit or Amazon.

For direct links to the fitness products I recommend, go to coconutsandkettlebells .com/bookresources.

THE EXTRAS

While these items aren't needed to complete the workouts in the Coconuts and Kettlebells Fitness Plan, here are a few extra fitness tools you may find valuable when doing workouts at home.

1. FOAM ROLLER

Foam rollers are cylinders of high-density foam that allow you to do self-massage on your muscles and soft tissue. Using the weight of your body, foam rolling can be used to increase blood flow and loosen up tight muscles prior to activity, or to work out tightness and areas of pain post-workout. It's also a great technique for opening the thoracic spine. I recommend purchasing The Grid from TriggerPoint Therapy, as it's durable and won't compress over time. If you're on a budget, a simple high-density foam roller will do the trick.

2. MASSAGE STICK

Much like foam rollers, massage sticks allow you to do self-massage on your muscles and soft tissue. However, instead of using your body weight, you apply pressure by manipulating the stick across a muscle. Massage sticks are great for working out "kinks" or tightness in the neck, quads, calves, and IT (iliotibial) band. The Stick and Addaday are my two favorite brands; however, you can find many different varieties at sporting good stores or from online retailers like Amazon.

3. PLYO BOX

A plyometric (plyo) box is a versatile piece of equipment that can be used for strength and plyometric exercises. You can use it to perform movements like step-ups, elevated push-ups, and box jumps. I recommend getting a 3-in-1 plyo box, which is the most stable and can be positioned on different sides to create a variety of heights. Both wood and cushioned plyo boxes are available from online retailers like CFF Fit. If you're on a budget, fixed or adjustable plyo boxes can be found in a variety of heights at sporting good stores or from online retailers like Amazon.

WHAT TO EAT BEFORE AND AFTER YOUR WORKOUTS

As long as you're consuming nutrient-dense foods and eating sufficient calories, your body will have the resources it needs to support your workouts. This doesn't mean what you eat before and after your workouts is irrelevant; it simply means the strategies you use will depend on your lifestyle and schedule. To help you figure out what is going to work best for you, here are some general workout nutrition guidelines.

PRE-WORKOUT NUTRITION

The food you consume before your workout helps to ward off hunger and sustain your energy levels during your workout. Your pre-workout meal can be the last meal you ate or a small snack consumed shortly before your workout. Let's look at your three main options for pre-workout meal timing.

Option 1: Train while fasting

You work out first thing in the morning before breakfast and do not eat beforehand. This works great for people who need to work out very early, and when they work out, and for people who are more prone to GI distress during workouts. As long as you've supplied your body with sufficient calories the day before and are doing a workout from this book or similar (under an hour), this is a great option to experiment with.

Option 2: Consume a small snack 30 to 60 minutes before your workout

You work out in the morning before breakfast or several hours after a meal. While the exact timing will be individual to you, if it's been at least 3 to 4 hours since you ate a meal, eating a small snack 30 to 60 minutes prior to your workout can help boost your energy and performance.

Option 3: Consume a meal 2 to 3 hours before your workout

You work out midmorning, midafternoon, or at night after a meal. Working out 2 to 3 hours after one of your typical meals (breakfast, lunch, or dinner) gives your body enough time to digest your food and will leave you feeling energized and ready to go.

PRE-WORKOUT SNACK OPTIONS

When eating a pre-workout snack, start with a small serving of protein and add a high-quality source of fat and/or carbohydrates, depending on your individual needs and what makes you feel best during your workouts. Adjust your serving size according to how much time you have until your workout, how hungry you are, and the length of your upcoming workout.

If you tend to thrive following a higher-fat approach, try:

- 1 hard-boiled egg with sliced avocado or a few nuts
- 1 or 2 Bacon-Wrapped Eggs (page 146)
- Small serving of Apple, Avocado, and Chicken Salad (page 177)

If you tend to thrive following a higher-carbohydrate approach, try:

- 1 hard-boiled egg with fresh fruit
- 1 or 2 Chocolate-Cherry Energy Bites (page 172)
- Small serving of Apple Bacon Sweet Potato Hash (page 140)

POST-WORKOUT NUTRITION

After a workout, your body kick-starts a number of physiological processes in order to return to a resting state and create adaptations so it can handle the same amount of stress more easily in the future. During this time, the body becomes a nutrient-processing powerhouse, as replenishing and repairing muscle tissue requires a variety of resources. While it was once assumed that you must eat within thirty minutes of completing a workout to give the body what it needs, recent research has shown that for the majority of people, the magic isn't in the timing. What matters are the total calories and nutrients you eat throughout the day.

In other words, your post-workout meal is an opportunity to add to your overall intake of protein, carbohydrates, and fat, which will supply your body with the resources it needs to recover from your workouts.

What and how much you eat after a workout will depend on when your last meal was, and the volume and intensity of your training. Here are some basic guidelines to follow when creating a template that works for you.

Option 1: Consume a post-workout snack

If you ate a meal a couple of hours prior to your workout, a small post-workout snack is a great way to get in necessary nutrients and will hold you over until your next meal.

Option 2: Consume a post-workout meal

If your pre-workout meal was several hours before your workout or was a small one, eating a post-workout meal afterward is a good idea. If you worked out first thing in the morning and didn't eat beforehand, make it a priority to get in a sufficient meal shortly after your workout.

SHOULD YOU EAT MORE CARBS OR PROTEIN?

When doing longer, higher-intensity workouts, your need for carbohydrates increases. Because of this, you'll want to include a good whack of carbohydrates in your post-workout snack or meal. As a general guideline, start with a 2:1 ratio of carbohydrates to protein. This means that if you consume 20 grams of protein, you'll want to consume 40 grams (or more) of carbohydrates. When doing shorter or strength-focused workouts, focus on consuming sufficient protein post-workout. While you'll still want to consume carbohydrates, intentionally upping your intake is less important.

POST-WORKOUT SNACK OPTIONS

When eating a post-workout snack, include whole-food sources of protein and carbohydrates. Good sources of protein include those that are high in essential amino acids, such as meat, poultry, seafood, and eggs. For carbohydrates, you can choose from a variety of starchy vegetables and fruit, including potatoes, squash, plantains, bananas, apples, and berries. Here are a few ideas for post-workout snack combinations:

- 1 or 2 hard-boiled eggs plus fresh fruit

- Meat (such as shredded cooked chicken or roast beef) plus an apple

- Chicken-Sage Meatballs (page 206) plus a baked sweet potato

- On the go? Try grass-fed jerky plus dried fruit and nuts

When Nutrient Timing *Is* Important

*T*here are two special cases when eating shortly after a workout is important. First, if you're training fasted, you'll want to consume your post-workout meal soon after your workout as it will have a direct impact on your body's ability to switch "on" muscle protein synthesis—or the rebuilding of muscle tissue. Second, if you're an endurance athlete or training multiple times a day, quickly restoring lost glycogen (carbohydrates) is critical to your next training session.

BUSTING POST-WORKOUT NUTRITION MYTHS

CONVENTIONAL WISDOM	THE EVIDENCE
"Protein shakes work best post-workout because they are easy to digest and fast-acting."	While protein shakes are convenient, there is no real evidence that shows protein powders, especially fast-acting ones, are superior to whole foods post-workout.
"You shouldn't eat fruit post-workout, as fructose is sent to the liver to be processed first. Instead, eat starchy carbohydrates, such as sweet potatoes."	Fruit is perfectly acceptable to eat post-workout. In fact, research suggests that consuming a combination of glucose and fructose is superior to other foods because it is better tolerated and just as effective at replenishing muscle glycogen over a 24-hour period. Rapid replenishment of muscle glycogen is important only if you train multiple times a day.
"Don't include fat in your post-workout meal, as it slows digestion and will inhibit muscle protein synthesis."	While fat does slow digestion, the speed at which your post-workout meal is digested is not as important as once thought. In fact, preliminary research suggests that fat does not get in the way of glycogen replenishment and may increase the utilization of amino acids for muscle protein synthesis.

THE 4-WEEK COCONUTS AND KETTLEBELLS FITNESS PLANS

The three 4-week plans included in this book are designed to help you improve your fitness according to the following experience levels:

- *Beginner:* You're relatively new to working out or have taken an extended period of time off (more than 6 months) from any exercise.

- *Intermediate:* You've been working out for at least 6 months and have experience with low- to medium-intensity training.

- *Advanced:* You've been working out for at least 8 to 12 months and have experience with high-intensity workouts and strength training.

When following one of the fitness plans, feel free to shift the workouts to different days according to what works best for your schedule. Also, no matter what your experience level is, modify the workouts if necessary. Many workouts come with Modified Workout Guidelines. In addition to the workouts prescribed in each plan, make sure to add restorative movement, such as mobility exercises or walking, one to three times a week (see page 276 for more information about restorative movement). You can do restorative movement on the days you work out or on rest days.

- For a complete list of workouts, categorized by estimated time to complete, see pages 308–329.

- For step-by-step instructions on how to perform each exercise listed in the workouts, see pages 291–304.

4-Week Beginner Fitness Plan

SUNDAY	MONDAY	TUESDAY	WEDNESDAY	THURSDAY	FRIDAY	SATURDAY	TIME
	Center Field 10 minutes (page 311)		Bear Hug 15 minutes (page 313)		Strong-Arm 15 minutes (page 316)		40 minutes
	Spicy Meatball 15 minutes (page 312)		Leggings 20 minutes (page 321)		Desert Island 10 minutes (page 309)		45 minutes
	Center Field 10 minutes (page 311)		Rear-Ended 20 minutes (page 320)		Strong-Arm 15 minutes (page 316)		45 minutes
	Ring the Bell 20 minutes (page 319)		Leggings 20 minutes (page 321)		Fire Starter 15 minutes (page 315)		55 minutes

4-Week Intermediate Fitness Plan

SUNDAY	MONDAY	TUESDAY	WEDNESDAY	THURSDAY	FRIDAY	SATURDAY	TIME
	Leggings 20 minutes (page 321)		Bear Hug 15 minutes (page 313)		Muscle Tee 20 minutes (page 322)	Don't Let Go 10 minutes (page 310)	65 minutes
	Stella-r 15 minutes (page 314)		Gripping 20 minutes (page 323)		Rear-Ended 20 minutes (page 320)	Moving Day 10 minutes (page 311)	65 minutes
	Leggings 20 minutes (page 321)		Ring the Bell 20 minutes (page 319)		Muscle Tee 20 minutes (page 322)	Desert Island 10 minutes (page 309)	70 minutes
	Bruh 20 minutes (page 318)		Gripping 20 minutes (page 323)		Moved to Tears 30 minutes (page 325)	Center Field 10 minutes (page 311)	80 minutes

4-Week Advanced Fitness Plan

SUNDAY	MONDAY	TUESDAY	WEDNESDAY	THURSDAY	FRIDAY	SATURDAY	TIME
	Full Strength 30 minutes (page 327)		Bear Hug 15 minutes (page 313)		No Filter 30 minutes (page 328)	What the 10 minutes (page 310)	85 minutes
	Fabulous 40 30 minutes (page 324)		Kettlebell Complex 30 minutes (page 329)		Big Time 10 minutes (page 308)	Strong-Arm 15 minutes (page 316)	85 minutes
	Full Strength 30 minutes (page 327)		Rear-Ended 20 minutes (page 320)		No Filter 30 minutes (page 328)	Desert Island 10 minutes (page 309)	90 minutes
	Tower of Terror 30 minutes (page 326)		Kettlebell Complex 30 minutes (page 329)		Stella-r 15 minutes (page 314)	Leggings 20 minutes (page 321)	95 minutes

THE EXERCISES

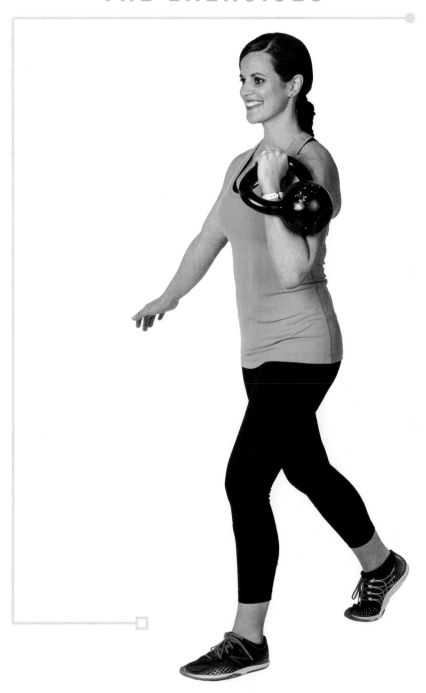

SHOULDER SWINGS

Front/Back

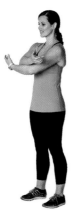 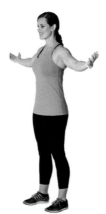

Up/Down

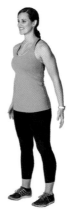 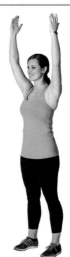

1. Keeping your shoulders completely relaxed and your elbows soft, swing your arms across the front of your body with your palms facing up.

2. Swing your arms open to a comfortable position that provides a light stretch in your chest. Repeat.

1. Keeping your shoulders completely relaxed and your elbows soft, swing your arms down by your side and slightly behind you.

2. Swing your arms up overhead to a comfortable position that provides a light stretch in your shoulders. Repeat.

KICKS

Front/Back

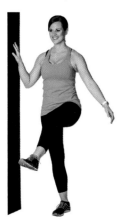 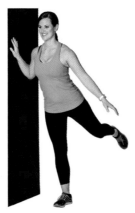

Side/Side

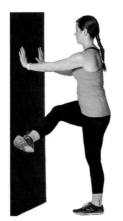 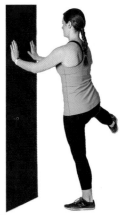

1. Using the wall for stability, lightly kick one foot forward in front of your body. Keep your ankle and knee soft.

2. Swing your leg backward to a comfortable position that provides a light stretch in your hip. Repeat as necessary and perform with the opposite leg.

1. Using the wall for stability, lightly kick one foot across your body in front of you. Keep your ankle and knee soft.

2. Swing your leg open to the opposite side to a comfortable position until you feel a light stretch in your groin. Repeat as necessary and perform with the opposite leg.

LYING KNEE TO CHEST

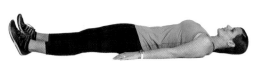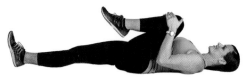

1. Lie flat on your back with your legs extended and your hands resting by your sides.

2. Lift one knee up toward your chest and gently pull your knee toward your body with your hands until you feel a comfortable stretch. Hold for 1 second.

3. Let go of your knee and place your leg back on the ground. Immediately perform the same movement with the opposite leg. Repeat.

INCHWORM

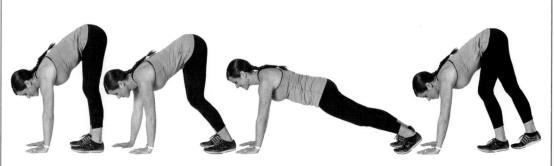

1. Start standing, then place your hands on the ground directly in front of you. Slightly bend your knees if necessary.

2. Slowly walk your hands forward until your body is in an extended plank position.

3. Once in a plank position, begin to slowly walk your feet back toward your hands. Repeat.

BEAR CRAWL

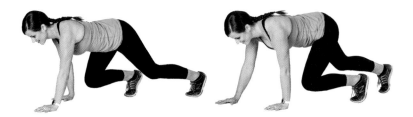

1. Start on your hands and knees so your hands are just underneath your shoulders and your knees are just underneath your hips. Place the balls of your feet on the ground and raise your knees off the ground so your torso is parallel with the ground.

2. To initiate the movement, pick up your left hand and your right foot, move them forward at the same time, and place them on the ground. When moving forward, keep your core tight and your spine neutral.

3. Perform with the opposite hand and foot. Repeat.

BODYWEIGHT SQUAT

Modification: Quarter Squat

What Not to Do: Caving Your Knees Inward

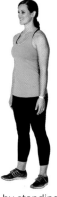
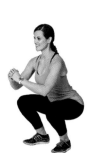
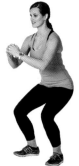
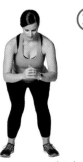

1. Begin by standing with your feet about shoulder-width apart.

2. To initiate the squat, shoot your hips back and down as if you're sitting in a chair. As you descend, keep your chest up and your knees in line with your toes. Continue to descend until your hip joint is in line with your knee joint and your upper leg is parallel with the ground.

3. To stand, extend at the knees and hips at the same, driving your hips open with your glutes.

If you experience pain going to full depth or lack the strength to do a full bodyweight squat, perform a quarter squat. To perform the quarter squat, stop a quarter of the way down while following the same cues and technique for the bodyweight squat.

A common mistake that people make when performing the bodyweight squat is letting their knees cave inward and dropping their chest forward. Instead, keep your feet turned slightly out, and think about spreading the floor with your feet to keep your knees in line with your toes.

FRONT PLANK

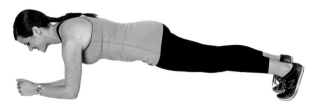

1. Start on your hands and knees. Place your elbows on the ground just underneath your shoulders and extend your legs behind you to place your toes on the ground. Your feet should be about shoulder-width apart.

2. Hold this position by maintaining complete tension in your core. In this position, make sure your spine is neutral and your hips do not sag toward the floor or rise up in the air.

GLUTE BRIDGE

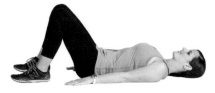 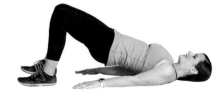

1. Lie on your back with your knees bent and your hands resting by your sides with your palms facing down.

2. Slowly lift your hips up off the ground by pressing your heels into the ground and driving your hips open with your glutes. Keep your spine neutral as you move. The movement should come from the hips, not the low back.

3. Squeeze your glutes at the top and hold for 1 to 2 seconds. Lower your hips back to the ground.

MOUNTAIN CLIMBER

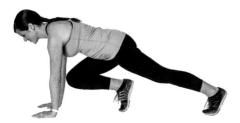

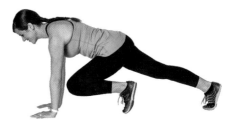

1. Start in an extended plank position with your wrists just underneath your shoulders.

2. Drive your right knee up to your chest and lightly tap your foot on the ground.

3. As you extend your right leg back to the starting position, do a small hop and simultaneously drive your left knee up to your chest. Lightly tap your left foot on the ground. Repeat.

REVERSE LUNGE

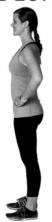

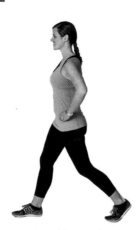

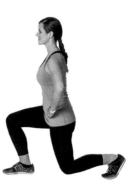

1. Start standing with your feet about hip-width apart.

2. Take a comfortable step backward with one foot and lower your hips toward the ground until your knee lightly grazes the ground. At the bottom of the lunge, both knees should be at about a 90-degree angle. While doing the movement, keep your ribs stacked over your hips and maintain a neutral spine.

3. To return to the start, pull your body up and forward with the leading leg and place your foot back underneath your body. Focus on engaging your glutes and driving through the heel. Repeat with the opposite leg.

PUSH-UP

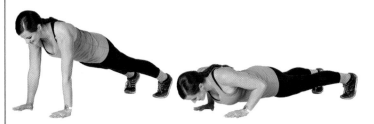

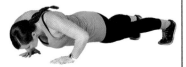

1. Start in an extended plank position with your wrists just underneath your shoulders.

2. Keeping your elbows at about a 30- to 45-degree angle with your torso, lower your body to the ground. While descending, keep your spine neutral and maintain tension in your core. At the bottom of the push-up, think about retracting your shoulder blades or pulling them together.

3. Push your body back up to start, moving your body as one unit.

A common mistake that people make when doing the push-up is letting their elbows flare out at a 90-degree angle. Instead, keep your elbows at a 30- to 45-degree angle with your torso when lowering your body to the ground.

Modification: Elevated Push-Up or Wall Push-Up

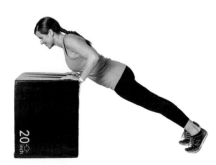

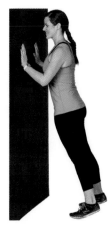

Elevated Push-Up: Place your hands on a secure step, box, or table, and perform the push-up as described. The more elevated your hands are, the easier it will be to perform the push-up.

Wall Push-Up: Stand directly in front of the wall with your feet about shoulder width apart. Place your hands on the wall so that your thumbs are even with your chest. Keeping your hands on the wall, take a step back until your arms are fully extended. Lower your body toward the wall, keeping your elbows in and your core tight. Retract your shoulder blades (bring them together) at the bottom of the push-up. To return to start, push your body away from the wall until your arms are fully extended.

SQUAT THRUST

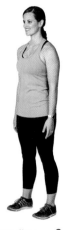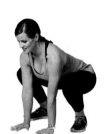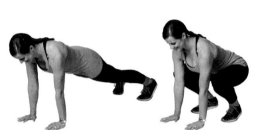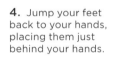

1. Start standing with your feet about shoulder-width apart.

2. Bending at the knees to squat down, place your hands on the ground just in front of your feet. Keep your spine neutral, making sure not to round your back.

3. Jump both feet back into an extended plank position.

4. Jump your feet back to your hands, placing them just behind your hands.

5. Stand up.

WALKING LUNGE

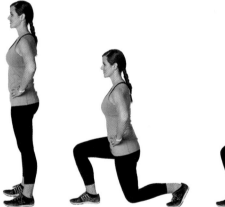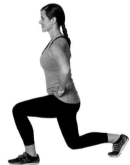

1. Start standing with your feet about hip-width apart.

2. Take a comfortable step forward with one foot and lower your hips toward the ground until your knee lightly grazes the ground. At the bottom of the lunge, both knees should be at about a 90-degree angle. While doing the movement, keep your ribs stacked over your hips and maintain a neutral spine.

3. To return to start, pull your body up and forward with your leading leg. Focus on engaging your glutes and driving through the heel.

4. Immediately take a step forward with the opposite leg and repeat.

ONE-ARM KETTLEBELL BENT-OVER ROW

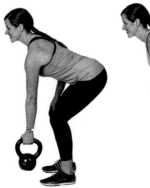

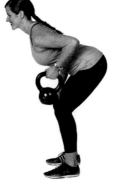

1. Stand holding a kettlebell at your side with your feet about hip-width apart.

2. Hinging at the hips, bend forward until your upper body is at about a 45-degree angle to the floor. Let the kettlebell hang directly in front of you and place the opposite hand on your knee for support.

3. Maintaining a neutral spine, row the kettlebell up toward your chest. Keep your elbow close to your torso and retract your shoulder blade at the top (pull it toward the center of your body).

4. Lower the weight back to start. Perform the set number of repetitions and repeat with the opposite arm.

KETTLEBELL DEADLIFT

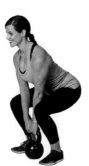

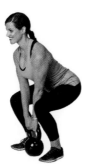

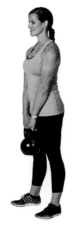

1. Stand with your feet about shoulder-width apart and a kettlebell directly underneath you between your feet.

2. Hinging at the hips and keeping a neutral spine, bend down and grab the kettlebell with both hands. While in this position, retract your shoulder blades (pull them together) to "load" your lats with tension.

3. Extending at the knees and hips simultaneously, stand up with the kettlebell. At the top, think about squeezing your glutes.

4. Return the kettlebell back to the floor by pushing your butt back and hinging at the hips.

ONE-ARM KETTLEBELL FARMER'S WALK

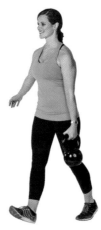

1. Stand tall with a kettlebell in one hand directly at your side.

2. Keeping your hips and shoulders square, slowly walk forward. While walking, keep your shoulders packed (down and back) and maintain tension in your core. Do not let the kettlebell rest on your body as you walk.

3. To turn around, set the weight down, turn to face the opposite direction, and pick the weight back up with the same arm. Repeat with the opposite arm.

GOBLET CLEAN

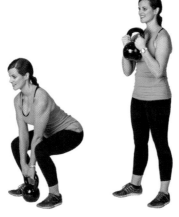

1. Stand with your feet about shoulder-width apart and a kettlebell directly underneath you between your feet.

2. Hinging at the hips and keeping a neutral spine, bend down and grab the kettlebell with both hands.

3. Powering through the hips, stand up quickly to launch the kettlebell straight up. Use your hands to guide the kettlebell, keeping it close to your body.

4. Once the kettlebell reaches chest height and begins to float, quickly rotate or "pop" your elbows down. Your grip will now be on the sides of the handle.

5. To lower the kettlebell back to the floor, hinge at the hips and rotate your hands back to the top of the handle.

GOBLET SQUAT

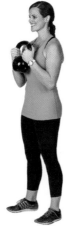

1. Stand tall and hold a kettlebell by the horns (the sides) in front of your chest. Your feet should be about shoulder-width apart.

2. To initiate the squat, shoot your hips back and down like you're sitting in a chair. As you descend, keep your chest up and your knees in line with your toes. Lower yourself to a depth that feels comfortable and within your range of motion. Your elbows should track inside of your knees at the bottom of the squat.

3. To stand, squeeze your glutes and extend at the knees and hips at the same time.

KETTLEBELL SWING

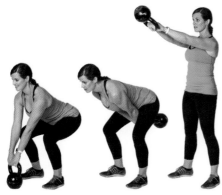

What Not to Do: Squatting During the Swing

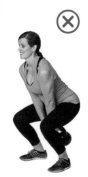

A common mistake that people make when performing the kettlebell swing is treating the swing like a squat. In the squat, you shoot your hips back and down as if you were sitting in a chair. To perform the kettlebell swing, think about pushing your butt back and hinging at the hips, and let your hips power the movement.

1. Stand with your feet shoulder-width apart and a kettlebell about a foot in front of you. Hinging at the hips and keeping a neutral spine, bend down and grab the kettlebell.

2. To initiate the swing, hike the kettlebell back and up between your legs. Your legs will slightly straighten in this position.

3. Powering through the hips, quickly stand up and swing the kettlebell up in front of your body to about eye level. Your arms will simply guide the kettlebell as it floats up.

4. At the top of the movement, your abdominal muscles and glutes should visibly contract. To help you do this, blow your breath out when the kettlebell reaches the top, which will create tension in your core.

5. Drive the kettlebell back down and up underneath you and repeat. When you're done, pause slightly at the bottom of the swing and place the kettlebell back on the ground in front of you.

ONE-ARM KETTLEBELL PUSH PRESS

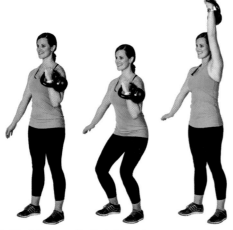

What Not to Do: Hiking Shoulder

A common mistake that people make when performing the push press is hiking their shoulder when pressing the kettlebell overhead. Instead, think about driving the movement with your hips, and keeping your shoulder down and away from your ear when performing the movement.

1. Stand tall holding a kettlebell in the racked position with your feet about shoulder-width apart.

2. To initiate the movement, dip slightly at the knees and use the power from your hips to drive the kettlebell straight overhead. Your wrist should rotate forward as the kettlebell floats up.

3. Once the kettlebell stops floating, use your strength to press the kettlebell up the final distance. Lock the kettlebell in the overhead position and stand up.

4. Keeping your elbow close to your body, return the kettlebell back to the racked position. Perform the set number of repetitions and repeat with the opposite arm.

ONE-ARM KETTLEBELL REVERSE LUNGE

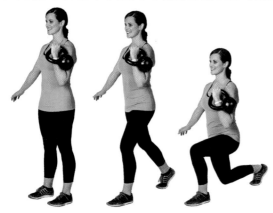

Watch Your Wrist!

When holding the kettlebell in the racked position, make sure your wrist is stacked over your forearm. There should be no "break" in your wrist. To facilitate this, hold the kettlebell by grabbing the corner of the handle that is closest to you and let the kettlebell rest in the soft spot on the back of your forearm. Hold the kettlebell close to your body and keep your elbow in.

1. Stand tall holding a kettlebell in the racked position with your feet hip-width apart.

2. Take a comfortable step backward with the same leg as the arm holding the kettlebell. Lower your hips toward the ground until your knee lightly grazes the ground. At the bottom of the lunge, both knees should be at about a 90-degree angle. While doing the movement, keep your ribs stacked over your hips and maintain a neutral spine.

3. To return to start, pull your body up and forward with the leading leg and place your foot back underneath your body. Focus on engaging your glutes and driving through the heel. Perform the set number of repetitions and repeat with the opposite leg.

WALL ANKLE MOBILIZATION

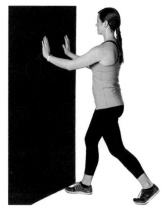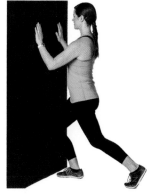

1. Start standing in front of the wall. Stagger your feet so your front toe is touching the wall and your opposite leg is comfortably behind you while on the ball of your foot. Place your hands on the wall in front of your chest.

2. Moving from the ankle, rock your body forward until your knee touches the wall.

3. Progressively move your body back away from the wall and repeat this movement, stopping just before you can no longer rock forward and touch your knee on the wall without raising your heel off the ground. Perform 2 or 3 sets of 10 to 12 "rocks" forward in this position. Repeat with the opposite foot.

WALL SQUAT

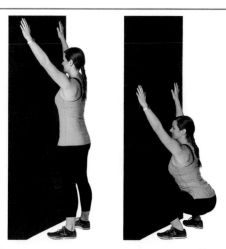

1. Start facing the wall with your feet slightly wider than shoulder-width apart. Your feet should be about 3 to 5 inches away from the wall. Place your hands up overhead so they are lightly touching the wall.

2. Squat down as far as you can, maintaining this position. With each repetition, you should be able to go down slightly farther. The goal is to eventually be able to perform a full squat in this position without leaning forward and hitting the wall or falling backward.

3. As you progress in your mobility, move closer and closer to the wall until your toes are touching the wall. Perform 2 or 3 sets of 10 to 12 repetitions.

THORACIC TWIST

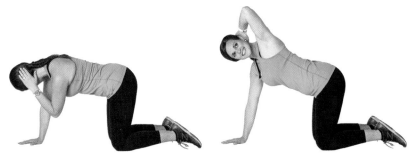

1. Start on all fours with your wrists just underneath your shoulders and your knees directly underneath your hips.

2. Place one hand on the back of your head and rotate your upper back so your elbow is pointing down.

3. Keeping your hips square and a small arch in your back, slowly rotate your elbow directly up until you feel a light stretch in your shoulder and upper back. Return to start by rotating your elbow back down so it points in the space between your opposite arm and torso. Perform 2 or 3 sets of 10 to 12 repetitions. Repeat with the opposite arm.

WALL SLIDE

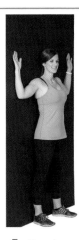

1. Stand up against the wall facing away from the wall, and lean back onto the wall so that your hips, back, and shoulders are flat against the wall.

2. Place your arms against the wall with your hands pointed up and elbows slightly bent.

3. Pressing your upper arms against the wall, slowly slide your arms up as far as you can while maintaining complete contact with the wall. As you move upward, be careful not to shrug your shoulders or arch your lower back.

4. Once you have extended your arms up as far as possible, slowly bring your arms back down as far as you can while maintaining pressure against the wall. Think about keeping your shoulder blades packed (pulled back and down) as you descend.

5. As your mobility improves, try to increase your range of motion and keep your elbows against the wall. Perform 8 to 10 repetitions.

THE WORKOUTS

All the workouts in the Coconuts and Kettlebells Fitness Plan are designed to be effective, engaging, and fun. Each workout incorporates a variety of functional movements, which allow you to get in a high-quality workout in a short period of time. To complete the workouts, the only tools you need are your body and kettlebells. This makes the workouts accessible and easy to do at home or at the gym.

To help you quickly find a workout that fits your needs, the workouts are organized by estimated time to complete. The exact time it will take you to complete a workout will depend on a variety of factors, so each section is labeled as "X minutes or less," where X is the estimated maximum amount of time it will take you to complete the workout. In each section, conditioning workouts are listed first and strength workouts are listed second. Some workouts also come with modified workout guidelines, which you can follow based on your experience level or how you're feeling on a particular day. The modified guidelines may slightly decrease the time it takes you to complete the workout, so take this into account when putting together your template.

CHOOSING THE RIGHT WEIGHTS

For conditioning workouts, use moderate loads that you can move at a steady pace. You should be able to move the weight with ease but feel challenged during the workout. For strength workouts, use heavier loads that push you in the workout. In general, the lower the repetitions, the heavier the weight you'll use. The time estimate given for each workout assumes you are using weights that are appropriate for the workout. If you find you finish a workout way before the estimated time, it's a good sign you may need to increase the weight(s) you use for a specific workout.

WARM UP

Warming up primes the body for movement. By gradually raising core body temperature, increasing blood flow, and improving overall flexibility and mobility, you'll be able to get the most out of your workout and reduce the risk of injury. Here's a list of activities you can to do to warm up before a workout:

1. Use a foam roller or massage stick to warm up your muscles and work out any "kinks" or areas of tightness you may be experiencing.

2. Complete 4 or 5 minutes of Dynamic Warm-Up Movements (see page 292). Do each exercise for at least 1 minute.

3. Spend at least 5 minutes performing the movements listed in the workout. For example, if you're doing a workout that has a series of movements, perform 3 to 5 repetitions of each exercise listed in the workout at a steady pace. If doing a strength workout, gradually work up to using the weight(s) you plan to use in the workout.

COOL DOWN

Cooling down gradually brings the body back to a resting state and aids in the removal of waste products, such as lactic acid. This can improve mobility and flexibility and support muscle recovery. Here's a list of activities you can do to cool down after a workout:

1. Perform 3 to 5 minutes of continuous low-intensity movement like walking.

2. Use a foam roller or massage stick to work out any "kinks" or areas of tightness you may be experiencing.

3. Do some light stretching.

DEFINING SETS, REPS, AND ROUNDS

To make sure you're in the know on the lingo, here's a quick diagram of what it means when talking sets, repetitions, and rounds:

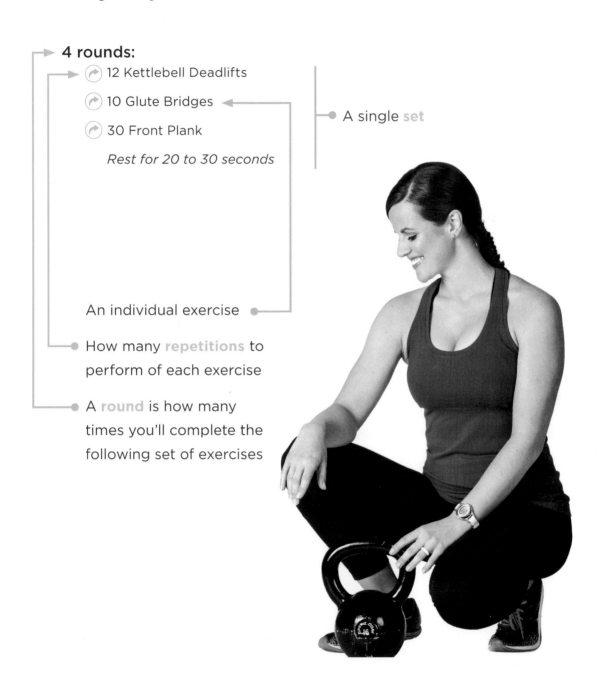

4 rounds:

- 12 Kettlebell Deadlifts
- 10 Glute Bridges
- 30 Front Plank

  Rest for 20 to 30 seconds

A single set

An individual exercise

How many **repetitions** to perform of each exercise

A **round** is how many times you'll complete the following set of exercises

BIG TIME

CONDITIONING WORKOUT

For each exercise, perform 8 rounds of 20 seconds on/10 seconds off intervals. Perform as many repetitions as possible during the 20-second "on" period. Rest for 90 seconds between the two sets.

THE WORKOUT:

8 rounds:

↻ Bodyweight Squats

8 rounds:

↻ Squat Thrusts

MODIFIED WORKOUT GUIDELINES:

Perform 6 rounds of each set. During each 20-second "on" period, move at a steady pace.

DESERT ISLAND

CONDITIONING WORKOUT

Perform the workout as fast as good form allows. Rest 90 seconds and perform a second round in reverse (starting with 1 Bodyweight Squat, 9 Kettlebell Swings).

THE WORKOUT:

- ↱ 1 Kettlebell Swing, 9 Bodyweight Squats
- ↱ 2 Kettlebell Swings, 8 Bodyweight Squats
- ↱ 3 Kettlebell Swings, 7 Bodyweight Squats
- ↱ 4 Kettlebell Swings, 6 Bodyweight Squats
- ↱ 5 Kettlebell Swings, 5 Bodyweight Squats
- ↱ 6 Kettlebell Swings, 4 Bodyweight Squats
- ↱ 7 Kettlebell Swings, 3 Bodyweight Squats
- ↱ 8 Kettlebell Swings, 2 Bodyweight Squats
- ↱ 9 Kettlebell Swings, 1 Bodyweight Squat

WHAT THE

CONDITIONING WORKOUT

Complete the workout using 15 seconds on/15 seconds off intervals. Perform as many repetitions as possible in 15 seconds for each exercise listed in the workout. Rest for 15 seconds before moving on to the next exercise.

THE WORKOUT:

4 rounds:

- ⟳ Kettlebell Swing
- ⟳ Mountain Climbers
- ⟳ Goblet Clean
- ⟳ Reverse Lunge (alternating legs)
- ⟳ Kettlebell Deadlift

DON'T LET GO

CONDITIONING WORKOUT

Perform the exercises listed in the workout every minute on the minute (EMOM) for 10 minutes. Perform the repetitions as fast as good form allows.

THE WORKOUT:

EMOM for 10 minutes:

- ⟳ 6 Kettlebell Deadlifts
- ⟳ 6 Goblet Cleans
- ⟳ 6 Goblet Squats

MOVING DAY

STRENGTH WORKOUT

Perform the repetitions slow and controlled. Choose a weight for each exercise that challenges you and allows you to push yourself but doesn't compromise form.

THE WORKOUT:

4 rounds:

- ↪ 10 Kettlebell Deadlifts
- ↪ 10 Push-Ups
- ↪ 8 One-Arm Kettlebell Bent-Over Rows (each arm)

Rest for 30 to 45 seconds

CENTER FIELD

STRENGTH WORKOUT

Perform the repetitions slow and controlled. Choose a weight for each exercise that challenges you and allows you to push yourself but doesn't compromise form.

THE WORKOUT:

4 rounds:

- ↪ 10 Goblet Squats
- ↪ 10 One-Arm Kettlebell Reverse Lunges (each leg)
- ↪ :30 Front Plank

Rest for 30 to 45 seconds

SPICY MEATBALL

CONDITIONING WORKOUT

For the first set, complete the workout using 20 seconds on/20 seconds off intervals. Perform as many repetitions as possible in 20 seconds for each exercise listed in the workout. Rest for 20 seconds before moving on to the next exercise. For the second set, perform as many repetitions as possible (AMRAP) of the exercise listed in 2 minutes. Rest for 2 minutes between the two sets.

THE WORKOUT:

4 rounds:

⤳ Goblet Cleans

⤳ Reverse Lunges (alternating legs)

⤳ Kettlebell Swings

⤳ Front Plank

2-minute AMRAP:

⤳ Squat Thrusts

BEAR HUG

CONDITIONING WORKOUT

Perform as many repetitions as possible in the allotted time. When the 30 seconds are up, move immediately to the next exercise.

THE WORKOUT:

5 rounds:

⟳ :30 Squat Thrusts

⟳ :30 Walking Lunges

⟳ :30 Bear Crawls

⟳ :30 Bodyweight Squats

Rest for 60 seconds

MODIFIED WORKOUT GUIDELINES:

Perform 4 rounds of the workout.

STELLA-R

CONDITIONING WORKOUT

Complete as many rounds as possible (AMRAP) in 15 minutes. Perform the repetitions as fast as good form allows.

THE WORKOUT:

15-minute AMRAP:

⟳ 4 Push-Ups

⟳ 8 Reverse Lunges (each leg)

⟳ 12 Goblet Cleans

⟳ 16 Mountain Climbers (each leg)

⟳ 20 Kettlebell Swings

MODIFIED WORKOUT GUIDELINES:

Complete a 12-minute AMRAP.

FIRE STARTER

CONDITIONING WORKOUT

Perform the workout as fast as good form allows.

THE WORKOUT:

5 rounds:

- 10 Squat Thrusts
- 8 One-Arm Kettlebell Push Presses (each arm)
- 10 Bodyweight Squats
- 8 One-Arm Kettlebell Reverse Lunges (each leg)
- 10 Mountain Climbers (each leg)

Rest for 30 seconds

MODIFIED WORKOUT GUIDELINES:

Perform 4 rounds of the workout. Rest for 45 seconds after each round.

STRONG-ARM

STRENGTH WORKOUT

For the first set, perform the repetitions slow and controlled. Choose a weight for each exercise that challenges you and allows you to push yourself but doesn't compromise form. For the second set, complete the set amount of repetitions in as little time as possible. Rest as needed between the two sets.

THE WORKOUT:

4 rounds:

↷ 8 One-Arm Kettlebell Push Presses (each arm)

↷ 8 One-Arm Kettlebell Bent-Over Rows (each arm)

↷ :30 One-Arm Kettlebell Farmer's Walk (right arm)

↷ :30 One-Arm Kettlebell Farmer's Walk (left arm)

Rest for 30 to 45 seconds

For time:

↷ 50 Goblet Cleans

WALK THE PLANK

STRENGTH WORKOUT

Perform the repetitions slow and controlled. Choose a weight for each exercise that challenges you and allows you to push yourself but doesn't compromise form. Rest as needed between the two sets.

THE WORKOUT:

3 rounds:

↱ 12 Goblet Squats

↱ 10 One-Arm Kettlebell Reverse Lunges (each side)

↱ :30 Front Plank

Rest for 20 to 30 seconds

4 rounds:

↱ 12 Kettlebell Deadlifts

↱ 10 Glute Bridges

↱ :30 Front Plank

Rest for 20 to 30 seconds

MODIFIED WORKOUT GUIDELINES:

Perform 3 rounds of the second set.

BRUH

CONDITIONING WORKOUT

Perform as many rounds as possible (AMRAP) in the time designated for each set. Move as fast as good form allows. Rest for 90 seconds between each set.

THE WORKOUT:

6-minute AMRAP:

- 5 Squat Thrusts
- 10 Kettlebell Swings
- 15 Bodyweight Squats

5-minute AMRAP:

- 5 One-Arm Kettlebell Push Presses (right arm)
- 5 One-Arm Kettlebell Reverse Lunges (right leg)
- 5 One-Arm Kettlebell Push Presses (left arm)
- 5 One-Arm Kettlebell Reverse Lunges (left leg)

6-minute AMRAP:

- 5 Push-Ups
- 10 Goblet Cleans
- 15 Mountain Climbers (each leg)

MODIFIED WORKOUT GUIDELINES:

Perform each set as a 5-minute AMRAP. Rest for 2 minutes between each set.

RING THE BELL

CONDITIONING WORKOUT

Complete the workout using 30 seconds on/30 seconds off intervals. Perform as many repetitions as possible in 30 seconds for each exercise listed in the workout. Rest for 30 seconds before moving on to the next exercise.

THE WORKOUT:

4 rounds:

- Goblet Cleans
- One-Arm Kettlebell Reverse Lunges (right leg)
- Kettlebell Swings
- One-Arm Kettlebell Reverse Lunges (left leg)
- Kettlebell Deadlifts

REAR-ENDED

CONDITIONING WORKOUT

Perform as many repetitions as possible in the allotted time. When the 45 seconds is up, move immediately to the next exercise.

THE WORKOUT:

5 rounds:

- ↱ :45 Squat Thrusts

- ↱ :45 Reverse Lunges (alternating legs)

- ↱ :45 Bodyweight Squats

- ↱ :45 Glute Bridges

Rest for 60 seconds

LEGGINGS

STRENGTH WORKOUT

For the first two sets, perform the repetitions slow and controlled. Choose a weight for each exercise that challenges you and allows you to push yourself but doesn't compromise form. For the third set, complete the set amount of repetitions in as little time as possible. Rest as needed between each set in the workout.

THE WORKOUT:

4 rounds:

⟳ 10 Goblet Squats

⟳ 10 One-Arm Kettlebell Reverse Lunges (each leg)

Rest for 30 to 45 seconds

3 rounds:

⟳ :30 Glute Bridges

⟳ :30 One-Arm Kettlebell Farmer's Walk (right arm)

⟳ :30 One-Arm Kettlebell Farmer's Walk (left arm)

Rest for 30 seconds

For time:

⟳ 50 Kettlebell Swings

MODIFIED WORKOUT GUIDELINES:

For the first set, perform 3 rounds. For the last set, perform 30 repetitions.

MUSCLE TEE

STRENGTH WORKOUT

For the first two sets, perform the repetitions slow and controlled. Choose a weight for each exercise that challenges you and allows you to push yourself but doesn't compromise form. For the third set, complete the set amount of repetitions in as little time as possible. Rest as needed between each set in the workout.

THE WORKOUT:

4 rounds:

↱ 10 Kettlebell Deadlifts

↱ 8 One-Arm Kettlebell Push Presses (each side)

↱ :30 Front Plank

Rest for 30 to 45 seconds

4 rounds:

↱ :20 Push-Ups

↱ :20 One-Arm Kettlebell Bent-Over Rows (right arm)

↱ :20 One-Arm Kettlebell Bent-Over Rows (left arm)

Rest for 30 seconds

For time:

↱ 50 Bodyweight Squats

MODIFIED WORKOUT GUIDELINES:

For the first set, perform 3 rounds. For the last set, perform 30 repetitions.

GRIPPING

STRENGTH WORKOUT

Perform the repetitions slow and controlled. Use one kettlebell for the entire workout. Try to move continuously during each round, pausing only to change your grip. Choose a weight that pushes you throughout the set but doesn't compromise form.

THE WORKOUT:

7 rounds:

↱ 5 Kettlebell Deadlifts

↱ 5 Goblet Cleans

↱ 5 Goblet Squats

↱ 5 One-Arm Kettlebell Push Presses (right arm)

↱ 5 One-Arm Kettlebell Reverse Lunges (right arm)

↱ 5 One-Arm Kettlebell Push Presses (left arm)

↱ 5 One-Arm Kettlebell Reverse Lunges (left arm)

Rest for 60 to 90 seconds

MODIFIED WORKOUT GUIDELINES:

Perform 5 rounds of the workout.

FABULOUS 40

CONDITIONING WORKOUT

Perform the workout at a steady pace. Move only as fast as good form allows.

THE WORKOUT:

- 40 Kettlebell Swings
- 40 Bodyweight Squats
- 40 Walking Lunges (each leg)
- 40 Goblet Cleans
- 40 Bear Crawls (each leg)
- 40 Push-Ups
- 40 Squat Thrusts
- 40 Reverse Lunges (each leg)
- 40 Mountain Climbers (each leg)
- 40 Kettlebell Swings

MODIFIED WORKOUT GUIDELINES:

Perform 25 repetitions of each exercise.

MOVED TO TEARS

CONDITIONING WORKOUT

For the first set, perform the repetitions at a steady pace in the allotted time. When the 45 seconds are up, move immediately to the next exercise. For the second set, perform the number of repetitions for each exercise listed in the workout before moving to the next set of repetitions. (Example: 10 Kettlebell Swings, 10 Mountain Climbers, 10 Bodyweight Squats; 20 Kettlebell Swings, 20 Mountain Climbers, and so on.) Move as fast as good form allows. Rest for 2 to 3 minutes between the two sets.

THE WORKOUT:

4 rounds:

↱ :45 Goblet Cleans

↱ :45 One-Arm Kettlebell Farmer's Walk (right arm)

↱ :45 One-Arm Kettlebell Farmer's Walk (left arm)

↱ :45 Walking Lunges

↱ :45 Bear Crawls

Rest for 45 seconds

For time:

10–20–30–20–10

↱ Kettlebell Swings

↱ Mountain Climbers

↱ Bodyweight Squats

MODIFIED WORKOUT GUIDELINES:

Perform 3 rounds of the first set.

TOWER OF TERROR

CONDITIONING WORKOUT

Perform the workout as a building ladder (like "The 12 Days of Christmas" song). Example: 1 Running Sprint; 2 Reverse Lunges, 1 Running Sprint; 3 Push-Ups, 2 Reverse Lunges, 1 Running Sprint, and so on. For exercises performed on both sides, one repetition is counted when you perform a repetition on one side. Move as fast as good form allows.

THE WORKOUT:

- 1 10-second Running Sprint (5 seconds out, tap the ground, 5 seconds back)
- 2 Reverse Lunges
- 3 Push-Ups
- 4 Squat Thrusts
- 5 Kettlebell Deadlifts
- 6 Walking Lunges
- 7 Kettlebell Swings
- 8 Bear Crawls
- 9 Bodyweight Squats
- 10 Mountain Climbers
- 11 Goblet Cleans
- 12 Glute Bridges

MODIFIED WORKOUT GUIDELINES:

Perform the workout up to 10 Mountain Climbers.

FULL STRENGTH

STRENGTH WORKOUT

For the first two sets, perform the repetitions slow and controlled. Choose a weight for each exercise that challenges you and allows you to push yourself for the given rep range, but doesn't compromise form. For the third set, perform the number of repetitions for each exercise listed in the workout before moving to the next set of repetitions. Move as fast as good form allows. Rest as needed between each set in the workout.

THE WORKOUT:

4 rounds:

⟳ 8 to 10 Kettlebell Deadlifts

⟳ 8 to 10 One-Arm Kettlebell Reverse Lunges (each leg)

⟳ 10 Glute Bridges

⟳ :20 Front Plank

Rest for 30 to 45 seconds

4 rounds:

⟳ 8 to 10 One-Arm Kettlebell Push Presses (each arm)

⟳ 8 to 10 One-Arm Kettlebell Bent-Over Rows (each arm)

⟳ 8 to 10 Push-Ups

⟳ :20 Front Plank

Rest for 30 to 45 seconds

For time:

10-8-6-4-2

⟳ Kettlebell Swings

⟳ Squat Thrusts

⟳ Bodyweight Squats

MODIFIED WORKOUT GUIDELINES:

Perform 3 rounds of the first two sets.

STRENGTH WORKOUT

For each set, perform the repetitions at a steady pace and with control. Choose a weight for each exercise that challenges you and allows you to push yourself but doesn't compromise form. Rest as needed between each set in the workout.

THE WORKOUT:

4 rounds:

⟳ 20 Goblet Cleans

Rest for 20 seconds, then:

⟳ 10 One-Arm Kettlebell Reverse Lunges (each leg)

⟳ 8 One-Arm Kettlebell Push Presses (each arm)

Rest for 30 to 45 seconds

4 rounds:

⟳ 20 Kettlebell Swings

Rest for 20 seconds, then:

⟳ 10 Goblet Squats

⟳ 8 One-Arm Kettlebell Bent-Over Rows (each arm)

Rest for 30 to 45 seconds

3 rounds:

⟳ :30 One-Arm Kettlebell Farmer's Walk (right arm)

⟳ :30 One-Arm Kettlebell Farmer's Walk (left arm)

⟳ :30 Glute Bridges

MODIFIED WORKOUT GUIDELINES:

Perform 3 rounds of the first 2 sets.

KETTLEBELL COMPLEX

STRENGTH WORKOUT

Perform the repetitions slow and controlled. Use one kettlebell for the entire workout. Try to move continuously during each round, only pausing to change your grip. Choose a weight that pushes you throughout the workout but doesn't compromise form.

THE WORKOUT:

4 rounds:

Complete 6 to 8 complex repetitions (1 complex repetition = 1 repetition of each exercise in the order listed below):

- 1 Kettlebell Deadlift
- 1 Goblet Clean
- 1 Goblet Squat
- 1 One-Arm Kettlebell Push Press (right arm)
- 1 One-Arm Kettlebell Reverse Lunge (right leg)
- 1 One-Arm Kettlebell Bent-Over Row (right arm)
- 1 One-Arm Kettlebell Push Press (left arm)
- 1 One-Arm Kettlebell Reverse Lunge (left leg)
- 1 One-Arm Kettlebell Bent-Over Row (left arm)

Rest for 2 minutes after each round

MODIFIED WORKOUT GUIDELINES:

Perform 3 rounds of the workout.

A Final Word of Encouragement

*E*ven with all the information and resources at your fingertips, approaching health and fitness in a new way can be intimidating. If you're feeling overwhelmed, remember that health is a journey, *not* a destination. Instead of being consumed by all the changes you want to make, ask yourself *What's my next step?* Focus on the one or two things you can do today that will prepare you for tomorrow. Over time, what once seemed hard will become your new way of existing, and you'll begin to achieve your goals.

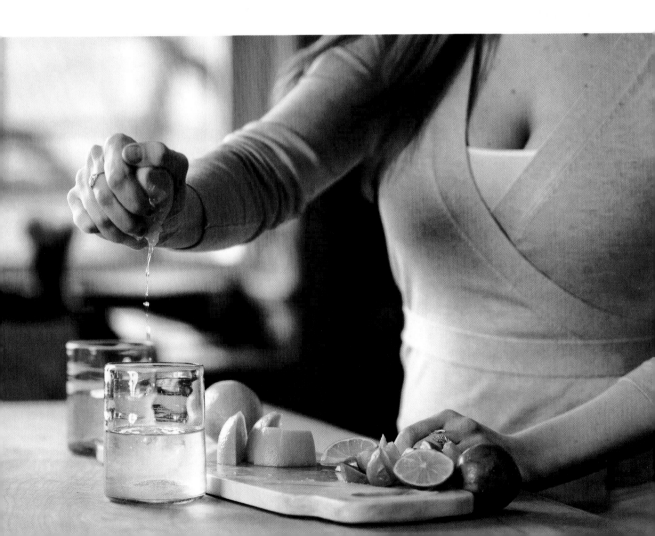

GRATITUDE

First and foremost, thank you to *Jim and Elaine Flauaus* for your steadfast love, care, and prayers. You're the reason I have always had an unwavering confidence that has allowed me to pursue my dreams.

To our agent, *John Maas*, thank you for fighting for us. We are forever grateful for your vision and direction. This book wouldn't be what it is without you.

Thank you to our editor, *Cassie Jones*. You allowed us to fulfill our dreams with this book, and put up with our numerous requests and changes. Thanks for being on our side.

To our food photographer, *Alena Haurylik*, thank you for your willingness to work with us to get the perfect shot for each dish. We are so grateful for your diligence, patience, and attention to detail. Thank you to *Teresa Robertson*, our friend and lifestyle photographer, and *Matt Godfrey*, our fitness photographer. You all helped us bring our vision to life.

Thank you to the *Well-Fed Women podcast community*. We are honored to be doing life with you, and your support means the world to us.

To the two women who have been encouraging me my entire life, my sister, *Hannah Wardrop*, and my best friend, *Rachel Thun*, thank you for letting me unload stress and talk about writing this book for years.

Thank you to my daughter, *Stella girl*. Because of you, my entire outlook on life and my body has transformed. You are my greatest teacher to date.

And last, thank you to my husband, *Ken Tarr*. Without you, this book wouldn't have happened. Thank you for putting Stella and me first, and for being selfless day in and day out. You're the best thing that's ever happened to me.

Noelle

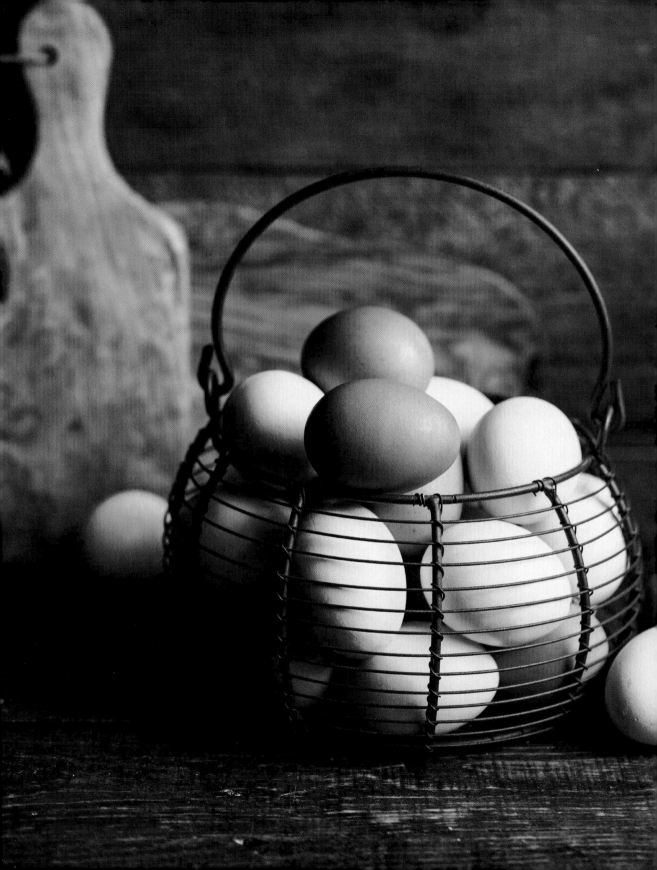

RESOURCES

For direct links to all the recommend brands and products referenced in this book, visit coconutsandkettlebells.com/bookresources.

NOELLE'S WEBSITES
coconutsandkettlebells.com
strongfromhome.com

STEFANI'S WEBSITES
paleoforwomen.com
paleoweightlossforwomen.com
pcosunlocked.com
clearskinunlocked.com

PRODUCTS WE LOVE
Epic Bar: epicbar.com
Frontier Co-op: frontiercoop.com
Jackson's Honest: jacksonshonest.com
Kettle & Fire: kettleandfire.com
Mountain Rose Herbs: mountainroseherbs.com
Ona Treats: onatreats.com
Organicville: organicvillefoods.com
Paleovalley: paleovalley.com
Primal Kitchen: primalkitchen.com
Redmond Real Salt: realsalt.com
RXBAR: rxbar.com
Selina Naturally (Celtic Sea Salt):
    selinanaturally.com
Siete Foods: sietefoods.com
Simple Mills: simplemills.com
Tropical Traditions: tropicaltraditions.com
Vital Proteins: Vitalproteins.com
Wild Foods Company: wildfoods.co

FOR FURTHER EDUCATION
National Strength and Conditioning Association:
    nsca.com
Nutritional Therapy Association:
    nutritionaltherapy.com
StrongFirst: strongfirst.com

OUR FAVORITE FOOD RESOURCES
Eat Wild: eatwild.com
Environmental Working Group: ewg.com
Local Harvest: localharvest.org
National Farmers Market Directory: nfmd.org
USDA Farmers Market Directory:
    http://search.ams.usda.gov/farmersmarkets

ONLINE FOOD RETAILERS
Radiant Life: radiantlife.com
Thrive Market: thrivemarket.com
Vitacost: vitacost.com
Vital Choice: vitalchoice.com

FOR QUALITY MOVEMENT TOOLS
CFF Fit: cfffit.com
Dragon Door: dragondoor.com

RECOMMENDED READING
The Autoimmune Wellness Handbook by Mickey
    Trescott, NTP, and Angie Alt, NTC, CHC
Hashimoto's Protocol by Izabella Wentz, PharmD
The Paleo Approach by Sarah Ballantyne, PhD
*Why Do I Still Have Thyroid Symptoms When My
    Lab Tests Are Normal?* and *Why Isn't My Brain
    Working?* by Datis Kharrazian, DHSc, DC, MS
Wired to Eat by Robb Wolf

NOTES

2. THE BIG FOUR INFLAMMATORY FOODS

1. David R. Jacobs., Myron D. Gross, and Linda C. Tapsell, "Food Synergy: An Operational Concept for Understanding Nutrition," *American Journal of Clinical Nutrition* 89, no. 5 (May 1, 2009): 1543S–1548S, https://doi.org/10.3945/ajcn.2009.26736B.

2. Alessio Fasano, "Leaky Gut and Autoimmune Diseases," *Clinical Reviews in Allergy & Immunology* 32, no. 1 (2007), https://crohnsdad.files.wordpress.com/2011/12/clin-rev-allerg-immunol-leaky-gutautoimmunity.pdf.

3. Kazumi Maruyama, Tomoe Oshima, and Kenji Ohyama, "Exposure to Exogenous Estrogen Through Intake of Commercial Milk Produced from Pregnant Cows," *Pediatrics International: Official Journal of the Japan Pediatric Society* 52, no. 1 (February 2010): 33–38, https://doi.org/10.1111/j.1442-200X.2009.02890.x.

4. Stefania La Terra, Vita Maria Marino, Mario Manenti, Giuseppe Licitra, and Stefania Carpino, "Increasing Pasture Intakes Enhances Polyunsaturated Fatty Acids and Lipophilic Antioxidants in Plasma and Milk of Dairy Cows Fed Total Mix Ration," *Dairy Science & Technology* 90, no. 6 (September 1, 2010): 687–98. https://doi.org/10.1051/dst/2010100.

5. T. R. Dhiman, G. R. Anand, L. D. Satter, and M. W. Pariza, "Conjugated Linoleic Acid Content of Milk from Cows Fed Different Diets," *Journal of Dairy Science* 82, no. 10 (October 1999): 2146–56, https://doi.org/10.3168/jds.S00220302(99)75458-5.

6. P. M. Kris-Etherton, Denise Shaffer Taylor, Shaomei Yu-Poth, Peter Huth, Kristin Moriarty, Valerie Fishell, Rebecca L. Hargrove, Guixiang Zhao, and Terry D. Etherton, "Polyunsaturated Fatty Acids in the Food Chain in the United States,," *American Journal of Clinical Nutrition* 71, no. 1 (January 1, 2000): 179S–188S, https://doi.org/10.1093/ajcn/71.1.179S.

7. Ibid.

8. A. P. Simopoulous, "The Importance of the Ratio of Omega-6/omega-3 Essential Fatty Acids," *Biomedicine & Pharmacotherapy = Biomedecine & Pharmacotherapie* 56, no. 8 (October 2002): 365–79.

9. Stephan Guyenet, "Seed Oils and Body Fatness—A Problematic Revisit," accessed February 8, 2018, http://wholehealthsource.blogspot.com/2011/08/seed-oils-and-body-fatness-problematic.html.

10. These statistics have been compiled and discussed at length by Paul Jaminet in his *Perfect Health Diet: Regain Health* and *Lose Weight by Eating the Way You Were Meant to Eat* (New York: Scribner Book Company), 2012.

11. Simopoulos, "The Importance of the Ratio of Omega-6/omega-3 Essential Fatty Acids."

12. P. Mohanty, W. Hamouda, R. Garg, A. Aljada, H. Ghanim, and P. Dandona, "Glucose Challenge Stimulates Reactive Oxygen Species (ROS) Generation by Leucocytes," *Journal of Clinical Endocrinology and Metabolism* 85, no. 8 (August 2000): 2970–73, https://doi.org/10.1210/jcem.85.8.6854.

13. Albert Sanchez, J. L. Reeser, H. S. Lau, P. Y. Yahiku, R. E. Willard, P. J. McMillan, S. Y. Cho, A. R. Magie, and U. D. Register. "Role of Sugars in Human Neutrophilic Phagocytosis." *American Journal of Clinical Nutrition* 26, no. 11 (November 1, 1973): 1180–84, https://doi.org/10.1093/ajcn/26.11.1180.

14. Magalie Lenoir, Fuschia Serre, Lauriane Cantin, and Serge H. Ahmed, "Intense Sweetness Surpasses Cocaine Reward," *PloS One* 2, no. 8 (August 1, 2007): e698, https://doi.org/10.1371/journal.pone.0000698.

15. Terry L. Davidson, Ashley A. Martin, Kiely Clark, and Susan E. Swithers, "Intake of High-Intensity Sweeteners Alters the Ability of Sweet Taste to Signal Caloric Consequences: Implications for the Learned Control of Energy and Body Weight Regulation," *Quarterly Journal of Experimental Psychology (2006)* 64, no. 7 (July 2011): 1430–41, https://doi.org/10.1080/17470218.2011.552729.

16. Susan E. Swithers and Terry L. Davidson, "A Role for Sweet Taste: Calorie Predictive Relations in Energy Regulation by Rats," *Behavioral Neuroscience* 122, no. 1 (February 2008): 161–73, https://doi.org/10.1037/0735-7044.122.1.161.

17. Mohamed B. Abou Donia, Eman M. El-Masry, Ali A. Abdel-Rahman, Roger E. McLendon, and Susan S. Schiffman, "Splenda Alters Gut Microflora and Increases Intestinal P-Glycoprotein and Cytochrome P-450 in Male Rats," *Journal of Toxicology and Environmental Health. Part A* 71, no. 21 (2008): 1415–29, https://doi.org/10.1080/15287390802328630.

5. LIVING WITH HEALTH, HAPPINESS, AND FREEDOM

1. Joseph Ratliff, Jose O. Leite, Ryan de Ogburn, Michael J. Puglisi, Jaci VanHeest, and Maria Luz Fernandez, "Consuming Eggs for Breakfast Influences Plasma Glucose and Ghrelin, While Reducing Energy Intake during the next 24 Hours in Adult Men," *Nutrition Research* 30, no. 2 (February 2010): 96–103, https://doi.org/10.1016/j.nutres.2010.01.002.

2. Jillon S. Vander Wal, Jorene M. Marth, Pramod Khosla, K.-L. Catherine Jen, and Nikhil V. Dhurandhar, "Short-Term Effect of Eggs on Satiety in Overweight and Obese Subjects," *Journal of the American College of Nutrition* 24, no. 6 (December 2005): 510–15.

3. A. J. Tomiyama, J. M. Hunger, J. Nguyen-Cuu, and C. Wells, "Misclassification of Cardiometabolic Health When Using Body Mass Index Categories in NHANES 2005–2012," *International Journal of Obesity* 40, no. 5 (May 2016): 883–86, https://doi.org/10.1038/ijo.2016.17.

6. THE MEAL PLANS

1. Andrew Schneider, "Tests Show Most Store Honey Isn't Honey," Food Safety News, November 7, 2011, http://www.foodsafetynews.com/2011/11/tests-show-most-store-honey-isnt-honey/.

2. Randy D. Shaver, "By-Products Feedstuffs in Dairy Cattle Diets in the Upper Midwest," *UW Extension*, n.d., 1–17.

3. S. K. Duckett, J. P. S. Neel, J. P. Fontenot, and W. M. Clapham, "Effects of Winter Stocker Growth Rate and Finishing System on: III. Tissue Proximate, Fatty Acid, Vitamin, and Cholesterol Content," *Journal of Animal Science* 87, no. 9 (September 2009): 2961–70., https://doi.org/10.2527/jas.2009-1850.

4. A. Tolan, Jean Robertson, C. R. Orton, M. J. Head, A. A. Christie, and Barbara A. Millburn, "Studies on the Composition of Food: 5. The Chemical Composition of Eggs Produced Under Battery, Deep Litter and Free Rage Conditions," *British Journal of Nutrition* 31, no. 2 (March 1974): 185–200, https://doi.org/10.1079/BJN19740024.

5. Cheryl Long and Tabitha Alterman, "Meet Real Free-Range Eggs." Mother Earth News, November 2007, https://www.motherearthnews.com/real-food/free-range-eggs-zmaz07onzgoe#axzz32HhyWebs.

6. Harvard Center for Health and the Global Environment, "Lesson Plans & Activities: Healthy and Sustainable Food The Lowdown on Local Food," https://chge.hsph.harvard.edu/lesson-plans-activities-healthy-and-sustainable-food-lowdown-local-food.

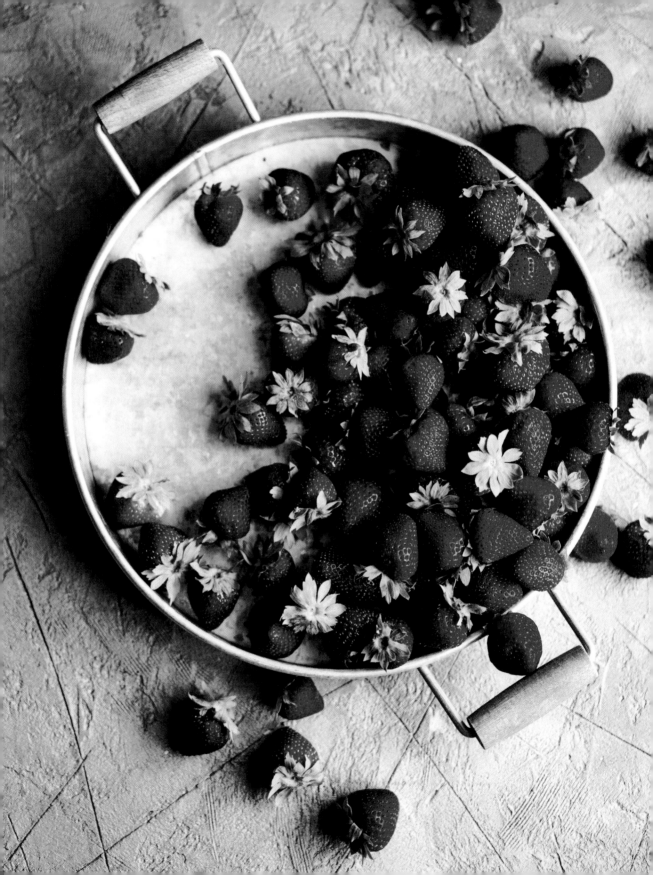

RECIPE QUICK REFERENCE BY DIETARY NEED

As a reminder, all the recipes in this book are gluten-free, dairy-free, and peanut-free. Always double-check the ingredients of items you've purchased when making recipes to make sure they're free of potential allergens.

Breakfast

RECIPE	EGG-FREE	NIGHTSHADE-FREE	NUT-FREE	VEGETARIAN	PAGE NUMBER
Breakfast Smoothie Trio	✓	✓	✓ (Cherry-Spinach Smoothie)	✓	135
Superfood Coconut Chai Latte	✓	✓	✓		136
Raspberry-Coconut Smoothie Bowl	✓	✓		✓	138
Apple Bacon Sweet Potato Hash	✓	✓	✓		140
Twice-Baked Breakfast Sweet Potatoes		✓	✓		142
Spinach, Tomato, and Mushroom Frittata			✓	✓	144
Bacon-Wrapped Eggs		✓	✓		146
Kale and Bacon Breakfast Skillet	✓	✓	✓		148
Fluffy Coconut Pancakes		✓		✓	150
Cinnamon Vanilla N'Oatmeal	✓	✓		✓	152
Pumpkin Breakfast Muffins		✓	✓	✓	154

Sides and Snacks

RECIPE	EGG-FREE	NIGHTSHADE-FREE	NUT-FREE	VEGETARIAN	PAGE NUMBER
Creamy Mashed Cauliflower	✓	✓	✓	✓	157
Savory Sweet Potato Wedges	✓		✓	✓	158
Parsnip and Carrot Fries	✓	✓	✓	✓	160
Bacon-Wrapped Asparagus Bundles	✓	✓	✓		162
Lemon-Garlic Roasted Broccoli	✓	✓	✓	✓	163
Rosemary Roasted Potatoes	✓		✓	✓	164
Zucchini-Tomato Sauté	✓		✓	✓	166
Jalapeño-Lime Cauliflower Rice	✓		✓	✓	167
Easy Apple "Cookies"	✓	✓		✓	168
Baked Plantain Chips	✓		✓	✓	170
Chocolate-Cherry Energy Bites	✓	✓		✓	172
Cinnamon-Toasted Coconut "Chips"	✓	✓	✓	✓	173
Spiced Rosemary Roasted Nuts	✓			✓	174

Salads, Dressings, and Dips

RECIPE	EGG-FREE	NIGHTSHADE-FREE	NUT-FREE	VEGETARIAN	PAGE NUMBER
Apple, Avocado, and Chicken Salad	✓	✓	✓		177
Chili-Lime Shrimp Salad	✓		✓		178
Roasted Beets and Berries Salad	✓	✓		✓	180
Strawberry Cobb Salad					182
Buffalo Chicken Dip			✓ (if ranch dressing is made with nut-free oil)		183
Everyone's Favorite Guacamole	✓		✓	✓	184
Mango-Jalapeño Salsa	✓		✓	✓	185
Avocado Butter	✓	✓	✓	✓	186
Simple Homemade Mayonnaise		✓ (if using nightshade-free Dijon mustard)	✓ (if using avocado oil)	✓	188
Cranberry-Apple Relish	✓	✓		✓	190
Raspberry Apple Cider Vinaigrette	✓	✓	✓	✓	191
Dairy-Free Ranch Dressing		✓ (if the mayo was made with nightshade-free Dijon mustard)	✓ (if the mayo was made with avocado oil)	✓	192
Honey-Lime Dressing	✓	✓	✓	✓	193

Main Dishes

RECIPE	EGG-FREE	NIGHTSHADE-FREE	NUT-FREE	VEGETARIAN	PAGE NUMBER
Spiced Potato Soup	✓			✓ (if using vegetable broth)	196
Baked Ratatouille	✓		✓	✓	198
Apple-Chicken Skillet	✓	✓	✓		200
Baked Sriracha Chicken Wings	✓		✓		202
Slow Cooker Chicken	✓		✓		204
Chicken-Sage Meatballs		✓			206
Bacon-Guacamole Chicken Rolls	✓		✓		207
Cilantro-Lime Turkey Burgers	✓ (without mayo)		✓		208
Classic Italian Turkey Meatballs					209
Bacon-Liver Meatballs	✓		✓		211
Asian Beef Stir-Fry	✓		✓		212
Zucchini-Beef Taco Skillet	✓		✓		214
Slow Cooker Garlic-Thyme Pot Roast	✓		✓		216
Shepherd's Pie	✓		✓		218

RECIPE	EGG-FREE	NIGHTSHADE-FREE	NUT-FREE	VEGETARIAN	PAGE NUMBER
Grilled Balsamic Flank Steak	✓	✓	✓		220
Homemade Bone Broth	✓	✓	✓		222
Sweet Potato Chipotle Bison Sliders	✓		✓		224
Slow Cooker Bison Chili	✓		✓		226
Pan-Seared Lamb Chops with Sage-Apple-Mint Puree	✓	✓	✓		228
Moroccan Lamb Meatballs	✓		✓		230
Oven-Roasted Spareribs	✓		✓		232
Balsamic Wine Pork Chops	✓	✓	✓		234
Firecracker Salmon	✓		✓		236
Coconut Macadamia Nut–Crusted Mahi mahi	✓	✓			238
Shrimp and Cabbage Stir-Fry	✓		✓		239
Thai Coconut Curry Shrimp	✓		✓		240
Caribbean Grilled Tuna Steaks	✓		✓		242

Treats

RECIPE	EGG-FREE	NIGHTSHADE-FREE	NUT-FREE	VEGETARIAN	PAGE NUMBER
Chocolate Coconut Bombs	✓	✓	✓	✓	245
Salted Dark Chocolate Almond Butter Cups	✓	✓		✓	246
Whipped Coconut Cream	✓	✓	✓	✓	248
Dark Chocolate Mug Cake		✓	✓	✓	250
Homemade Chocolate Shell Topping	✓	✓	✓	✓	252
Banana Split Pops	✓	✓	✓ (without the chopped walnuts)	✓	254
Chocolate-Covered Strawberry Ice Pops	✓	✓	✓ (without the nut topping)	✓	256
Almond Shortbread Cookies	✓	✓		✓	258
No-Bake Almond-Coconut Cookie Bars	✓	✓		✓	260
Lemon-Raspberry Mini Cheesecakes	✓	✓		✓	262
Avocado Chocolate Mousse	✓	✓		✓	264
Watermelon-Lime Gummies	✓	✓	✓		266

VISUAL RECIPE INDEX

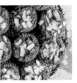

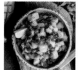

Slow Cooker
Garlic-Thyme
Pot Roast
216

Shepherd's
Pie
218

Grilled
Balsamic
Flank Steak
220

Homemade
Bone Broth
222

Sweet Potato
Chipotle Bison
Sliders
224

Slow Cooker
Bison Chili
226

Pan-Seared
Lamb Chops
228

Moroccan
Lamb
Meatballs
230

Oven-Roasted
Spareribs
232

Balsamic
Wine Pork
Chops
234

Firecracker
Salmon
236

Coconut
Macadamia Nut–
Crusted Mahimahi
238

Shrimp and
Cabbage
Stir-Fry
239

Thai Coconut
Curry Shrimp
240

Caribbean
Grilled Tuna
Steaks
242

CHAPTER
11

TREATS

Chocolate
Coconut
Bombs
245

Salted Dark
Chocolate Almond
Butter Cups
246

Whipped
Coconut
Cream
248

Dark
Chocolate
Mug Cake
250

Homemade
Chocolate
Shell Topping
252

Banana Split
Pops
254

Chocolate-
Covered
Strawberry
Ice Pops
256

Almond
Shortbread
Cookies
258

No-Bake
Almond-
Coconut
Cookie Bars
260

Lemon-
Raspberry
Mini
Cheesecakes
262

Avocado
Chocolate
Mousse
264

Watermelon-
Lime
Gummies
266

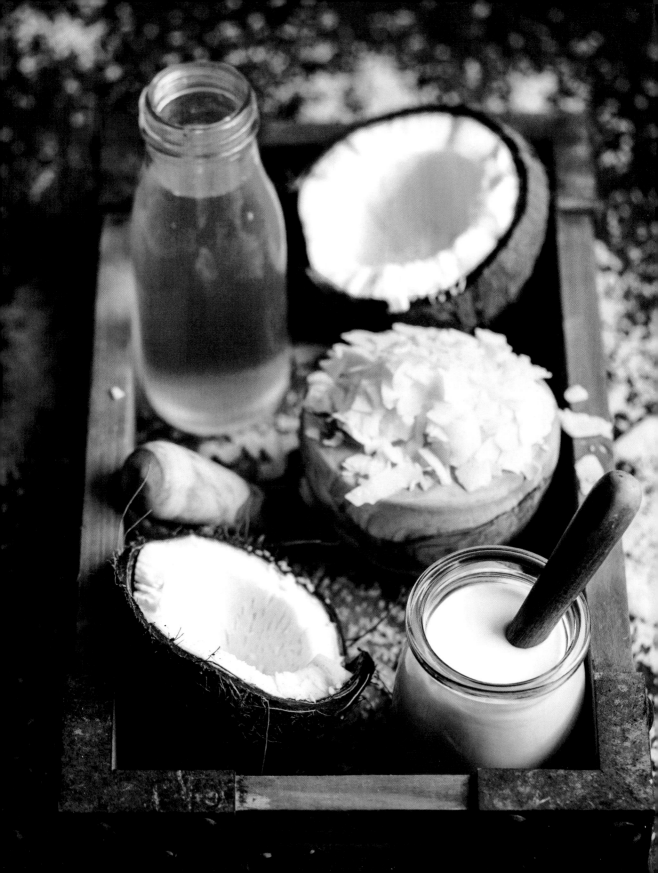

INDEX

NOTE: Page references in *italics* refer to photos of recipes.